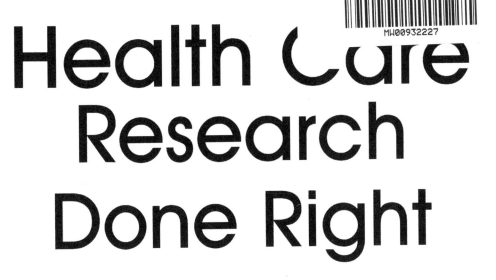

Health Care Research Done Right

A Journal Editor Shares Practical Tips and Techniques for High Quality and Efficiency

Kathleen A. Fairman

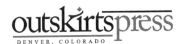

outskirtspress

DENVER, COLORADO

Acknowledgements

A project of this kind inevitably requires the help, support, and—perhaps most of all—patience of many people. This one is no exception. Fred Curtiss, Editor-in-Chief of the *Journal of Managed Care Pharmacy*, deserves special thanks for his uncompromising attention to detail and integrity, from which I have learned a great deal. Many years before my arrival at the journal, Fred instituted procedures that have been instrumental in advancing its quality and reputation during the past decade. Without his attention to excellence, mine would not have been possible. And, at the risk of beginning a sentence with "I'd like to thank the Academy," I *would* like to thank the Academy of Managed Care Pharmacy for its support and for sharing the vision of a "toolkit" that researchers could use to improve their work. Thanks also to coworkers Carol Blumentritt, Jennifer Booker, and Sheila Macho for their support and especially to "Marvelous Margie" Hunter for graphic design consultation and for unlocking the mysteries of the .tif file.

Many professionals, along with students and researchers whom they supervise, graciously donated their time to review book chapters. I owe a great deal to the insightful comments of the following talented individuals (listed in alphabetical order by organization name):

- Suprat Saely, PharmD, BCPS, **Detroit Receiving Hospital, Detroit Medical Center**
- Candice Garwood, PharmD, BCPS, **Eugene Applebaum College of Pharmacy and Health Sciences, Wayne State University**
- Mark Jackson, BScPhm, BComm, RPh, and Cathi Li, **Green Shield Canada**
- Mary E. Costantino, BS, PhD, and Karen Worley, PhD, **Humana Inc.**
- Frederic R. Curtiss, PhD, RPh, CEBS, *Journal of Managed Care Pharmacy*
- Roseann S. Gammal, PharmD candidate, and Linda M. Spooner, PharmD, BCPS, **Massachusetts College of Pharmacy and Health Sciences**
- Brenda R. Motheral, MBA, PhD, **Pharmacy Benefit Management Institute**
- Patrick P. Gleason, PharmD, FCCP, BCPS; Jill A. Phillips, RPh; and Catherine I. Starner, PharmD, BCPS, CGP, **Prime Therapeutics**

- Jeremy Schafer, PharmD, MBA, and Alexandra Tungol, PharmD, **Prime Therapeutics**
- Justin B. Dickerson, MBA, and Robert L. Ohsfeldt, PhD, **Texas A&M Health Science Center**
- Mitchell J. Barnett, PharmD, MS; Quang Vinh Bui, PharmD; and Chandra L. Steenhoek, PharmD, **Touro University College of Pharmacy**
- Thomas N. Hill, PharmD candidate; Stephen J. Kogut, PhD, MBA; Brian J. Kurt, PharmD candidate; and Kristina E. Ward, BS, PharmD, BCPS, **University of Rhode Island College of Pharmacy**
- Roy E. Mock, RPh, BCPS, BCOP, **University of Washington**
- Norman V. Carroll, PhD, and Nantana Kaisaeng, BPharm, MBA, MHA, **Virginia Commonwealth University**
- Peter Whittaker, PhD, **Wayne State University**

These reviewers asked thoughtful questions, pointed out areas of ambiguity, and identified important topics that I had missed. Their work improved this book immeasurably. Any remaining errors or omissions are, of course, my own.

Although I am grateful to all the teachers from whom I have been privileged to learn over the years, I would like to acknowledge several in particular: Shap Wolf and the late Morrie Axelrod of the Arizona State University (ASU) Survey Research Laboratory, who carefully trained me in survey research methods, and Mary Benin, also of ASU, who made statistical theory and practice clear to me for the first time.

Finally, thanks go to my husband, Michael, and our three children, Matt, James, and Jonah—stalwart souls who assisted in identifying historical examples, did extra household chores, and endured culinary mishaps including our new family legend, "Wrote-Too-Long Stew." James also spent many hours researching public domain artwork for illustrations, assisting with the book's index, and carrying out a much-needed reorganization of project files.

Thanks to all of you for your support and hard work!

Table of Contents

Foreword

Health Care Research Done Right is a much needed book that is appealing to a wide audience. Journal editors can embrace this book as a wealth of essential suggestions for authors in need of guidance to improve the quality of their writing, avoid mathematical errors, make the distinction between association and causation, and describe their results accurately and without overstatement. Faculty members responsible for teaching graduate and aspiring undergraduate students will be thankful for the opportunity to use this book in coursework to develop skills in conducting and reporting research and in literature evaluation. Students will appreciate the book's practical examples, many of which were drawn from the author's experience as Associate Editor and Senior Methodology Reviewer for the *Journal of Managed Care Pharmacy*. And, all will appreciate the book's style, which is interesting, easy to read, and unique in the field of books intended to help writers and researchers. This book is so comprehensive that it can be the primary reference in a course for undergraduate or graduate students and can be described with the entirely plausible tagline that "it's in there," full of the practical tips and perspectives to help students and professionals attain success as researchers, writers, and reviewers.

Much of this book is must-read for almost all those engaged in health care research in any role. The suggestions in Chapters 5 and 6 to help avoid common mistakes in basic and advanced data analysis will be useful to all researchers, not just data "mechanics," in making their work products more accurate and more credible. In addition to the key critical points that the author makes regarding statistics and methods, including the "sensible analysis" checklist, there are many helpful perspectives for authors that are presented in this book such as appreciation of peer reviewers as customers who notice when researchers ignore reasonable feedback and requests. In the pursuit of excellence, authors can help themselves be more successful by approaching peer review with the expectation of obtaining suggestions and guidance to assist in making their published manuscripts more readable and useful. It is so very important that authors think of their "customers" (readers) in their description of research methods and in the presentation and interpretation of results.

The context of the book is a field in need of continuous quality improvement to support today's emphasis on evidence-based decision making and comparative effectiveness research. With the increasing volume of published and unpublished information, including an average of more than 70,000 new citations *per month* in MEDLINE/PubMed in 2011, all readers will appreciate the guidance in this book for evaluation of the quality of evidence. The author uses practical examples to help explain the multitude of threats to internal and external validity. The combination of examples, list of confounding factors, and the summary of principles of causation and principles underlying guidelines for rating quality of evidence, is helpful for researchers and authors in the proper presentation and interpretation of study results and for reviewers and readers in judging the quality of the evidence and therefore the value of the research. There are also helpful tips for filtering the often overwhelming amount of information that is available on a given subject.

Practical, useful, understandable, and fun to read. There is a lot to like in this book. In addition to covering seemingly mundane subjects such as the common problem of inaccuracy in the published literature in an interesting way, the author is very sincere in the perspective that there is much at stake in conducting research correctly and reporting the results clearly and accurately. In all fields and particularly in the biosciences, poorly conducted research or incorrectly reported results can cause harm. This book is an inspiration for excellence in the conduct of research and in reporting results in a manner that improves comprehension for readers and thereby makes the writer/researcher more successful.

Frederic R. Curtiss, PhD, RPh, CEBS
Editor-in-Chief
Journal of Managed Care Pharmacy

CHAPTER 1
The Case for Excellence

"When I was a kid, everyone wanted to be a rock and roll star. But if you really want to do something creative, fun and stimulating, then science is as good as it gets."—Research neurologist Richard Ransohoff[1]

"Accuracy of statement is one of the first elements of truth; inaccuracy is a near kin to falsehood."—American theologian Tryon Edwards[2]

Fifteen years ago, when I was a research manager for a large managed care company, our staff met with a pharmaceutical company representative whom I will call "Sam." Sam had requested the meeting to encourage us to compare his company's product, Drug A, with its competitors using our pharmacy claims (billing) data. Naturally, Sam was enthusiastic about Drug A and believed that the proposed study would demonstrate its superiority on a number of dimensions. We advised Sam that we could perform the study in exchange for compensation but that we could promise neither specific results nor publication. Sam's response startled all of us. He chuckled and winked broadly. "Don't worry," he said knowingly. "We can get 'ya published." In other words, Sam apparently had access to at least one avenue to publication and was assuring us that we could take advantage of the opportunity—*if* we produced findings favorable to Drug A.[3] (For the record, we turned him down.)

In many fields of study, researchers make choices about where to attempt publication. There are "top tier" journals, the ones to which most researchers in academia or industry aspire. Publication in one of these journals assures professional attention and potentially even better remuneration or promotional opportunities. These are the high-prestige journals in their fields, the journals with the highest "impact factors" (a standard measure of the number of times that their articles are cited), the journals "where the cool kids play," as a friend of mine describes it. But, typically, these "better" journals demand a high-quality product—a research question that has clear relevance for the target audience, a carefully performed data collection process, valid methods that are clearly presented in the study report, a discussion that explains the study findings in the context of previous and future work, and a manuscript prepared according to the standards of the International Committee of Medical Journal Editors.[4]

In contrast, a researcher who submits to a less selective journal, such as the one that Sam may have had in mind for Drug A, generally faces a less demanding proposition. Publication in one of these journals doesn't carry the same prestige, but it's easier. A lower-quality study is publishable. The research question might be selected to prove a commercial or political point that is advantageous to the study sponsor rather than to advance knowledge in the field. The study methods might be invalid or not described clearly enough to facilitate replication of the study by others. The study report itself might reflect a careless approach to the work—for example, mathematical errors, or text that does not match to tables.

The review process might differ as well. Reviewers might ask fewer questions. A researcher who chooses to ignore all or most reviewer comments might be published despite making minimal or no changes to his or her work. For researchers whose study sponsor is willing to pay the fees for "rapid review" or "page charges" that are assessed by some journals, work is published relatively quickly and easily. Some study sponsors will even pay for medical writers who will do much of the "grunt work" on behalf of a named author, such as gathering references or drafting initial versions of the text.

It's possible to accumulate an impressively long list of publications this way. But is that the best path for *you*? What choices will you make about the quality of the work that you produce?

Excellence or Mediocrity: It's Your Choice

When researchers choose *excellence*, they make decisions that will enhance the credibility and usefulness of their findings *for those who will read or use their work*. Members of the research audience, who may be broadly described as "information users" or "readers," need *high-quality evidence*. An *excellent* research project is focused throughout the entire process—from the first gleam of an idea through the final project report—on *meeting that need*.

Excellence should be distinguished from perfection. As we shall see in Chapter 3, there is no perfect research design or project; instead, most choices in research involve tradeoffs. But it is important to make those tradeoffs completely clear to information users, so that they understand the strengths and weaknesses of the work and can make an informed decision about applying its findings in their own settings. That is why clarity in reporting study methods and results is a key component of excellence, as explained in Chapter 10.

To understand how excellence works in practice, think about all the steps in a typical research project. Choices begin immediately and continue throughout the process, even for researchers who don't intend to publish their work. For example, when beginning a project, a researcher can choose whether to search published information to determine what is already known about the topic and to learn about the methods used by others—or can simply forge ahead without this valuable information to "save time." Prior to analyzing a dataset, a researcher can choose to take the (usually brief) time necessary to develop an *a priori* data analysis plan—or can begin with no plan except to explore the data and modify the analyses multiple times to reach a desired conclusion. (I have previously called this behavior "fishing, trapping, and cruelty to numbers."[5]) When writing a study report, a researcher can choose to present the methods and findings in a clear, step-by-step fashion—or can adopt a "black box" approach that leaves the reader feeling bewildered about the accuracy and applicability of the results.[5] Many such choices are made by researchers, both in academia and in other settings, on a daily basis. I know, because as a journal editor, I've seen the consequences both of poor choices and of good ones.

Complicating the task of making good choices is the easy availability of secondary-source databases and high-speed computing capabilities, which have made it possible for a researcher to repeat the same analysis literally hundreds of times in a single week using slightly different methods each time. Additionally, the convenience of personal computers, which permit researchers to work with nearly complete independence instead of in groups using a single mainframe computer as they did of necessity 20 or 30 years ago, has reduced the amount of feedback provided routinely during the research process (except in those departments and companies that have wisely incorporated feedback mechanisms into their procedures). Exacerbating this challenge is lack of oversight that occurs because, in this technically complex age, many researchers report to supervisors who are not researchers themselves or who do not have—and cannot be expected to have—expertise in the topic areas of every researcher whom they supervise. To this mix, add pressure to produce certain findings—whether for commercial, political, ideological, or competitive reasons—and it can *seem* nearly impossible even to identify the best techniques for producing high-quality work, let alone use them consistently.

So, why bother? Why aim for excellence when, sometimes, just "getting by" and producing the answer that "everybody wants to hear" (or, maybe, that your employer wants to hear) is good enough? In my experience, which includes 25 years in health care research in both the public and private sectors and five years as a research journal editor, there are **four good reasons** to care—a great deal—about the quality of your work.

First and foremost, *the job of a researcher is to produce accurate information.* This task is nothing short of a high calling, because the quality of the information that you produce can have a profound effect on the well-being of your family, friends, people whom you have never met, and maybe even generations to come, depending on your topic and findings. In their seminal book, *The Craft of Research*, Booth, Colomb, and Williams (2008) observe that research

> *"is a profoundly social activity that connects you both to those who will use your research and to those who might benefit—or suffer—from that use. But it also connects you and your readers to everyone whose research you used and beyond them to everyone whose research they used."*[6]

These connections, Booth et al. argue, have important ethical implications:

> *"In short, when you report your research ethically, you join a community in a search for some common good. When you respect sources, preserve and acknowledge data that run against your results, assert claims only as strongly as warranted, acknowledge the limits of your certainty, and meet all the other ethical obligations on your report, you move beyond gaining a grade or other material goods—you earn the larger benefit that comes from creating a bond with your readers. You discover that research focused on the best interests of others is also in your own."*[6]

In contrast, when the quality of work is poor—for example, when data are presented selectively to favor a specific desired conclusion, when calculations are performed incorrectly, when a survey response rate is so low that the results reflect the views of a small and nonrepresentative group—decisions are made based on bad information. And, as the keen observations of Booth et al. suggest, bad information, which in turn leads to bad decisions, has the potential to cause harm—some of which may not be immediately apparent to the researcher who caused it. (We'll see examples throughout this book.)

Striving for excellence is the better and more ethical path.

Second, it is *strategically advantageous* to be "part of the solution" rather than "part of the problem." What is "the problem"? The quality of published research in multiple areas of study is widely recognized as far from ideal. In the health care field, a phenomenon that was described by knowledgeable observers as "the scandal of poor medical research" in 1994 and as "the scandal of poor epidemiological research" in 2004 has spawned considerable attention to what is wrong with health care research and how to fix it.[7] As Chapter 10 explains, much of "what is wrong" is lack of transparency and clarity in the explanations of study methods and findings that appear in published articles. As an important part of "the solution," the **E**nhancing the **QUA**lity and **T**ransparency **O**f health **R**esearch (EQUATOR) network, formed in 2006, promulgates standards for health care research reporting that have been adopted by numerous research journals, including top-tier publications.[8] Similar efforts to enhance the quality and transparency of published work are ongoing in many fields.[9]

These developments have an important implication for you: the researcher who knows how to conduct and present research accurately and transparently will increasingly be viewed as a credible source of evidence. And credibility is no small thing because a researcher with a good reputation won't just keep up with the curve—he or she will help to *lead* it. Viewed more broadly from a societal perspective, research leaders who have chosen excellence become role models for other researchers, thereby increasing the quality of evidence exponentially.

Third, in this age of *rapid dissemination of information*—made even more rapid in recent years with the development of "social media," such as Facebook and Twitter—bad news travels fast. As the examples in Chapter 2 illustrate with painful clarity, the reputations of well-intentioned and talented researchers have been damaged by failure to maintain simple systems and patterns of behavior that facilitate prompt identification and correction of data problems. Researchers who are aware of how to prevent errors—and, more importantly, how to detect and fix errors when they do occur—retain their good reputations even in the face of controversy.

Fourth, if you receive *difficult feedback*—either formally from a journal peer reviewer or informally from a fellow worker or student—and are tempted to ignore it and seek an easier route to dissemination of your work, there is something that you should know. When the reviewers whose comments you ignored see the work published—either in the journal for which they reviewed, in another journal that was willing to allow you to ignore reviewer input, or on a nonpeer-reviewed website—they see your name on the article and know who you are. They remember your paper and what they said about it. If they gave you reasonable feedback and you failed to respond to it, they know that, too. And, if they see commercial sponsorship of your work, they may suspect that the sponsorship was related to your decision to ignore their comments. Even if they are wrong about your motives, that is not a good reputation to have. (There's a better way to handle tough feedback; see Chapter 9.)

As associate editor of the *Journal of Managed Care Pharmacy* (*JMCP*), which is selective in publication and uses extensive quality-improvement procedures to encourage excellence by authors and peer reviewers,[10] I occasionally field complaints from authors who say that the process of producing high-quality work is difficult and ask why we make it "too hard." They are asking the wrong question. Instead of asking why some journals insist on high-quality work, they should be identifying ways to improve their techniques so that they can be *both* effective *and* efficient in responding to feedback—*and* publish in those higher-quality journals. In other words, the *right* question is "how can I produce excellent work, at a lower cost in time and/or money?"

> ## Key Points: Aiming for Excellence
>
> ❖ Health care research has a profound effect on information users and on society as a whole.
> ❖ Efforts to improve research are ongoing in multiple fields—it is wise to be "part of the solution" and not "part of the problem."
> ❖ Researchers with reputations for credibility often become leaders.
> ❖ Peer reviewers notice when researchers ignore reasonable feedback.
> ❖ It is easier than you may think to do a great job—you don't have to choose between excellence and efficiency!

It is to this crucial question that this book is directed. Happily, the answer is that once you learn the right techniques and habits, and practice them faithfully, you'll find that it is actually much *easier* than you think to do a *great* job on a research project. High quality *and* efficiency—what's not to like about that?

How This Book Can Help

The need for this book first became clear to me more than a decade ago while working for the managed care company, which at that time was trying to develop its research function and become a thought leader in the industry. It didn't take many new hires for my supervisor and I to realize that the majority of graduates from advanced degree programs at the masters and doctoral levels, although knowledgeable in their fields, lacked basic skills needed to do the work that they had been hired to do. In some instances, the researchers were aware of *what* needed to be done—for example, perform a sensitivity analysis or redraw a sample in response to a journal peer reviewer's concern—but not *how* to do it in a reasonable period of time. That is, they were missing "tricks of the trade" necessary to perform the work efficiently. So they tended to dismiss suggestions for improvement as "too hard" and unfortunately sometimes gave up too quickly on a publishable manuscript. In other instances, the researchers lacked understanding of principles that are covered only briefly (if at all) in statistics and methods classes but used frequently in practical research applications, such as appropriate methods for percentage comparisons, weighting for sample stratification, cumulative type I ("false positive") error, and regression to the mean. (Don't worry if you are unfamiliar with these terms; they are covered in Chapter 5.)

We saw the other side of the coin, too—professionals who were unsure of whether research results were valid but needed to make decisions based on them. Like the researchers, these information users were skilled in their fields, but they did not know how to distinguish high-quality from low-quality studies. Faced with the inconsistent reports that are ubiquitous in a body of literature based on study designs with varying degrees of rigor, some would rely on "gut instinct" or a suboptimal assessment process that the *JMCP* editors have previously described as the "whodunnit" approach—that is, assuming that if research appeared in a reputable journal, was written by well-known authors, or was funded by a noncommercial source, it must be valid.[11]

Regardless of whether you are an information producer or an information user, if you are like many recent or not-so-recent graduates of advanced degree programs whom I have encountered over the years, one or more of the following statements may apply to you:

- **You are unsure about practical research applications.** You like your field. You like exploring interesting questions. But you are not sure how the techniques that you were taught in statistics and methods classes "fit together" to help you answer the questions that you care about. You might even have taken those classes early in your graduate school education to "get them over with," making them a distant memory now.
- **You're busy!** "Multitask" has become your middle name. You're a student trying to conduct a research project while taking other classes or working part time,

or you're a research professional engaged in multiple studies simultaneously. But no one has ever shown you how to organize your research plans, files, and work products to make this juggling act easier.

- **Important information is sometimes unavailable.** You have been asked questions about how your research was conducted that you were either unable to answer or relied on memory to answer because you lacked an efficient system to access the information promptly.

- **It's too difficult to respond to some feedback.** You received feedback about your research that you dismissed because responding to it would require reconstructing a data analysis, which seemed too hard.

- **You took basic math a *long* time ago.** The journal to which you submitted your work requires a descriptive data table, but your graduate school instruction focused primarily on "advanced" statistical techniques and you are unsure of how to proceed. Or, you have been told that you performed or presented basic descriptive calculations incorrectly, but you did not understand or know how to respond to the feedback.

- **You need more information about surveys.** You would like accurate information about what your target population is really thinking, but you have little or no formal coursework in survey research.

- **You are not sure about secondary-source data.** You currently use one or more databases consisting of information, such as medical claims, survey data, or test scores, that you did not actually collect yourself. In fact, you are not sure how or by whom the data were collected, and have never thought about whether this lack of information is a problem.

- **You are unsure of quality standards.** You are sometimes asked to review and comment on the work of others but are not always sure of the standards by which their work should be judged.

- **You *use* research information, but you are not a researcher.** In the course of your work, you are sometimes presented with "research evidence" of the need for a particular decision or policy change. But you are not sure about whether the evidence is valid and, sometimes, the evidence provided by one source directly conflicts with that provided by another. You need to be able to filter out the junk from the good science—the information that you can rely on.

If any of these characteristics apply, you need help "filling the gaps" between what you know and what you need to know to do your job more effectively and efficiently. In response to this need, I developed and taught "crash courses" on basic, practical research skills for professionals and recent graduates in health care. I use much of this teaching material in my current role as a journal editor. Drawing on this experience, this book is a collection of practical tips and techniques to help you do your work better and faster.

In this book, you will learn how to:

> - Set up and maintain a *simple* tracking system that will permit you to respond *quickly and easily* to requests for information and changes, even when those requests are unreasonable or involve a major redesign (Chapter 2)
> - *Plan your research well* at the start to avoid problems later in the process (Chapters 3 and 4)
> - Perform and describe an accurate *literature review* (Chapter 4)
> - *Avoid common mistakes* in basic and advanced data analysis so that your work is *credible* to those who will use it (Chapters 5 and 6)
> - *Understand and use appropriately* secondary data sources, such as pharmacy and medical claims (billing) data (Chapter 7)
> - Collect data directly from your target population by writing and administering an effective and accurate *survey* (Chapter 8)
> - *Incorporate feedback* that you receive from others—whether it is positive or negative—to produce an improved work product (Chapter 9)
> - Respond *politely but effectively* when you are asked to conduct research incorrectly (Chapter 9)
> - *Report your work* accurately, clearly, and transparently, so that information users understand what you did and what it means for them (Chapter 10)
> - Assess the *quality* of research evidence (Chapters 3 and 10)

A few notes on what this book is *not*. This book is not an in-depth guide to every aspect of a research study, mostly because excellent resources for many project stages are already available. Booth et al.'s *The Craft of Research*[6] and Kate Turabian's *A Manual for Writers*[12] are detailed guides to help researchers find a topic, formulate questions, find information sources, create logically sound and credible arguments, and write effectively about the work and its implications. Jane Miller's *The Chicago Guide to Writing about Numbers*[13] and *The Chicago Guide to Writing about Multivariate Analysis*[14] provide detailed guidance on the presentation of quantitative information and are "standout" resources for their clarity and the helpful summary checklists at the end of each chapter. Where applicable, I refer interested readers to these and other resources for in-depth or technical discussion of certain topics. In that sense, this book is both a "road map"—a guide to help you find available information—and a source of new information.

A few notes on what I assume about you: The book assumes upper-level undergraduate or graduate-level training. I assume that you have taken at least one basic statistics class and probably (but not necessarily) at least one advanced statistics class. I assume coursework in your field of interest, no matter what that might be. The examples in the book are drawn from multiple fields, and the basic principles have widespread application. I also assume some coursework in or experience with writing, especially research papers. I do *not* assume extensive working knowledge of basic mathematics because, in my experience, "simple" mathematical operations are often more difficult than advanced statistics for graduate-level researchers, most of whom took basic mathematics many years ago.

First, we turn in Chapter 2 to the systematic organization, processing, and verification of research data. We begin with two examples of prominent researchers who didn't follow simple documentation procedures—and ended up paying a high price for their mistake.

References

1. My research career: lessons learned. Spotlight on: Richard Ransohoff, MD. January 24, 2011. Available at: http://www.principalinvestigators.org/no-61-sharing-my-secrets-a-spotlight-on-dr-richard-ransohoff-md/.

2. Quotations by Tyron Edwards. Available at: http://www.andiquote.co.za/authors/Tyron_Edwards.html.

3. Since that time, mounting evidence has suggested that inappropriate influence over the process of generating and publishing medical research is widespread. See, for example:

   - Fairman KA, Curtiss FR. What should be done about bias and misconduct in clinical trials? *J Manag Care Pharm.* 2009;15(2):154-60. Available at: http://www.amcp.org/data/jmcp/154-160.pdf.
   - Fugh-Berman A. The corporate coauthor. *J Gen Intern Med.* 2005;20(6):546-48.
   - Lee K, Bacchetti P, Sim I. Publication of clinical trials supporting successful new drug applications: a literature analysis. *PLoS Med.* 2008;5(9):e191.
   - Martinson BC, Anderson MS, de Vries R. Scientists behaving badly. *Nature.* 2005;435(7043):737-38.
   - Sismondo S. Ghost management: how much of the medical literature is shaped behind the scenes by the pharmaceutical industry? *PLos Med.* 2007;4(9):e286.
   - Rising K, Bacchetti P, Bero L. Reporting bias in drug trials submitted to the Food and Drug Administration: review of publication and presentation. *PLoS Med.* 2008;5(11):e217.
   - Turner EH, Matthew AM, Linardatos E, Tell RA, Rosenthal R. Selective publication of antidepressant trials and its influence on apparent efficacy. *N Engl J Med.* 2008;358(3):252-60.

4. International Committee of Medical Journal Editors. Available at: http://www.icmje.org/.

5. Fairman KA. Differentiating effective data mining from fishing, trapping, and cruelty to numbers. *J Manag Care Pharm.* 2007;13(6):517-27. Available at: http://www.amcp.org/data/jmcp/pages%20517-27.pdf.

6. Booth WC, Colomb GG, Williams JM. *The Craft of Research. Third Edition.* Chicago, IL: University of Chicago Press; 2008: quotations pp. 273, 276.

7. See for example:
   - Altman DG. The scandal of poor medical research. *BMJ.* 1994;308:283-84.

- Altman DG. Poor-quality medical research: what can journals do? *JAMA.* 2002;287(21):2765-67.
- von Elm E, Egger M. The scandal of poor epidemiological research: reporting guidelines are needed for observational epidemiology. *BMJ.* 2004;329:868-69.

8. EQUATOR network. Available at: www.equator-network.org.
9. See, for example:

- Cumming G, Fidler F, Leonard M, et al. Statistical reform in psychology: is anything changing? *Psychol Sci.* 2007;18:230-32.
- Curran-Everett D, Benos DJ. Guidelines for reporting statistics in journals published by the American Physiological Society: the sequel. *Adv Physiol Educ.* 2007;31:295-98.
- Ding K, Hu P. Research studies in two health education journals, 1988-1997: targets and methodologies. *The International Electronic Journal of Health Education.* 1999;2(3):101-10.
- Fidler F, Thomason N, Cumming G, Finch S, Leeman J. Editors can lead researchers to confidence intervals, but can't make them think: statistical reform lessons from medicine. *Psychol Sci.* 2004;15(2):119-26.
- Jerome RN. Further developing the profession's research mentality. *J Med Libr Assoc.* 2008;96(4):287-88.
- Kitchenbaum BA, Pfleeger SL, Pickard LM, et al. Preliminary guidelines for empirical research in software engineering. National Research Council of Canada. January 2001. Available at: http://nparc.cisti-icist.nrc-cnrc.gc.ca/npsi/ctrl?action=rtdoc&an=8914084.
- Tooley J. The quality of educational research: a perspective from Great Britain. *Peabody Journal of Education.* 2001;76:122-40.
- Volker MA. Reporting effect sizes estimates in school psychology research. *Psychology in the Schools.* 2006;43(6):653-72.
- Wacker JG. A conceptual understanding of requirements for theory-building research: guidelines for scientific theory building. *Journal of Supply Chain Management.* 2008;44(3):5-15.

10. Credit for the quality monitoring and improvement measures used by the *Journal of Managed Pharmacy* is owed to its Editor-in-Chief, Frederic R. Curtiss, PhD, RPh, CEBS, who implemented these initiatives beginning in 2002.
11. Fairman KA, Curtiss FR. Rethinking the 'whodunnit' approach to assessing the quality of health care research—a call to focus on the evidence in evidence-based practice.

J Manag Care Pharm. 2008;14(7):661-74. Available at: http://www.amcp.org/data/jmcp/661-674_FairmanCurtiss-Final.pdf.

12. Turabian KL. *A Manual for Writers of Research Papers, Theses, and Dissertations. Seventh Edition.* Chicago, IL: University of Chicago Press; 2007.

13. Miller JE. *The Chicago Guide to Writing about Numbers.* Chicago, IL: University of Chicago Press; 2004.

14. Miller JE. *The Chicago Guide to Writing about Multivariate Analysis.* Chicago, IL: University of Chicago Press; 2005.

CHAPTER 2

A Documentation System to Increase Accuracy *and* Efficiency

"Everyone bought the numbers; no one checked the math."—1996 comment on the revelation that wildly popular 1985 research findings on the economic effects of divorce were actually the result of data processing errors made by a graduate student.[1,2]

"The dog ate global warming."—2009 comment on the revelation that the raw data necessary to verify the extensively publicized "hockey stick" graph of a recent sharp rise in global temperatures had either been lost or discarded by the research unit that produced it.[3,4]

"J'accuse: Many of the medical research papers you read will be wrong, not as a result of methodologic flaws, poor design, or inappropriate statistics, but because of typing errors."—Biostatistician Andrew Vickers[5]

> **What You Will Learn in Chapter 2**
>
> ✓ How good documentation practices can *protect* your reputation, your time, and your sanity
>
> ✓ How to implement *five simple but essential practices* that will allow you to catch problems in your data analysis *before* they cause damage
>
> ✓ How making changes to your data analysis in response to feedback can be *easy*
>
> ✓ How to use your project documentation to provide information that most journals consider *essential*

Don't Let This Happen to You: Why You Should Care About Documentation

In 1986, when I had just finished my master's degree in sociology, Lenore Weitzman was considered a hero by many graduate students, including me. She was living the dream of using sociological research to change the world for the better. Published in 1985, Weitzman's "groundbreaking" book, *The Divorce Revolution*, had captivated the nation with "hard evidence" of what activists had long suspected: after a divorce, men walked away with most of the wealth, leaving their hapless wives and children destitute in a process known to sociologists as the "feminization of poverty."[2] Weitzman's study of California's no-fault divorce process, which had been signed into law by then Governor Ronald Reagan in 1969, found that the "standard of living" (a ratio of income to needs) for women in the Los Angeles area declined by an astonishing 73% after divorce, while their former husbands enjoyed a 42% increase on the same measure.[1,2]

The so-called "73/42" figure quickly became, according to a 1996 Associated Press news account, "one of the most widely quoted statistics in recent history" and "the centerpiece" for criticisms of no-fault divorce laws.[2] In 1986, Weitzman's book won the American Sociological Association's "Distinguished Contribution to Scholarship" award.[6] In the same year, Weitzman highlighted the 73/42 statistic in Congressional testimony.[7] In less than nine years following its publication, the book was cited in 348 social science articles, 250 law review articles, 85 newspaper articles, 25 national magazine articles, and 24 cases brought before appellate and state supreme courts.[6] Reviews of the book, appearing in 22 social science journals, 12 law journals, and 10 national popular press publications, concluded almost universally that Weitzman's work indicated an urgent need for divorce law reform to mitigate the "disastrous" effects of no-fault divorce on women and children.[6] Weitzman herself recalled in 1996 that as a result of the 73/42 statistic and other findings described in the book, 14 new divorce laws were passed in the state of California alone.[8]

But in 1996, a problem even more shocking than the original 73/42 statistic became public: Weitzman's numbers were wrong, apparently the result of errors made by one or more graduate students or employees who performed the data analyses under her supervision.[2,8] Social Science Research Council sociologist Richard Peterson, who obtained access to Weitzman's stored data files about ten years after the book's publication, began comparing the computer data with the original (paper) surveys. Peterson found numerous errors, among them that "over 450 variables were incorrectly coded for 67 [of Weitzman's 228] cases because they had been merged into the file using incorrect ID numbers."[6] After producing a corrected file, a task made more difficult "because Weitzman did not explain how she handled a variety of measurement problems" and statistical calculations, Peterson reported that using Weitzman's primary outcome measure, the ratio of income to needs, he found a 27% decline in standard of living for women and a 10% increase for men.[*]

---

[*] The appropriateness of Weitzman's standard-of-living measure has also been disputed, but that disagreement falls outside the scope of this chapter. See Braver S, O'Connell D. *Divorced Dads: Shattering the Myths.* New York: Tarcher/Putnam; 1998.

Peterson's devastating summary conclusion was that "it is clear that the results reported in *The Divorce Revolution* for the change in the average standard of living are in error. They could not have been derived from the data and methods described in the book."[6] Although disputing some details of Peterson's analysis, Weitzman acknowledged the error in the much-quoted statistic in a 1996 interview with the Associated Press: "I'm responsible—I reported it."[2]

More recently, negative consequences of problems in the handling and storage of data were experienced by scientists at the University of East Anglia's (UEA) Climatic Research Unit (CRU), which in late 2009 revealed that raw data necessary to replicate their extensively publicized findings about human-caused global warming had been discarded, probably when the CRU moved to a new building in the 1980s.[4,9] CRU had for several years failed to comply with Freedom of Information Act requests for the raw data because, the CRU website explained, it no longer had them. The originally collected data had been cleaned by the CRU "for homogeneity issues" to adjust for disparate data collection conditions at various weather stations throughout the world, producing a "value-added" dataset. However, data storage limitations "meant that we were not able to keep the multiple sources [of data] … We, therefore, do not hold the original raw data but only the value-added (i.e. quality controlled and homogenized) data."[9]

In the highly politicized "climate" surrounding global warming theory, the CRU's announcement, coupled with the contents of the infamous "climategate" emails that were "hacked" from the UEA's computer system and disseminated on the Internet in November 2009, prompted a flood of accusations about CRU's work.[3,10] These included allegations that CRU knew of serious problems with the data but chose to use them anyway and that CRU's claim of inadequate storage capacity was "balderdash."[3,10] The vehemence of the controversy was understandable; the political stakes were (and at this writing are) remarkably high. As one British news account observed, the "CRU is the world's leading centre for reconstructing past climate and temperatures. Climate change sceptics have long been keen to examine exactly how its data were compiled. That is now impossible."[4] A scientist who had unsuccessfully tried to obtain the raw data through a Freedom of Information request complained that "the CRU is basically saying, 'Trust us'. So much for settling questions and resolving debates with science."[4]

Yet, news accounts published at the height of the controversy suggested a surprising explanation for the CRU's announcement—that the fundamental problem leading to the loss of the data was not dishonesty, but disorganization. Interviews with sympathetic colleagues of Phil Jones, the internationally known UEA climatologist most closely identified with global warming research, suggested that what appeared to be a nefarious intent to suppress information was attributable to data collection and storage procedures that were, in Jones' February 2010 self-assessment, "not acceptable."[10] BBC environmental analyst Roger Harrabin reported that Jones' office was

> " ... piled high with paper, fragments from over the years, tens of thousands of pieces of paper, and [colleagues] suspect what happened was he took in the raw data to a central database and then let the pieces of paper go because he never realized that 20 years later he would be held to account over them."[11]

An independent panel of academic scientists reached a similar conclusion in April 2010, describing the CRU staff as "a small group of dedicated if slightly disorganised researchers who were ill-prepared for being the focus of public attention."[12] Although concluding that the "sole aim" of the CRU researchers was "to establish as robust a record of temperatures in recent centuries as possible" and that all work published by the CRU "was accompanied by detailed descriptions of uncertainties and ... appropriate caveats," the panel reached a devastating, albeit kindly stated, conclusion about the consequences of the CRU's disorganization on the field of climate science:

> "With very noisy data sets a great deal of judgement has to be used. Decisions have to be made on whether to omit pieces of data that appear to be aberrant. These are all matters of experience and judgement. ... Under such circumstances there must be an obligation on researchers to document the judgemental decisions they have made so that the work can in principle be replicated by others. ... **CRU accepts with hindsight that they should have devoted more attention in the past to archiving data and algorithms and recording exactly what they did. At the time the work was done, they had no idea that these data would assume the importance they have today and that the Unit would have to answer detailed inquiries on earlier work.**" (emphasis added)[12]

A House of Commons investigative panel similarly concluded in March 2010 that

> "... we can sympathise with Professor Jones, who must have found it frustrating

*to handle requests for data that he knew—or perceived—were motivated by a desire simply to undermine his work. … However, climate science is a matter of great importance and the quality of the science should be irreproachable. **We therefore consider that climate scientists should take steps to make available all the data that support their work (including raw data) and full methodological workings (including the computer codes). Had both been available, many of the problems at UEA could have been avoided.**" (emphasis added)[13]*

Notably, both Weitzman and Jones have argued that, while their procedures for storing and processing data were clearly suboptimal, the fundamental validity of their findings is unaffected.[8,10] Both assert that the missing or erroneous data represent only a small portion of a much larger body of work in support of their conclusions.[8,10] They might be right.

But, for the purposes of illustrating the importance of good documentation practices, these assertions are beside the point. Both Weitzman and Jones found themselves accused—in remarkably unflattering terms—of stonewalling to protect their findings and even of lying to the public.[3,14] Both found themselves in the unfortunate and permanent position of being unable to defend or engage in scientific discourse about their conclusions, because some of the information necessary to do so is gone and cannot be recovered. Moreover, body of work aside, there is no question that errors of this magnitude diminish the fundamental credibility of the researchers involved and, ultimately, of the findings that they produce. In other words, even if highly publicized mistakes have no *real* effect on scientific validity, the *perceived* effect does enough damage to make the experience painful. You do not want this to happen to you.

And, as we shall see in the rest of this chapter, it doesn't have to.

An Easy and Effective Project Documentation System

In 2000, a coauthor and I received feedback from the peer reviewers of a health policy journal that ultimately published our work, a retrospective analysis of an administrative health care claims database for a large health plan.[15] One peer reviewer commented that our sampling decision to exclude enrollees whose benefits had changed during the study period might have been problematic. The reviewer asked us to conduct sensitivity analyses in which we would rerun the data, this time including those enrollees, and determine if the exclusion had any effect on our findings.

It had been about three months since the paper had been initially submitted which, in the busy world of most data analysts, might as well have been 100 years. We remembered almost nothing of our procedures, having conducted many data analyses on different topics since submitting the paper to the journal. The work involved returning to the initial stage of pulling the sample, reprocessing the claims using the larger group, then replicating eight data tables and two figures. Nonetheless, the entire process took just a few hours (plus computer run time and transcription of the statistical output into new tables for the journal reviewers). Why so easy? Because we had used a remarkably simple but effective documentation system, the task of locating and rerunning the necessary files was painless and efficient.

Documentation System: Five Steps

A. Verify data that are received from others.

Total active time (per file received): 30-60 minutes. (Note: Active time is "hands on" time, excluding computer run time. The time commitment is greater when manual data entry must be verified, e.g., when paper survey results have been coded and entered by hand.)

B. Track work files by name.

Total active time (per day): 5 to 10 minutes.

C. For each manuscript or work product, produce a publication tracking record that summarizes the source of each data table or figure.

Total active time (per work product, e.g., per article or presentation): 30-60 minutes.

D. Annotate computer program file as you work.

Total active time: After an initial learning curve, assuming that this activity is routinely incorporated into programming activities, the added time should be negligible.

E. Use a work product review system that is never overlooked, no matter how urgent the need for the research results.

Total active time (per research project): 1 hour for analyst to prepare "package" for review; 1-4 hours for completion of review, depending on scope and complexity of project.

A. Verify Data That Are Received From Others

Whenever a data file is received from any source, verify that the file contents are accurate. Although the specific verification process will depend on the type of file and the topic of the research, the general idea is to ensure that the file actually contains what it is purported to contain *before* you use it. Examples of good verification practices are shown in Table 2A.

Table 2A
Suggested Procedures to Verify Incoming Data

Verification Element and Process	To Catch These Common Sources of Error
Number of cases • Ask the file source how many cases the file contains, and verify the case count in the file that you received. • Check case count not just overall, but per unit of time (e.g., by month).	• File transmission errors (e.g., computer problems) • Human error (e.g., file source sends the wrong file) • Incomplete dataset (e.g., data were supposed to be reported for entire calendar year, but the twelfth month contains only a few cases)
Key findings • For example, if the file includes survey data, ask the file source to calculate frequencies on several of the survey responses. If the file contains cost information, ask the file source to calculate mean values for several cost fields. • Then, run the same analyses yourself and ensure that you get the same answers that your file source reported to you.	• Miscommunication about file contents (e.g., how the fields are coded, location of fields in the file) • Miscommunication about how to interpret the fields in the file
Matching summary and detail records in separate files • For example, if File A contains a record of expenditures for individual purchases and File B summarizes those purchases to the person level, verify a few purchase fields to determine that the individual purchases in File A sum to the totals shown in File B.	• Miscommunications about the contents of files • Matching errors (e.g., inadvertently matching records for one person to records for an entirely different person because of a programming error) • Identification number discrepancies (e.g., same person has two different identifiers or same identifier is associated with two different people)
Requested characteristics • If you asked that specific characteristics be used for file creation, verify that every case in the file has those characteristics. For example, if you requested a file of persons aged 64 years or younger with at least two purchases from Store A in 2008, verify that each person in the file meets the specified age and purchasing criteria.	• Miscommunication about project specifications • Human error in file creation • Changes in coding (e.g., Store A has two different identifiers, but you knew about only one of them)
Matching across files • If you will be using multiple files, verify that data match across files as they should. For example, if you have been told that the identifiers match (e.g., the same identifying numbers in File A and File B refer to the same person) verify that cases with matching identifiers in both Files A and B have the same date of birth, gender, age, or any other information that you have.	• Miscommunication about the contents of multiple files • Human errors that occur in file creation (e.g., file creator accidentally assigns the same identifier to two different people)

Table 2A *(continued)*
Suggested Procedures to Verify Incoming Data

Verification Element and Process	To Catch These Common Sources of Error
Modification of previous work • If your work modifies a study previously published by you or someone else, first verify/replicate the work (or a few key analyses), then perform the modifications.	• Misunderstanding of previously published work • Inadvertent replication of an error in the previously published work (e.g., procedure was described incorrectly in the publication)
Keying accuracy • If data were manually keyed (e.g., from hard copy surveys) verify all (preferable) or a sample of data to verify that the results appearing in the survey match the data. • Check for "nonsense" values (e.g., age = 493, days of therapy is a negative number)	• Typographical errors • Misunderstanding of the "code book" (keying instructions) by one or more data entry staff

[a] One client with whom I have worked combined these checks with data exploration (Chapter 7, Table 7B) in a single checklist. This approach has the advantage of simplicity because the analyst uses only a single tool; however, data verification should be performed immediately upon receipt of the data, whereas data exploration can take place over a longer period of time.

Note that not all of these verification steps will be necessary for every project. (An important exception is that you should *always* verify the number of cases when you receive a file to detect human- or computer-caused file transmission errors.) Additionally, it is possible that some verification steps not listed here will be necessary. The key is to spend a little time thinking about how to ensure accurate communication about what the data files contain for your particular project. Note also that if computing capacity or "run time" is a problem, you can usually verify a subsample of cases and accomplish the same goal.

If you are wondering why anyone would perform steps to detect errors so obvious that they shouldn't ever happen, please consider **two key points**. **First**, most serious errors *are* obvious. Although in a perfect world these errors would not happen, they unfortunately happen anyway. Complete error prevention is impossible in a world of fallible human beings; the point of verification is to prevent the errors that inevitably *will* occur from affecting the integrity of your project. **Second**, most verification steps involve simple frequencies or crosstabulations that take only a few minutes to perform. *It is not necessary to use complex analytic procedures. The key point is simply to verify that you and your file source have the same understanding about what the file contains.*

A "real-life" example may be helpful. I once worked on a project in which we studied "tiered" prescription drug benefits. In a three-tiered benefit, patients pay the smallest amount for generic drugs, a higher amount for "preferred" brand drugs, and the highest amount for "nonpreferred" brand drugs. To conduct our analyses, we received a file of drug claims (billing data) in which we could identify each drug. We also received a separate file showing the status—generic, preferred, or nonpreferred—for each drug. Our first step was to verify that the files matched. That is, for each generic drug claim, we checked to be sure that the patient paid the generic cost-sharing amount; for preferred brands, we checked for the preferred brand amount, and so on. To our dismay, at the initial verification step, we realized that the copayments did *not* match consistently. An investigation revealed that the discrepancy was caused by two problems. First, some products had changed tiers (i.e., from preferred to nonpreferred status or vice versa) during the study period, an issue that we identified by running simple crosstabulations on the copayment match rates by month for each drug. We realized that we had to set up a separate analytic category for drugs with a tier status change during the study period. Second, conversations with employees who had provided the files revealed that the term "preferred" was not consistent with the nomenclature that they used in processing and storing the data and was, therefore, not clear to them; thus, the data that we had received did not match our project specifications. We had to use more specific terminology to communicate our file requests. As time-consuming as the investigation was, it was far better than discovering the discrepancy after running the analyses and writing the report or, worse yet, not discovering it at all and publishing erroneous information.

B. Track Work Files by Name

If you are like most researchers, during the course of any project you work with multiple data files—sometimes *many* files—and you often need to access file information quickly. Typically, you will encounter circumstances that require you to repeat a step in the analysis. These might include responding to questions from journal peer reviewers or from information users (i.e., those who will use or make decisions based upon your results); correcting mistakes made by you or others; making changes to an *a priori* analysis plan; or encountering unexpected data quality problems. Or, you might wish to carry out a follow-up analysis of your previously published work, which requires that you analyze data files with which you last worked a long time ago. Additionally, if you are writing either an article for a peer reviewed journal or a paper for submission to a teacher or mentor, you will need to explain your analytic procedures systematically (usually step-by-step) in the methods section of the study report.

If you are currently a student, the lapsed time from initial work product to receipt of feedback from a teacher or mentor is usually much shorter than it will be after graduation. Still, you need to be able to answer questions, make changes if your teacher/mentor deems them advisable, and even avoid those middle-of-the-night "oh m'gosh, is my analysis all wrong?" moments of panic.

A file tracking system makes carrying out these important tasks much easier. An example of the system is shown in Table 2B. The logic of the system is simple. For each data file, you will make a record of how, when, and by what computer program it was produced.

Table 2B
Sample Data File Tracking Chart

Project: Three-tier utilization analysis
Subdirectory: c:\spss\three_tier

Description	Name of Program	Run Date	Name of Data File Created
Raw data received from Halls-of-Learning University on 03.05.09; created SPSS system file. Confirmed n=10,016 cases with Mary Smith at HLU.	read1.sps	03.10.09	T3_survey1.sav
Recoded invalid incomes for 6 families	clean1.sps	03.15.09	T3_master1.sav
Recoded gender=unknown for 12 respondents using manual search of eligibility records	clean2.sps	03.16.09	T3_master2.sav
Recoded missing data for question 3 using comments on questionnaire—5 respondents	clean3.sps	03.17.09	T3_master3.sav
Classified chronic diseases (questions 5-10) into categories	chronic1.sps	03.18.09	chronic_class.sav

Although the system is easy to use, it requires consistent application. That is, use it for *every* data file, *every* day. Additionally, to facilitate data access, maintain all study computer files in a single location in a subdirectory with an informative name. For example, the subdirectory name "three_tier" is much more informative than "research" or "study" in helping you and others determine the location of the data files.

If possible, it is advisable to maintain backup copies of data files on a centralized drive that is accessible to all members of a department or research group, again using an informative subdirectory name. If, for any reason, the primary data analyst is unable to fulfill his or her duties, any member of the team will be able to use the tracking record and files to perform analyses. (Of course, all members of the research team should be bound by appropriate confidentiality agreements, and the drive should be secured by password protection or another similar method to protect the privacy of research subjects.)

C. Publication Tracking Record

Before submitting a document for publication, either to a peer-reviewed journal or for Internet posting, produce a record that you will use for internal tracking purposes, summarizing the source of each data table or figure in the publication. You will use this information, along with the file tracking system, to respond to questions from information users or peer reviewers about how your data analyses were performed. An example is shown in Table 2C.

Table 2C
Sample Publication Tracking Chart

Project: Three-tier utilization analysis
Subdirectory: c:\spss\three_tier
Submitted to: *Journal of Managed Care Pharmacy*
Submission date: July 3, 2010

Location in Publication	Statistic Produced	Name of Program and Output File	Run Date	Data File
Page 3	20% of drug claims in 2008 were for third-tier medications	claim_profile.sps claim_profile.doc	06.15.10	T3_master3.sav
Page 8	Table 1 demographic characteristics	demographics.sps demograph4.doc	06.20.10	T3_patient1.sav
Page 8	Table 1 clinical characteristics for sample overall	clinical1.sps clinical6.doc	06.20.10	T3_clinical2.sav
Page 8	Table 1 clinical characteristics for patients with chronic illness	chronic1.sps chronic1.doc	06.21.10	chronic_class.sav
Page 9	Table 2 outcomes for all patients and for patients with chronic illness	outcomes1.sps outcomes1b.doc	06.22.10	T3_master4.sav
Page 10	Table 3 regression analyses	logistic.sps logistic.spo	06.23.10	T3_master4.sav

Note that using the publication tracking record and computer files stored in a centralized location, even a data analyst who has not previously been involved with the project, or who completed the work months before and no longer remembers it, can easily locate and replicate the necessary files if questions arise or changes are necessary. In a more common scenario, a graduate student who is bogged down in final exams or a busy researcher trying to juggle multiple projects simultaneously can address questions or make changes without having to rely on memory or on "trial and error" (i.e., testing files to determine which is the right one), which can waste a great deal of time.

D. Computer Output Annotation

As the data analyst works, he or she should record, in the computer program and/or output (depending on the software used), notes that explain the logic and steps in the program to someone unfamiliar with its details. The annotations are intended to facilitate the work product review that will be performed by an internal peer reviewer prior to release of the information (see E below). Additionally, the notes are helpful to the data analyst who returns to the program at a later date, either for modification or to answer questions, but who no longer remembers it well. To facilitate later understanding of the study methods if necessary—for example, if a question is asked about the rationale for a sampling decision or a request is made to replicate the project using new data—it is *much* better to *document* decisions about changes in the study protocol in writing, rather than relying on memory. The documentation does not have to be complex or lengthy; for example, "Removed Clinic A from study sample because Clinic A's physicians failed to attend all project training sessions and n of patients=3."

Explanations of the annotation process are shown in Table 2D. Annotations might include something like the following examples:

This job creates an age group variable and calculates termination rates for each age category; name of job is agegrp.sps located in compliance study subdirectory; KAF.

Look back 180 days before therapy initiation date; determine if antinauseant was used during that time.

Identify the earliest and latest dates of antidepressant drug use based on sorted fill dates.

Table 2D
Computer Output Annotation

What the Analyst Should Do	Why the Analyst Should Do It
General rule of thumb: The computer output should contain all the information necessary for a person who is unfamiliar with the program to verify that the work product matches specifications and was done correctly.	• Following this rule of thumb will make the processes of verifying and, if necessary, replicating the work faster and easier for everyone.
At the start of the program, include a comment line describing the name of the computer program, what the program does, and the analyst's initials. For example: "This program calculates mean income by household category for input into standard of living analysis; name is hhincome.sps; KAF."	• Description of the program helps the internal peer reviewer to understand what he or she is looking for in the computer output file. • Inclusion of computer program name enables all staff – including those unfamiliar with the project – to locate the files easily at a later date. • Initials identify staff for follow-up questions.
At each stage of the program, write a brief description of what the code in that section does and any other information needed to understand the rationale for the code. For example: "Determine number of months from first diagnosis date to first drug treatment date; first diagnosis is earliest date with either a primary or secondary diagnosis of migraine; first treatment is date of first claim for Drug X."	• Description helps internal peer reviewer to understand what he or she is looking for. • Internal peer reviewer will check both the description of the code and the code itself against project specifications.
At each major step of the program, include a verification step documenting that the step was successful. • After recoding from one categorization method to another, crosstabulate the old variable against the new and make sure that the distributions across categories are as expected. • After performing multiple programming steps to generate a summary variable, list a sample of cases. The list should include the summary variable and the variables used to generate it. Use the list to verify that the summary variable was calculated according to specification. • Check that each category description matches data (e.g., for persons in an "age 18 to 24" category, the minimum age should be 18 and the maximum should be 24).	• Having verification in the output facilitates work product review; internal peer reviewer does not have to open data source and run separate analyses to verify accuracy. • Provides an easy way to check for programming errors. • Provides a check for unexpected patterns in the data (e.g., out-of-range codes or numerous missing values).
Include descriptive data, such as mean, median, minimum, maximum, and interquartile range, for all key study variables.	• Descriptive statistics help internal peer reviewer to verify that the statistical technique used was appropriate for the data. • Unexpected results (e.g., age = 350 years) point to coding or keying errors.

Note that the documentation does not have to be, and probably should not be, complicated or elaborate. Often a simple list of a sample of cases does the job well. For example, assume that the analyst has calculated (1) age at start date and end date of treatment, based on the patient's date of birth and the first and last pharmacy claim dates for a study drug of interest; and (2) total cost of treatment and total days of therapy based on the claim costs and days supply dispensed, respectively. The lists might look something like this:

Raw data file

Patient	Birth Date	Service Date	Cost	Days Supply
001	1969.07.03	2009.06.09	$100	30
001	1969.07.03	2009.07.10	$100	30
001	1969.07.03	2009.08.04	$100	30
001	1969.07.03	2009.09.15	$100	30
002	1999.03.16	2009.07.20	$250	90
002	1999.03.16	2010.01.10	$250	90

Summary data file

Patient	Age at start	Age at end	Total cost	Total days
001	39	40	$400	120
002	10	10	$500	180

E. Work Product Review System

Maintain and strictly enforce these two rules:

1. *Every* work product, and the computer programs that produced the data for that work product, must be reviewed and verified, in detail, by someone other than the original analyst—an internal peer reviewer.
2. The work product review *must* be completed prior to release of the information, no matter how urgent the need for the findings.

The job of the internal peer reviewer is to ensure that work products are accurate and have been produced according to specification. This role is *supportive, not adversarial*; responsibility for the quality of the work product rests with *both* the original data analyst and the internal peer reviewer. In a "small shop," the principal investigator and analyst may review each other's work. In a larger work group, multiple analysts can be cross-trained to perform internal peer reviews. Graduate students can review one another's work; this is *excellent* training.

The internal peer reviewer should have access to the following information:

1. Research proposal or protocol document, preferably with an *a priori* analysis plan (Chapter 4).
2. Data file tracking chart (Table 2B).
3. Publication tracking chart, if the work product is close to dissemination or submission for publication (Table 2C).
4. *Annotated* computer output (either paper or electronic) for each computer program that produced either the data files or the research findings (Table 2D), sorted in chronological order to facilitate the review process.
5. Summary results tables prepared by analyst (e.g., tables or figures that will be included in the final work product).
6. Data files in the centrally stored location, in case the internal peer reviewer needs to perform an analysis to address a question or concern.
7. Any other materials that might be needed to check the quality of the work— for example, if survey data have been used and manually keyed, the internal peer reviewer might ask the analyst to pull a sample of hard copy surveys for verification. (Manual keying should have been checked prior to this stage, but the internal reviewer may want to verify a sample of cases.)

After receiving the project materials, the internal peer reviewer should examine each step in sampling, data processing, calculation, and production of tables and figures to ensure that the work matches the study plan or, if it does not, verify that the change was intentional and not made in error. The internal peer reviewer should also track the sample from beginning to end of the process. For example, if there were 1,000 cases at the end of step 1, there should be 1,000 cases at the start of step 2. Similarly, the sample size should be checked after each sample inclusion or exclusion step to ensure that the expected number of cases is present in the sample at each stage of the process. Sample cases should never just "appear" or "disappear." This procedure is **necessary for two reasons. First**, unexpected gain or loss of cases probably indicates a flaw in the program logic or an unexpected data pattern. **Second,** a sample selection flow chart showing the number of cases included and removed at each major step of the sampling process is recommended in research-reporting guidelines and is a requirement of many journals (Chapter 10).

The internal peer reviewer should also check the accuracy of the code. Because not every reviewer is a "programming whiz," the inclusion of verification steps in the computer output itself (Table 2D) saves the internal reviewer a great deal of time and, potentially, frustration.

If the internal reviewer determines that the available documentation is insufficient to verify the accuracy of the work product, it is his or her responsibility to ask the analyst for the necessary information. It is important that the internal reviewer have the authority to request additional information and to suspend release of the study results, if necessary, until verification is complete. *An organizational culture that values accuracy is critical to the effectiveness of the process. A "rubber stamp" will do nothing to protect you or your fellow workers/ students from the threat of inadvertently releasing erroneous study findings.*

A summary data quality control checklist is in Table 2E.

Table 2E
Data Quality Control Summary Checklist

Verification
➢ Upon receipt of file, contents have been verified to ensure that they match specifications.
➢ Previously published analyses or results of known work are replicated before using the file.
➢ Manual keying of all (preferable) or a sample of cases has been checked for accuracy.

Documentation
➢ All study documents are stored in location(s) accessible to all members of the team.
➢ Files and subdirectories have been given informative names.
➢ Documentation is clear even to persons who are unfamiliar with or no longer remember the work.
➢ Computer output includes annotation indicating the program name, program task, run date (if not automatically generated by statistical software), and identity of analyst.
➢ Annotations throughout the computer output explain each major step.
➢ Each step in the analysis includes verification of accuracy.
➢ Number of cases is shown at each stage of the sampling process.
➢ Data file tracking chart has been maintained.
➢ Publication tracking chart has been created if work product is to be disseminated or submitted for publication.

Work Product Review
➢ Documentation is adequate to verify results.
➢ Work performed matches specifications (i.e., steps performed match study protocol and/or methods section of research report).
➢ Coding is accurate (i.e., no coding errors in the statistical program).
➢ Number of cases is accounted for through all stages of sampling and data processing.

Adapted with permission from Fairman KA. Peeking inside the statistical black box.[16]

Paper Versus Electronic Storage

It is considered *de rigueur* these days to rely primarily on electronic, rather than paper, files. However, paper has its place in project documentation for **several reasons. First**, some analysts may find it easier to keep a file tracking notebook located on their desks, in which they jot notes as they work, than to open up a computer document every time they want to make a file entry. **Second**, some documentation arrives in paper form—for example, a letter from a project sponsor requesting a change to an analysis or notes jotted down during a meeting. Information of this type is important and should be retained for use in the work product review process. **Third**, computers do crash from time to time, and files located on only a single desktop computer are at risk. *To a limited extent*, the choice of paper versus electronic storage should be made by the primary data analyst because he or she must be comfortable with the documentation system for it to be used consistently. However, a data analyst who wants to rely *solely* on electronic documentation should be instructed to (1) maintain letters or other hard-copy correspondence in a clearly marked binder or folder and (2) back up electronic study files daily. Compliance with these requirements should be monitored routinely and, if appropriate, included as part of job performance review protocols.

Do I *Have* To?

The work product review process seems cumbersome at first. However, with practice and the provision of a good "package" of materials by analysts to internal peer reviewers, it goes quickly. More importantly, as the following analysis of the 73/42 mistake shows, it can save you from the embarrassment of having to retract a research finding.

How Could the "73/42" Mistake Have Been Prevented?

In his article describing the reanalysis of Weitzman's data, Peterson recounts a remarkably lengthy process of trying to determine how the erroneous 73/42 statistic had been produced using the files that he had been told were the project data files ("one is an SPSS systems file and the other file contains the raw data").[6] Despite multiple attempts, he ultimately reported that "I have been unable to discover how Weitzman's results could have been obtained. The most likely explanation is that errors in her analysis of the data were responsible for producing her results."[6]

In response, Weitzman provided a fascinating and detailed account both of the sequence of events that led to the publication of the erroneous figure and of her fruitless attempt

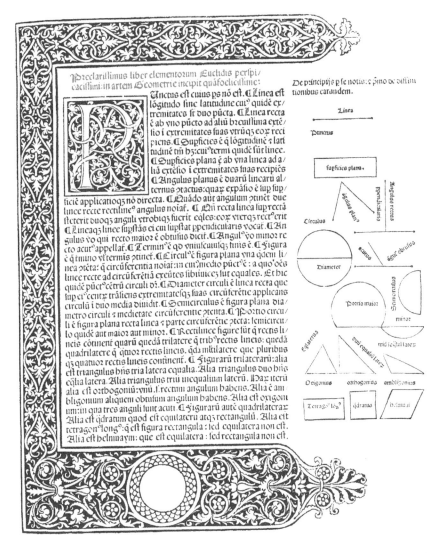

First page of Euclid's Elements, Campanus of Novara, 1482 (original manuscript, 1260). Widely considered to be among the most influential textbooks ever written, the *Elements* drew from several sources, including earlier translations of Euclid's work, and remained in use for many centuries. Euclidian geometry provides compelling evidence that an organizational system need not be complex to be effective. Although an infinite number of Euclidian proofs and theorems are possible, they are all based on a logical system describing a small number of simple spatial relationships, such as the intersection of lines. Source: Campanus of Novara. Available at: http://www.gap-system.org/~history/Biographies/Campanus.html. Public domain image from Wikimedia Commons.

to reconstruct the data analysis, which she described as a "very sad, time consuming, and frustrating experience."[8] As her explanation shows, **both the original error and the sequence of events that followed it were completely preventable.**

> Weitzman: *"The data collection was subcontracted to the UCLA Survey Research Center which did the interviews (in 1978), coded the data, and subjected them to a rather elaborate verification and retrieval procedure.... Changes to the original raw data file resulting from this data cleaning process were made by a series of programming statements on a master SPSS system file.* **The raw data file that is stored at the Murray Center** *[one of the files used in the Peterson analysis]* **is the original "dirty data" file and does not include these cleaning changes**.... *Unfortunately, the original* **cleaned** *master SPSS system file no longer exists."* (emphasis in original)[8]

Analysis: The publication tracking record (Table 2C) showing the name and run date of the computer program(s) that produced each study result, including the 73/42 statistic, would have prevented use of the wrong file by Peterson. Additionally, had there been a file tracking record (Table 2B), the data used for 73/42 could have been recreated easily despite the loss of the master SPSS file.

> Weitzman: *"Unfortunately, the original cleaned master SPSS system file no longer exists. I assumed it was being copied and reformatted as I moved for job changes and fellowships ... With each move, new programmers worked on the files to accommodate different computer systems. ... I know now (but did not know then) that the original master SPSS system file that I used for my book had been lost or damaged at some point and was not included among these files. The SPSS system file that I thought was the master SPSS system file was the result of the merging of many smaller subfiles that had been created for specific analyses."*[8]

Analysis: Weitzman describes 4 separate moves to institutions with 4 different computer systems, clearly a challenge. However, her sample comprised only 228 people, making it likely that the final master file used in the analyses that were published in the book could have been placed onto a floppy disk (the common data medium at the time), enabling Weitzman to personally retain the data. Additionally, even if the data would not have fit on a floppy or other medium that Weitzman could transport herself, verifying the data at each transfer (Table 2A), a task that would have taken little time to complete with such a small number of cases, would have prevented the loss of the file. Finally, failing these precautions, the publication tracking record (Table 2C) would have made the loss of the data file immediately apparent the very first time that anyone tried to replicate or answer questions about the study results, enabling an earlier (and likely more successful) search at the various institutions for the missing information.

> Weitzman: *"I now report, with chagrin, that I myself had questioned the 73 percent decline in women's post-divorce standard of living when the figure was first computed and asked my computer expert on three separate occasions to verify it. He said he had done so, with the same result, and I accepted that."*[8]

Analysis: **Ouch.** With a systematic work product review process in place, either Weitzman or a designated supervisor would have reviewed the code and computer output and identified the 73/42 mistake before it was published. ***Weitzman's difficult experience illustrates the inadequacy of asking an analyst to verify his or her own results. As a quality assurance method, that approach simply does not work.***

> Weitzman: *"When questions were raised about the 73/42 percent statistic I went back to what I believed was the master SPSS system file to rerun the analysis. ... When I could not replicate the analyses in my book with what I had mistakenly assumed was the archived master SPSS system file, I hired an independent consultant ... to help me untangle what had happened. ... But she could not do this without an accurate data file to work with. We then went back to the original questionnaires and recoded a random sample of about 25 percent of the cases. There were so many discrepancies between the questionnaires and the 'dirty data' raw data file, and between the questionnaires and the mismatched SPSS system file, that we finally abandoned the effort and left a warning to all future researchers that **both files at the Murray Center were so seriously flawed that they could not be used**."* (emphasis in original)[8]

Analysis: The process of checking questionnaires against the raw data file should have occurred as part of the data verification process immediately upon completion of keying (Table 2A).

Do Mistakes Like the 73/42 Error Really Happen Today?

Readers may be thinking something like this: "Both of the scenarios described in this chapter happened decades ago. Computing capabilities today are so much better now. Hasn't the availability of better technology virtually eliminated the problem of poor documentation? Do I *really* have to worry about any of this?"

As biostatistician Andrew Vickers observed in a 2006 commentary, the problem of the "garbage-in-garbage-out" effect in medical research is ongoing; he cites the example of a colleague who nearly published erroneous findings before Vickers checked a sample of data collection sheets against the electronic data file and found substantial and serious keying errors.[5] In fact, as Vickers points out, the "drop-down" interactive menu technology that became available in most statistical packages beginning in the 1990s has actually made the likelihood of error *worse*.[5] Although some packages permit the researcher to invoke an option that saves the programming statements from an interactive session to a separate file, the easily used interactive menu technology makes it tempting to ignore the all-important step of saving the statistical programming code. When a researcher foregoes this step, the programming work is largely irreproducible and cannot be verified.[5] Thus, the need for caution is generally *amplified*—not reduced—by the electronic "step savers" available to researchers today.

Summing Up: What Have We Learned?

Maintaining project documentation will never be the most interesting part of your day (or mine). But it is one of the most important. As Vickers notes:

> *"I have often had to fight with investigators to get them to implement ... simple [data] procedures and checks, most typically because they are thought to 'take too long.' Well, no lab scientist uses dirty equipment on the grounds that bottle washing is too time-consuming."*[5]

Although establishing the discipline of a documentation system can require a learning curve and perhaps more than a little persuasion of reluctant colleagues, the necessary time investment is more than offset by the gains in accuracy, ease of response to requests for information or changes, and—of no small importance—peace of mind.

In the next chapter, we delve into the topics of validity, confounding, and sound research design to set the stage for project planning. We begin in nineteenth-century London with a disease of "fearful virulence"[17] that spawned a decades-long process of discovery about disease transmission, as well as what is perhaps the most important epidemiological map in human history.

References

1. Workman M. Why child/spousal support guidelines are skyhigh. S.P.A.R.C. Undated. Available at http://deltabravo.net/custody/skyhigh.php.

2. Webster K. Post-divorce wealth gap was wrong, agrees author. May 17, 1996. *The Seattle Times.* Available at: http://community.seattletimes.nwsource.com/archive/?date=19960519&slug=2329984.

3. Michaels PJ. The dog ate global warming. *National Review Online.* September 23, 2009. Available at: http://www.nationalreview.com/articles/228291/dog-ate-global-warming/patrick-j-michaels.

4. Leake J. Climate change data dumped. *Times Online.* November 29, 2009.

5. Vickers AJ. Look at your garbage bin: it may be the only thing you need to know about statistics. November 3, 2006. Available at: http://www.medscape.com/viewarticle/546515.

6. Peterson RR. A re-evaluation of the economic consequences of divorce. *American Sociological Review.* 1996;61:528-36.

7. Peterson RR. Statistical errors, faulty conclusions, misguided policy: reply to Weitzman. *American Sociological Review.* 1996;61:539-40.

8. Weitzman LJ. The economic consequences of divorce are still unequal: comment on Peterson. *American Sociological Review.* 1996;61:537-38.

9. University of East Anglia, Climatic Research Unit. CRU data availability. Available at: http://www.cru.uea.ac.uk/cru/data/availability/.

10. Heffernan O. 'Climategate' scientist speaks out. *Nature News.* February 15, 2010. Available at: http://www.nature.com/news/2010/100215/full/news.2010.71.html.

11. Petre J. Climategate U-turn as scientist at centre of row admits: There has been no global warming since 1995. *Mail Online.* February 14, 2010. Available at: http://www.dailymail.co.uk/news/article-1250872/Climategate-U-turn-Astonishment-scientist-centre-global-warming-email-row-admits-data-organised.html.

12. Oxburgh R, Davies H, Emanuel K, et al. Report of the International Panel set up by the University of East Anglia to examine the research of the Climatic Research Unit. April 12, 2010. Available at: http://www.uea.ac.uk/mac/comm/media/press/CRUstatements/SAP.

13. House of Commons Science and Technology Committee. The disclosure of climate data from the Climatic Research Unit at the University of East Anglia. Eighth Report

of Session 2009-10. March 31, 2010. Available at: http://www.desmogblog.com/sites/ beta.desmogblog.com/files/phil%20jones%20house%20of%20commons%20report.pdf.

14. Rapp C. Lies, damned lies, and Lenore Weitzman. Undated. Available at: http://www. acbr.com/biglie.htm.

15. Motheral B, Fairman KA. Effect of a three-tier copay on pharmaceutical and other medical utilization. *Med Care*. 2001;39:1293-1304.

16. Fairman KA. Peeking inside the statistical black box: how to analyze quantitative information and get it right the first time. *J Manag Care Pharm*. 2007;13(1):70-74. Available at: http://www.ncbi.nlm.nih.gov/pubmed?term=fairman%20peeking%20 statistical%20black%20box.

17. Henry Mayhew quotes. Available at: http://www.brainyquote.com/quotes/quotes/h/ henrymayhe274379.html.

CHAPTER 3

Association, Causation, and the Hazards of Relying on Observation: The Importance of Good Research Design

"As there is no difference whatever, either in the houses or the people receiving the supply of the two Water Companies, or in any of the physical conditions with which they are surrounded, it is obvious that no experiment could have been devised which would more thoroughly test the effect of water supply on the progress of cholera than this, which circumstances placed ready made before the observer."—Epidemiological pioneer John Snow, describing in 1854 the methods of his landmark comparison of customers of companies that drew water from polluted versus nonpolluted sources[1]

"I'm afraid I have to make the same points I've made over and over. An epidemiologic relationship between glucose level and risk of cardiovascular events does not mean [that] lowering glucose levels with an intervention will have the desired effect. ... there are no shortcuts. We just don't know what we're doing until an adequate randomized trial is done."—Cardiologist Robert Califf, commenting on the surprising finding of the ACCORD (Action to Control Cardiovascular Risk in Diabetes) trial that intensive blood sugar control in type 2 diabetes, which

What You Will Learn in Chapter 3

✓ Why observational research is a valuable part of scientific progress—but often *just the beginning* of evidence-based decision making

✓ Which *common but flawed research designs* often lead to erroneous conclusions

✓ What *confounding* is and how it affects study validity

✓ What factors are most often used to assess the likelihood that an observed relationship is *causal*

✓ Why researchers sometimes encounter difficult *tradeoffs* in study design

✓ How to use observational evidence to meet the needs of information users—*without* "overinterpreting" the data

had been expected to reduce cardiovascular deaths, had actually increased the rate of mortality by 22%[2]

"People with white hair have higher mortality than people with other hair colors, but dyeing their hair black or blond is unlikely to improve their survival chances."—Research methodologist Jane Miller[3]

Do you think that public discourse today has become too mean-spirited? You might be right. But for historical perspective, consider the following political commentary, published on June 23, 1855:

> *"These unsavory persons, trembling for the conservation of their right to fatten upon the injury of their neighbors, came in a crowd, reeking with putrid grease, redolent of stinking bones, fresh from seething heaps of stercoraceous deposits to lay their 'case' before the Committee. They were eloquent upon the health-bestowing properties wafted in the air that had been enriched in its playful transit over depots of rotten bones, stinking fat, steaming dungheaps, and other accumulations of animal matter, decomposing into wealth..."*[4,5]

With these words, the editors of one of the most prestigious journals in international medical history, *The Lancet*, described the merchants who attended a March 1855 Parliamentary hearing on a proposed amendment to the *Nuisances Removal and Diseases Prevention Act* of 1846. Championed by politicians and scientists who favored the *miasma* ("bad air") theory of cholera transmission, the amendment would have imposed regulations on fume-emitting industries including knacker's yards, which processed animal carcasses, and manufacturers of soap, which at that time was made by a fat-rendering procedure that emitted unpleasant odors.[6]

The editorial marked a climactic point in one of the most vicious and, ultimately, important debates in the history of medicine. Editors of *The Lancet*—known as a "reformist" publication with a "zeal to counter the forces that undermine the values of medicine, be they political, social, or commercial"[7]—supported the amendment as well as the *miasma* theory of cholera transmission, and attacked physician John Snow, who had advanced the theory that cholera was caused by a "morbid poison entering the alimentary canal."[1] And it was no ordinary attack. The first in a series of *Lancet* editorials about Snow described his views as typifying "the crude opinions and hobbyistic dogmas of men whose perceptions are dimmed by the gloom of the den in which they think and move" and the debate over cholera transmission as "the misfortune of Medicine, in its conflict with the prejudices of society," to be "continually exposed to discomfiture, through the perverse, crotchetty, or treasonable behavior of certain of its own disciples."[4,5]

Of course, evidence would eventually prove *The Lancet* editors wrong about cholera transmission, if not about the merits of laws intended to reduce noxious fumes. By 1866, eight years after Snow's untimely death at 45 years of age, his theory of cholera transmission had become widely accepted by scientists.[8] And, in 1883, physician and bacteriologist Robert Koch discovered *Vibrio cholerae*.[8] Snow's "morbid poison" had been identified.

Perhaps the story of the conflict between John Snow and proponents of the *miasma* theory should be viewed as an account of science at its best—the power of a growing body of evidence forever changing viewpoints about the transmission of a deadly disease and ultimately, saving millions of lives through increasingly effective disease prevention initiatives. But if we stop there in our understanding of the historical account, we miss much of its significance for us today. What one contemporary epidemiologist described as Snow's "struggle to understand and control [cholera]"[1] is at its heart the story of a staunch refusal to accept cursory evidence and of a passion for working hard—to a degree that some contemporary researchers might find incredible, if not impossible—to provide better information to a public desperately in need of it.

Careful Observation and Scientific Progress:
The Hard Work of John Snow

In decrying Snow's theories as contrary to the "well-weighed decisions of [the] true representatives"[4] of science, the *Lancet* editors relied heavily on the work of "the accomplished head of the Statistics Department of the Register Office,"[4] William Farr. Rather than "deal with the causes of mortality," the *Lancet* editors noted, Farr had calculated "the rates of mortality in different districts," finding that

> "… there is a natural mortality which does not exceed 17 in 1000; that whensoever that rate is exceeded there are noxious and generally removable causes in operation, and therefore that any excess of deaths above this proportion ought to be the signal for applying the resources of science to the improvement of the health of the district."[4]

In other words, Farr had performed a relatively simple **cross-sectional** (single point-in-time) analysis of death rates by geographic area, observed an association between higher death rates and more intense concentrations of noxious odors, and concluded that the association equated to a causal mechanism.[8] Get rid of the sources of the odors, said prevailing wisdom based in part on Farr's results, and disease rates would decline.

Contrast Farr's simple analysis with the work performed by Snow over a period of at least 6 years: a painstaking and, in places in his detailed account, heartbreaking case-by-case record of disease transmissions, incubation periods, and deaths in various locations; an elaborate epidemiological map of London streets that today is considered a landmark in the history of public health; the identification of the now infamous "Broad Street pump" as a key source of infection; in-depth investigation of Broad Street pump use by nonresidents of the street who contracted cholera; and, perhaps the pinnacle of Snow's work, a statistical comparison of cholera mortality rates for customers of water companies that drew their water from polluted versus pure sources. Snow wrote of his natural experiment in 1854:

> "No fewer than three hundred thousand people of both sexes, of every age and occupation, and of every rank and station, from gentlefolks down to the very poor, were divided into two groups without their choice, and, in most cases, without their knowledge; one group being supplied with water containing the sewage of London, and, amongst it, whatever might have come from the cholera patients, the other group having water quite free from such impurity."[1]

Even this elegant and powerfully designed analysis required intense effort because many water consumers (e.g., renters) did not know the source of their water. "It would, indeed, have been almost impossible for me to complete the inquiry," Snow noted, "if I had not found that I could distinguish the water of the two companies with perfect certainty by a chemical test." That is, to eliminate the possibility of incorrectly categorizing each customer's water source (a problem known to epidemiologists as **misclassification of exposure**), Snow devised a simple test of the sodium content in each water sample to determine the water source with certainty.[1] Snow's hard work paid off in credible and actionable results: the cholera death rate for customers of the Southwark and Vauxhall company, which drew its water from the polluted Thames River, was 71 per 10,000 houses, compared with 5 per 10,000 houses for the Lambeth water company, which drew its

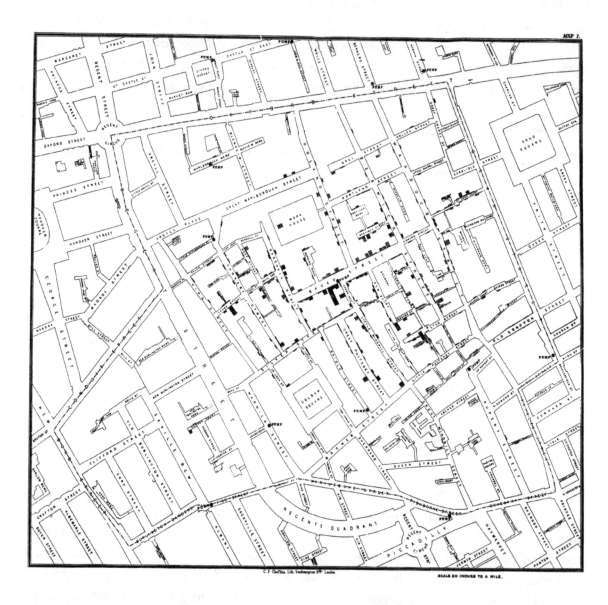

Map of cholera case clusters by location, streets of London, 1854. Drawn by then-controversial physician John Snow, the map is today considered a landmark in the history of public health.[1] Public domain image from Wikimedia Commons.

water from a purer upstream source.[1]

With this analysis, coupled with the findings of his Broad Street pump investigation, Snow had accomplished something that is critically important—but often profoundly challenging—in epidemiological research: he had established the *causal plausibility* of his hypothesized relationship between water impurity and cholera. Eventually, Farr "was much struck by" Snow's findings,[1] and in 1866, Farr issued a report publicly acknowledging water as the primary mode of cholera transmission and refuting the *miasma* theory.[8]

Observational Analysis: It's a Start

The outcome of Snow's battle against conventional wisdom provides a compelling illustration of a phenomenon that should be obvious in science, but is nonetheless sometimes forgotten: initial simple observations of natural phenomena are intriguing but can sometimes lead to erroneous conclusions. And, if results based *solely* on simple or unquestioned observation are used as a basis for decision making, the results can be costly or even dangerous to those involved. Contemporary examples of this phenomenon abound. Two within the past decade are standout examples of progression of knowledge from simple observation to rigorous testing—and, ultimately, to refutation of popular but erroneous opinion.

Disease management for seniors with chronic illness: a good idea, but it didn't work. The Medicare Health Support (MHS) project was a **randomized controlled trial** (RCT) initiated in 2005 by the Centers for Medicare & Medicaid Services (CMS) in response to the urgings of proponents of disease state management (DSM) for chronic care. DSM has many definitions; in the MHS project, it included patient education, 24-hour telephone advice lines staffed by nurses or pharmacists, referrals to community resources (e.g., Meals on Wheels), coordination with physicians, and medication adherence monitoring.[9-11] The idea underlying DSM is simple and sensible. Because patients with multiple chronic diseases may have difficulty navigating the health care system and/or understanding complex regimens of treatments and lifestyle recommendations (e.g., medication, diet, exercise), providing them with a readily available, user-friendly source of advice and information may improve their health, enhance quality of life, and reduce health care costs.[9] As one popular press account explained in 2006:

"... a patient might call the doctor in the morning with a concern. If the physician is delayed in returning the call, the patient might become worried and call an ambulance. Patient hotlines can address many concerns, alleviate the worry, and stop unneeded—and expensive—trips to the hospital."[10]

In advocating for the MHS as a way to "prove that disease management can be cost-effective at a national level with a Medicare population,"[10] proponents pointed to numerous *observational* studies, that is, studies in which the researcher does not assign subjects to treatments but instead measures, usually retrospectively, the events as they occurred without the researcher's involvement. In observational studies of patients who received DSM, the costs of DSM programs were more than offset by medical cost savings due to better patient outcomes, primarily reduced hospitalization rates.[11] Reports of return-on-investment (ROI) rates as high as 11-14 (meaning that for every $1 spent on the program, savings of $11 to $14 were realized) were common.[9] Yet, knowledgeable observers pointed out that the base of evidence for DSM was weak, consisting mostly of **two flawed study designs**.[11]

The **first** typical, flawed design was simple pre-intervention versus post-intervention (i.e., before versus after) analysis, in which patients who used DSM were sampled, and their pre-DSM versus post-DSM outcomes were compared. These *pre–post* analyses are vulnerable to a mathematical phenomenon known as *regression to the mean,*[12] in which high values (e.g., medical costs and utilization rates) are expected to decline naturally over time regardless of intervention (see Chapter 5 for an explanation of the mathematical cause of this phenomenon). The problem of regression to the mean was exacerbated in most DSM studies because participants were often chosen to receive DSM based on evidence of increased medical risk—for example, high medical expense or a recent hospital stay. In studies using this design, dramatic declines in medical costs and hospitalization rates following a DSM intervention were often erroneously attributed to the DSM, but in reality, they were mathematically entirely predictable with no intervention at all.[11,12]

The **second** typical design was a **cohort study** (i.e., a group comparison) of outcomes for an *intervention group* consisting of patients who had chosen DSM versus a *comparison group* of patients who either did not meet the clinical criteria for DSM (e.g., insufficient disease severity to qualify) or had opted not to participate. This design is vulnerable to *selection bias,* in which the observed outcomes are at least partially caused by a factor underlying intervention group selection rather than by the intervention itself. In other words, DSM researchers who thought that they were observing the effects of DSM were, in reality, sometimes observing nothing more than pre-existing group differences. Specifically, when patients who are more severely ill are especially likely to be referred to DSM, the opportunity for regression to the mean is greater in the DSM group than in a comparison group, making the DSM outcomes appear better than they actually are. Additionally, motivation to improve health may affect *both* receipt of the intervention (i.e., choice to use DSM) *and* health care outcomes (e.g., lower rates of hospital use). In studies using a cross-sectional design (e.g., comparing the two groups during a single six-month time period), DSM patients typically had better outcomes, but they may have been predisposed to better outcomes regardless of the intervention.

The effects of regression to the mean and selection bias on previous DSM research made the MHS, which randomized Medicare enrollees with diabetes or heart failure to DSM (**intervention group** or **treatment group**) versus no-DSM (**control group**), especially important. Random assignment into study groups (i.e., giving all clinically qualifying Medicare enrollees a known probability of selection into each group instead of allowing beneficiaries or their health care providers to determine group selection) made selection bias highly unlikely. And, having a control group effectively eliminated the problem of regression to the mean because natural mathematical trends would occur over time in both study groups. It seemed that DSM advocates would finally have the proof of effectiveness that they needed to expand DSM to chronic disease on a nationwide scale.

The problem was, the MHS evaluators found that DSM provided to Medicare beneficiaries didn't work—at least not well enough to fulfill the CMS contractual requirement that DSM "break even" financially (i.e., produce medical savings at least equal to the fees paid to DSM vendors) in the first year. Although the "break-even" requirement was remarkably modest compared with the previously reported ROI calculations, in June 2007 the CMS program evaluators announced that the fees paid (about $74 to $159 per participating beneficiary per month) had "far [exceeded] the savings produced."[13]

Two causes of the program failure are especially notable for research design. **First**, "only a small fraction" of hospitalizations and emergency room visits for the DSM patients were related to diabetes or heart failure, leaving the vendors with little opportunity to prevent disease-related inpatient care.[13] The evaluators pointed to regression to the mean as a key factor underlying this problem. That is, because the study groups were "regressing to the mean with fewer subsequent admissions for the condition that qualified beneficiaries for the program," DSM vendors "may have substantially overestimated" their ability to prevent hospitalizations, "**at least relative to a randomly matched comparison**

group also regressing-to-the-mean." (emphasis added)[9]

Second, after randomization, some Medicare beneficiaries chose *not* to receive DSM services despite having been assigned to the DSM group. Those who *did* actively engage in the DSM program were generally healthier than those who opted out. In other words, those who really needed the program and might have benefited from it were less likely to use it, giving the DSM vendors limited opportunity to effect *changes* in health-related behaviors.[13] Because the MHS design measured *changes* from the baseline period to the follow-up period for both groups, instead of comparing the groups using a methodologically weaker cross-sectional analysis of a single period of time, its results clearly revealed that the DSM participants did not experience greater *change* in health outcomes as a result of DSM, that is, relative to the control group.

ACCORD demonstrates potential dangers in relying solely on observation. In 2000, the *British Medical Journal* published a high-quality observational analysis of the relationship between hemoglobin A1c (a measure of average blood glucose over a two- to three-month period of time, commonly used as a measure of control of diabetes) and a variety of medical complications.[14] The study investigators, Stratton et al., classified patients with type 2 diabetes according to A1c level (i.e., better versus worse glucose control, with higher levels indicating worse control) using an appropriate "time-varying" method (i.e., accounting for changes in A1c over time). Cox regression analyses assessed the hazards of diabetic complications for patients at higher versus lower A1c levels, controlling for many relevant factors including demographics, smoking, cholesterol and triglyceride levels, presence/absence of urinary protein, and systolic blood pressure.

Results were both striking and exceptionally promising for patients with type 2 diabetes who wanted to avoid the potentially deadly complications of the disease. Each 1% reduction in mean A1c was associated with remarkable decreases in risks of diabetic complications—21% for diabetes-related death, 14% for myocardial infarction, and 37% for microvascular complications (e.g., diabetic retinopathy).[14] At the lowest A1c level measured in the study, less than 6%, which represents a normal (nondiabetic) A1c, the rates of diabetes-related death and diabetic complications per 1,000 were 5.5 and 24.9, respectively. In contrast, for those with A1c of 7% to less than 8%, the standard A1c target at the time,[15] the rate of diabetes-related death was 11.5 and the rate of diabetic complications was 43.6. Although cautioning that "it is important to realize that epidemiological associations cannot necessarily be transferred to clinical practice,"

Stratton et al. concluded that "any reduction in [A1c] is likely to reduce the risk of complications, with the lowest risk being in those with [A1c] values in the normal range (<6.0%)" and "the nearer to normal the [A1c] concentration the better."[14]

Although some clinicians subscribed to the "lower is better" view about A1c, which became increasingly popular in the years immediately following publication of the study by Stratton et al., appropriate recognition of the limitations of observational evidence to guide patient care was widespread.[16,17] As the National Heart Lung and Blood Institute (NHLBI) observed in 2010, despite the *association* between normal A1c and positive outcomes, no randomized trial had ever actually studied whether *treating* patients with type 2 diabetes to a normal A1c would produce the same, positive outcomes.[15] For this reason, in 2001 the NHLBI launched the Action to Control Cardiovascular Risk in Diabetes (ACCORD) trial, which randomized patients with type 2 diabetes and high risk of cardiovascular disease to "intensive" blood glucose-lowering, targeted to A1c less than 6% as suggested by Stratton et al.'s findings, or to "standard" treatment, targeted to A1c of 7.0%-7.9%.[15]

Unfortunately, the ACCORD trial did not produce the hypothesized finding that intensive glucose lowering would result in a lower death rate. In fact, it produced the opposite result: once subjected to the rigorous test of an RCT, the same intensive treatment that had looked so promising in high-quality observational analysis actually *increased* mortality by an estimated 3 deaths per 1,000 treated patients per year, or approximately 22%.[15] This unwelcome development, which led to an early cancellation of the "intensive" treatment "arm" (group) of the trial for patient safety reasons in February 2008,[18] "flummoxed"[2] experts worldwide. As of early 2011, numerous analyses of every conceivable reason for the higher-than-expected death rate had produced no explanation.[19] "Once again," noted one knowledgeable observer in 2008, "the most sound of scientific and biologic plausibility has been refuted by a large clinical-outcomes trial."[2]

Although the finding of a higher death rate with intensive glucose lowering was the first surprise to come out of ACCORD, it was not the last. A separate randomized analysis was performed in a subgroup of ACCORD sample subjects who had hypertension in addition to diabetes. The subgroup analysis assessed the effects of "intensive" drug treatment to reduce blood pressure to a level that was recommended by numerous major clinical guidelines despite what an ACCORD study report described as "a paucity of evidence from randomized clinical trials to support these recommendations."[20,21] Although the blood pressure target studied in ACCORD had been based on high-quality observational analysis, it produced no cardiovascular benefits for patients compared with a more relaxed blood pressure target, and it slightly increased the rates of "serious adverse events attributed to antihypertensive treatment."[21]

Quality of Evidence: Defined by Internal and External Validity

What do these examples teach us about quality of evidence? **Four key principles** can be remembered with the acronym WELD. **First**, producing high-quality evidence takes *Work*. Although simple associations are usually easily calculated, they are often misleading. **Second**, knowledge often *Evolves*; that is, early observations often yield to better evidence as a result of increasingly rigorous testing. **Third**, for ethical reasons, there may be *Limits* to our ability to test every theory, requiring us to do the best we can with the information we have. For example, no ethical researcher would randomize residents of a city to drink cholera-tainted water, although doing so might have been the most accurate test of John Snow's theory in nineteenth-century London; and the ACCORD investigators had no choice but to terminate the intensive treatment experiment after realizing that it was dangerous to some study participants. **Fourth**, and perhaps most important, our opinions about cause-and-effect, especially when based on simple observational analyses, are often wrong—as William Farr learned about his *miasma* cross-sectional analyses and the DSM proponents learned from the MHS experiment. So, in addition to appropriate humility about our opinions, we need *Design guidelines* to help us carry out and interpret appropriate tests of our suppositions using progressively stronger types of evidence.

Two key concepts in determining the accuracy and usability of a study—hallmarks of excellence as defined in Chapter 1—are **internal validity** and **external validity**. Internal validity, formally defined by Cook and Campbell (1979) as "the approximate validity with which we infer that a relationship between two variables is causal or that the absence of a relationship implies the absence of cause,"[22] refers to *appropriate inference*. That is, do the relationships among the variables measured in a study actually represent the causal construct that the investigator intended to assess? External validity, formally defined by Cook and Campbell as "the approximate validity with which we can infer that the presumed causal relationship can be generalized to and across alternate measures of the cause and effect and across different types of persons, settings, and times,"[22] refers to *applicability*. That is, are the results usable for the groups, settings, and purposes to which they likely will be applied?

The most helpful systems for rating quality of evidence address *both* external and internal validity. A user-friendly example, the Canadian Hypertension Education Program (CHEP) rating system, which is based on the more well-known Grading of Recommendations Assessment, Development, and Evaluation (GRADE) standards, is summarized in Table 3A.[23]

Table 3A
Summary of Principles Underlying Guidelines for Rating Quality of Evidence[a]

Rationale	Higher Scores	Lower Scores
Internal validity: To assess whether A causes B, an ideal design measures *only* the effect of A on B—without being affected by other factors, such as regression to the mean or selection bias.	"Adequate" RCT • "Allocation concealment" and "blinded assessment of outcomes"—neither the study subjects nor the investigators know who received treatment instead of placebo, making it unlikely that results are affected by enthusiasm for the treatment. • Intention-to-treat analysis—outcomes are assessed for all those assigned to intervention or control arm, not just for those who are sufficiently motivated or able to complete the protocol. • Adequate follow-up—dropout rate of less than 10% • Sufficient sample size[b] • Subgroup analyses planned *a priori* and few in number[c]	"Inadequate" RCT • Inadequate subgroup analyses (too many, underpowered, or not *a priori*)[b,c] • Observational study • Systematic review of evidence from multiple studies, especially if results of different studies are inconsistent
External validity: To assess the effect of an intervention or treatment in "real-world" use, an ideal study design represents the groups, circumstances, and purposes for which the intervention or treatment will be used.	• "Clinically important outcome" (e.g., death, stroke, myocardial infarction) • Study sample is representative of population in which the treatment will be used.	• "Validated surrogate" outcome—"RCTs have consistently demonstrated that improvement in the surrogate translates into a consistent and predictable improvement in the clinical end point"—gets a lower score than clinically important outcome. • "Unvalidated surrogate outcome" gets a lower score than validated surrogate. • Study sample differs from population in which intervention will be used (e.g., intervention has been tested only in young persons, but elderly will use the intervention).

Grades
- A = Adequate RCT or adequate subgroup analysis,[d] adequate sample, clinically important outcome, sample represents population in which treatment will be used.
- B = Adequate RCT or adequate subgroup analysis, adequate sample, *but* the study used a validated surrogate outcome or the sample does not represent the population.
- B = Equivocal RCT evidence, such as inadequate sample, *but* clinically important or validated surrogate outcome.
- C = Adequate RCT or adequate subgroup analysis, adequate sample, *but* unvalidated surrogate outcome.
- C = Observational design or inadequate RCT or subgroup analysis, adequate sample, clinically important outcome, sample represents population well.
- C = Observational design or inadequate RCT or subgroup analysis, adequate sample, *but* clinically validated surrogate or sample does not represent population.
- D = Either equivocal RCT evidence or observational evidence about an unvalidated surrogate.
- D = Observational study or inadequate RCT with inadequate sample size, regardless of external validity of outcome measure.

[a] Scores and grades are based on the Canadian Hypertension Education Program evidence-grading method as described by McAlister et al.[23]
[b] See Chapter 4 for a discussion of statistical power in study planning.
[c] See Chapter 5 for a discussion of cumulative type 1 error and "fishing expeditions."
[d] Adequate subgroup analysis was defined as "*a priori*, done within an adequate RCT, one of only a few tested, and there was sufficient sample size within the examined subgroup to detect a clinically important difference with power >80%."[23]
RCT = randomized controlled trial.

More About Observation and Causation:
What You See Isn't Always What You Get

Two patterns in the evidence-grading table are obvious. **First**, it is hard to get an "A." That is as it should be; the usefulness of research results can be compromised by many factors. **Second**, observational studies generally receive a much lower grade than do RCTs, reaffirming the lessons learned from the historical and contemporary examples presented earlier in the chapter. This pattern is unsurprising because numerous research guidelines all recommend randomized over observational designs for internal validity.[23,24] However, low-quality RCTs also receive low grades. For example, the effectiveness of a randomized design relies on *allocation concealment*—that is, hiding information about group assignment from investigators and their staff to eliminate human intervention in the group assignment process. Allocation might be concealed by placing group assignment information in opaque, sealed envelopes so that those who are processing subjects for study entry cannot see or act upon the allocation (e.g., by knowingly assigning sicker cases to the control group). If allocation is *not* effectively concealed, the benefits of randomization for internal validity are highly compromised, and the study earns a lower grade.

What is less obvious from the table is the critically important point that the preference for randomized over observational design is more than just methodological purism or a "wonky" interest in esoteric detail. As developers of evidence guidelines have pointed out, and as the ACCORD findings illustrated clearly, *the error of equating association with causation has sometimes led to suboptimal patient care and even to unnecessary deaths.*[25]

Why are RCTs so strongly preferred in evidence assessment guidelines? A key problem with observational designs is *confounding*, sometimes called "spurious association," in which a factor (C) is systematically related to both a predictor (A) and an outcome (B), causing an *association* between A and B that sometimes "tricks" us into believing that A caused B. William Farr's observational analysis of nineteenth-century London, which documented an association between bad odors and high death rates, is a good example. Crowded conditions in some parts of London *both* caused foul odors *and* facilitated the transmission of *Vibrio cholerae*. John Snow's testimony before Parliament that Farr's relationship between odors and disease was "coincidence" because "where there are open sewers you have mostly a number of people living together under such circumstances that they get fever ... and the general water supply in certain districts is also very bad"[6] opened him to enormous criticism from the *Lancet* editors—but he was right. The relationship between odors and cholera was indeed coincidental.

It is also *possible* that observations about the relationship between odors and cholera were affected by **surveillance bias**, sometimes called **detection bias**, in which the *reporting* of an outcome (but not the outcome itself) is systematically affected by an **independent variable** (predictor or explanatory variable) that is *thought* to influence the **dependent variable** (outcome).[26] That is, perhaps cholera cases were more likely to be noticed or reported in malodorous regions because officials or citizens were aware of (i.e., more likely to be watchful for) the "relationship" between odors and the disease. In health care research, surveillance bias may occur in the measurement of disease sequelae. For example, one might find a statistical association between diabetes and glaucoma partly because patients with diabetes are more likely to have regular eye examinations, increasing the likelihood of glaucoma detection.[26]

An interesting analysis of the hazards of confounding—described by its authors, Dormuth et al. (2009), as a "cautionary tale"—assessed the association between use of statin (cholesterol-lowering) medications and a wide variety of positive health outcomes.[27] The analysis was particularly important because numerous previous observational studies had found an association between medication adherence and positive health outcomes, leading naïve observers to suggest that implementing programs to improve medication adherence would yield health improvements in a cause-and-effect relationship. But after statistically adjusting for confounding factors in a high-quality multivariate analysis typical of this type of observational study, Dormuth et al. found a relationship between better adherence to statin treatment and reductions in negative outcomes that drug treatment could not possibly have prevented, such as burns, falls, poisoning, and accidents, as well as diseases unrelated to statin treatment, such as asthma and dental problems.[27] One likely explanation for the finding is the well-documented "healthy adherer effect," a phenomenon in which patients who comply with medical treatments are more likely than noncompliant patients to engage in other healthy behaviors, such as regular exercise, driving carefully, and fastening one's seat belt.[28] Because healthy behaviors cause *both* treatment adherence *and* positive health outcomes (e.g., fewer cardiovascular events and hospitalizations), simple observational comparisons of outcomes for adherent and nonadherent patients usually show an *association*, which is partially spurious, between greater adherence and better health.[29] In an analysis of the "healthy adherer effect" by Simpson et al. (2006), patients who were compliant with "beneficial drug therapy" were about half as likely to die as noncompliant patients. That finding sounds as if drug adherence produced mighty impressive results—except that patients with good adherence to *placebo* treatment experienced approximately the same mortality benefit![28]

The moral of these studies is that interpretation of observational analysis is often difficult at best. Findings might mean what you think they mean—or they might mean something else entirely. That is why, for isolation (unconfounded measurement) of the effect of any factor on the outcomes of interest, in general nothing beats a randomized design. When research subjects are properly randomized to different study conditions (e.g., DSM versus no DSM), they are highly unlikely to differ systematically on other confounding factors, making a conclusion that the independent variable caused the dependent variable much more supportable.

How Can We Learn from Observational Evidence? Principles of Causation and Value of Observation in Scientific Progress

As noted above, sometimes randomization is impossible for ethical or practical reasons. Additionally, as we shall see in more detail in the next section of the chapter, sometimes the available randomized evidence is flawed or limited. In these circumstances, observational evidence can provide important information. In gathering and interpreting observational data, threats to internal validity can be reduced by attention to principles of causation—that is, factors that can help determine the likelihood that the relationship between two factors is truly causal instead of spurious. Although descriptions of factors vary, the most common and classic (dating back to 1960s analyses of the relationship between smoking and lung cancer) are summarized in Table 3B.

> ### Key Points: Threats to Validity
>
> ❖ *Regression to the mean*: High values tend to decline over time regardless of intervention.
> ❖ *Confounding*: Factors systematically associated with both independent and dependent variables can "trick us" into confusing association with causation.
> ❖ Attention to *principles of causation*, especially plausibility, improves internal validity in observational analysis.
> ❖ *Threats to external validity* occur when study conditions or methods make the sample nonrepresentative of the target population.

Table 3B
Common Criteria for Assessing Causality of Relationships in Epidemiological Studies

A Relationship Is More Likely To Be Causal If It Shows …	Potential Pitfall	Example
Consistency: It is observed consistently in multiple studies.	A consistently observed association could represent nothing more than repeated use of the same flawed method.	Observational research consistently showed associations between DSM and large health care cost savings because of methodological weaknesses common in DSM studies prior to the MHS.
Strength: It is statistically strong (e.g., high correlation).	Spurious associations can be statistically strong when they are attributable to strongly causal confounders.	The number of fire trucks at a fire is strongly correlated with fire damage—but that is because both are caused by the size of the fire.[a]
Dose-response: Increasing "doses" (amounts) of the predictor factor are associated with increases in the outcome.	The form of the relationship should be examined carefully; changes could occur at particular threshold points, providing insight into the specific relationship between the predictor and the outcome.	Because consumer response to price is not rational and is instead triggered by emotional cues, a change in price from $10.98 to $10.99 is unlikely to cause a decline in purchasing behavior, whereas a change in price from $10.99 to $11.00 is more likely to reduce purchasing.[b]
Plausibility: A plausible explanation for the relationship is known.	Even if highly plausible, an association can still be misleading.	The association between normal A1c and positive outcomes for patients with type 2 diabetes (Stratton et al.)[14] was biologically plausible, but ACCORD suggested that treatment to normal A1c levels is unsafe for some patients with type 2 diabetes.
Temporality: The predictor precedes the outcome it is thought to cause (i.e., for A to cause B, A must precede B).	• If the predictor occurs repeatedly, predictors occurring prior to the start of the research study period can be missed in data collection. • Even temporally consistent relationships might not be causal.	• Medication nonadherence may repeat over time; an episode of nonadherence occurring in 2008 would be unmeasured in a study that begins in 2009. • The association between normal A1c and positive diabetes outcomes was temporal (i.e., measured using an appropriate time-varying method); nonetheless, it suggested a treatment approach that was ultimately refuted.

[a] This example was provided in an amusing and informative blog entry by consultant William Burns (1996).[32]
[b] One of many examples from *Predictably Irrational*, by behavioral economist Dan Ariely (2008).[33]
Sources:
Potischman and Weed. Causal criteria in nutritional epidemiology.[30]
Hill. The environment and disease: association or causation?[31]
ACCORD = Action to Control Cardiovascular Risk in Diabetes; A1c = hemoglobin A1c; DSM = disease state management; MHS = Medicare Health Support experiment.

Despite the limitations that sometimes occur in applying these principles to assess the internal validity of observational evidence, *the important role of observation in contributing to scientific progress should not be overlooked.* For example, as researchers Grimes and Schulz (2002) explained in a helpful guide to descriptive studies:

> *"... the results of a survey done in a Puerto Rican pharmaceutical factory indicated an exceptionally high prevalence of gynaecomastia among employees ... This finding led to the hypothesis that exposure to ambient [estrogen] dust in the plant might be the cause;* **serum concentrations of [estrogen] lent support to the hypothesis. After improvements in dust control in the factory, the epidemic disappeared.***"* (emphasis added)[34]

Note that the Puerto Rican study exhibited two of the principles shown in Table 3B, thereby greatly enhancing the usefulness of its findings. *Causal (biological) plausibility* was established with the measurement of serum estrogen levels. A *temporal relationship* was established when removal of the dust was followed by a decline in gynaecomastia. In this instance, an RCT—for example, exposing one group of employees to dust and leaving another group unexposed—would have been unethical and infeasible, as well as unnecessary in light of the compelling observational evidence.

Controversies over Study Methods:
What They Teach Us About Internal/External Validity "Tradeoffs"

One of the things that I like best about working as a methodologist is that most controversies over studies with a profound public policy or health care impact are methodological. That is, generally those who disagree with the results of a study are more likely to argue about the methods than about any other feature—and in many (but not all) instances, they are right. These controversies illustrate the importance of *thoughtful* consideration of *both* the internal and external validity of study methods before beginning a research project. Following is a description of a few such controversies, presented in order from least to most complex.

Randomization to inherently biased groups. A 1998 trial by Kiviluoto et al. compared laparoscopic cholecystectomy (sometimes called "minimally invasive" or "keyhole" surgery, LC) with open cholecystectomy (OC) in treating patients with acute cholecystitis.[35]

Results seemed remarkable. Among patients randomized to OC, major postoperative complications were observed in 23% and minor complications in 19%, compared with only a single case (3%) of minor complications in the LC group. However, an important detail mentioned only in the full study report, and not in the PubMed study abstract, was the qualification of the surgeons. Because LC was "technically demanding," the patients randomly assigned to LC received surgery performed by the study's investigators, who were experienced surgeons. In contrast, the OCs were performed mostly by senior surgical residents.[35] This methodological decision raised questions about whether the better outcomes for LC were attributable to the technique itself or to the surgical skills of the more experienced team, creating a potential problem for internal validity that was perhaps avoidable. Instead of assignment of all OCs to less experienced surgeons, perhaps all or a portion of OCs could have been assigned to the study investigators. If possible to assign only a portion of OCs to the study investigators, perhaps that group could have been assessed separately in an *a priori* subgroup analysis.

Concerns about randomization to biased comparator groups are common and often well-founded. For example, in the Multinational Etoricoxib and Diclofenac Arthritis Long-term (MEDAL) trial of a new pain reliever, in which one important safety outcome was cardiovascular events (a dangerous drug side effect), the control group drug was diclofenac. Editorialists pointed out that the choice of diclofenac as the control group drug was peculiar because it is not commonly used in the United States and has a higher cardiovascular risk than naproxen, which *is* commonly used.[36] They argued that the results of the MEDAL trial, which found that cardiovascular risk for the new pain reliever was comparable to that of diclofenac, were inherently flawed by the choice of a control group drug with an unnecessarily high cardiovascular risk level. Similar concerns have been raised about trials of antihypertensive medications.[37]

A related common issue is bias attributable to incomplete or flawed **blinding** within a randomized design. In an ideal design from the perspective of internal validity, neither the investigators nor the study subjects know whether subjects are receiving the treatment (intervention) or the control, to avoid biasing the results with enthusiasm for (or concerns about) the treatment. For this reason, drug trials typically use comparators (usually, but not always, including placebo) that look and taste/feel like each other (e.g., identical pills or injection schedules) so that blinding of investigators and subjects is maintained. Failure to blind can open an investigation—and policy decisions based on its results—to intense criticism. For example, a 2011 *Therapeutics Initiative* newsletter blasted the decision of

Health Canada (federal health administrator and regulator) to license dabigatran (a direct thrombin inhibitor) for stroke prevention in patients with nonvalvular atrial fibrillation, based primarily on the results of the Randomized Evaluation of Long-Term Anticoagulation Therapy (RELY) trial.[38] Although RELY was randomized, its comparison between dabigatran and warfarin (a standard anticoagulant drug) was *not* blinded, creating, according to the newsletter, a "high risk of bias."[38] Additionally, blinding is not always feasible. For example, it is obviously impossible to blind study subjects to treatment assignment in a comparison of drugs versus surgery, although it is both feasible and optimal to blind those who are responsible for assessing patient outcomes (e.g., based on the reading of x-rays or administration of a symptom inventory).

Selection effects prior to randomization. In the Justification for the Use of Statins in Prevention: an Intervention Trial Evaluating Rosuvastatin (JUPITER) study, "apparently healthy" individuals without high cholesterol but with elevated high-sensitivity C-reactive protein (hs-CRP), a biomarker for (indicator of) inflammation that has been associated with cardiac disease risk in observational research, were randomized to treatment with rosuvastatin (a cholesterol-lowering medication) or placebo.[39] The relationship hypothesized by the JUPITER investigators was supported: persons with elevated hs-CRP were less likely to suffer cardiovascular events if treated with rosuvastatin. Despite strong internal validity because of the randomized design, the trial has been wildly controversial, in large part because of the economic and clinical implications of treating young and disease-free people with chronic medication for a lifetime.[40]

Among the many reasons for the controversy were **sample exclusions made *before* randomization. First**, the sample was pre-screened for adherence using a 4-week "run-in" period in which potential study subjects were treated with placebo tablets, and only subjects who took more than 80% of their placebo tablets were permitted to continue to the randomization phase. **Second**, the list of exclusions for comorbidities (coexisting disease) was long and included many common conditions, such as diabetes, liver disease, uncontrolled hypertension, recent substance abuse, and inflammatory conditions including severe arthritis, lupus, and inflammatory bowel disease. Of 26,286 potential study participants, 19,323 (73.5%) were deemed clinically eligible to participate; and of those, an additional 1,521 (7.9%) were excluded for noncompliance during the run-in period, leaving 17,802, or only 67.7% of the original pool, who were randomized by the JUPITER investigators.[39,40]

These sampling decisions highlight the sometimes difficult tradeoffs that researchers must make between external and internal validity. For example, had the researchers included in the study sample partially adherent patients (those who took some but not all study pills), the internal validity of the trial would have been compromised—that is, for patients in whom rosuvastatin was ineffective, it would have been impossible to tell whether the problem was the drug or the nonadherence. However, in real-world practice, physicians routinely see patients who are only partially compliant and must decide how to treat them. Thus, the exclusion of patients with less than 80% adherence during the "run-in" period left unanswered important questions about the external validity of JUPITER findings for these patients. Would a patient with 75% adherence benefit from rosuvastatin? What about a patient with 60% adherence? Similarly, although patients with diabetes or uncontrolled hypertension are highly likely to be treated in routine clinical practice, their exclusion from the JUPITER trial means that we know little about whether the JUPITER treatment strategy is safe and effective for them. And, as it turns out, the exclusion of patients with diabetes from JUPITER was especially problematic because of a surprise finding in JUPITER that diabetes was slightly *more* likely to develop in patients treated with rosuvastatin versus placebo.[39] To avoid or mitigate these problems, perhaps patients with common conditions that could potentially compromise or complicate the effects of rosuvastatin treatment, including partial adherence, diabetes, or uncontrolled hypertension, should have been included in the trial but assessed separately in *a priori* subgroup analyses.

The Opportunity Scholarship Program: intention-to-treat a study subject who can't possibly receive the treatment. A fascinating and complex controversy occurred in 2008 following the announcement of early results from an RCT of the Opportunity Scholarship Program (OSP), which provided vouchers for up to $7,500 annually to the families of low-income children for the purpose of subsidizing private school education.[41,42] Study investigators at the U.S. Department of Education's Institute of Education Sciences (IES) randomized families who entered a voucher "lottery"—necessary because the number of families applying for a voucher far exceeded the number of vouchers available—to a voucher group (receipt of a voucher that could be applied to tuition, school fees, and transportation at a participating private school for up to five years) or to a control group (no voucher awarded). After three years of follow-up, researchers found no statistically significant differences in math scores, but the reading level of voucher kids was an average of approximately 3.1 months better than that of nonvoucher kids.[41] In the final study analysis based on four to five years of follow-up, students who won the voucher lottery did not have significantly higher math or reading test scores but were more likely to graduate from high school (82%) than students whose families had not won a voucher (70%).[41,42]

It doesn't sound as if the OSP had much effect on academic achievement as measured by test scores, does it? And the randomized design used by the IES was certainly first-rate for internal validity. But school choice advocates cried foul over the analytic technique, arguing that the best test of the OSP would have been measurement of the educational achievement of kids who actually *used* a voucher to attend private school.[43] In support of their point, they cited an appendix to the study report containing the results of an instrumental variable analysis* that estimated the effects of private school attendance on student achievement. That analysis showed that after accounting for baseline factors that predicted whether a family would *choose* a private school, kids who *attended* a private school had significantly better reading and math scores than those who attended a public school.

Perhaps anticipating criticism of the study method, or perhaps simply to explain it thoroughly, the IES authors provided a detailed methodological rationale in their clear and thorough study report. Because the OSP "does not compel students to actually use the scholarship or make them move from a public to a private school," the study "treatment" was defined as "the award or offer of" a scholarship, "which is all the Program can do."[41] Additionally, the IES investigators used a standard **intention-to-treat** method, in which the outcomes of the randomized groups are compared regardless of drop-outs or refusals to participate, instead of a **per protocol** method, in which results are analyzed for only those completing a program or treatment. In other words, the OSP study compared those who received a voucher with those who did not, *regardless of actual use of the voucher*.

In considering the OSP trial method, it is important to understand why studies of interventions in health care and public policy routinely use intention-to-treat analysis. In real life, one can't keep only the good outcomes (i.e., those who can tolerate a drug well enough to take it for the recommended treatment period, those who enroll in and stay in private school) and discard the suboptimal outcomes (e.g., dropouts). Suboptimal outcomes, regardless of whether they are caused by the actions of study subjects themselves, are

---

* Instrumental variable analysis, a technique intended to adjust for "unmeasured confounders"—that is, confounding factors that are not directly measured by the researcher—is discussed in more detail in Chapter 6. In the voucher study, a two-stage analysis was used. The first stage estimated "the likelihood that individual students attended a private school" during a specified time period (e.g., three years for the three-year study report). The second stage applied the likelihood estimate in a regression analysis that estimated the effect of private schooling. Notably, because 15% of *control* group kids attended a private school, usually paid for by an alternative scholarship, the instrumental variable analysis reflects the estimated effects of private school attendance for the sample overall, not just the voucher winners.

real outcomes. Thus, it does not make sense to exclude them in analysis. Additionally and more importantly, had the OSP study not used an intention-to-treat approach, it faced a very real threat of selection bias. That is, among those families that were *offered* a voucher, those that chose to *use* the voucher may have been more motivated to achieve academic success than nonusing families. Had the researchers limited the intervention group to families using the voucher, they would have been comparing a fully randomized group (the nonvoucher control group, which presumably contained both highly motivated and less motivated families) with a partially randomized, probably more highly motivated *subgroup* of voucher families who chose and stayed in private school. Thus, excluding those who failed to enter and complete a specific amount of education in a private school would have threatened internal validity by compromising randomization.

However, the appropriateness of the intention-to-treat approach taken by the IES researchers for *internal* validity masked two serious and related concerns about the design's *external* validity. First was the ability to access the treatment, and second was dropout from data collection.

Accessibility and external validity in the OSP. Of families who were offered an OSP voucher, 25% did not use it in any program year, and 34% used it "during some but not all" of the years.[41] When families who did not use the voucher at any time during the third program year were asked about their decision in a survey, 22% said that there was no available space in the private school that they wanted their child to attend, and 21% said that they had moved away from the Washington, DC area, where the private schools were located.[41] Additionally, many private schools included in the study (38% in the first year of the program, 46% in the second year) cost more than the $7,500 voucher maximum, up to nearly $30,000.[41] The *maximum* income for voucher-eligible families was 180% of federal poverty level, or $38,160 for a family of four in 2008,[42,44] making it unlikely that the additional tuition could be absorbed by a voucher family.

Thus, it appears that many study families were, in essence, assigned to receive an intervention that did not actually apply to them, an important external validity problem. In other words, it makes little sense to randomize a family to receive a piece of paper saying that they have an opportunity that, in reality, they have no way to access and then measure whether the piece of paper helped them. In this respect, the method violated the study objective, which was to measure the effect of *opportunity* to receive a private school education on student outcomes.

It should be noted that the IES authors performed a standard statistical adjustment for nonparticipation in an intervention, the "Bloom Adjustment," in which the estimated programmatic effect (difference between intervention and control groups) is divided by the intervention group uptake rate (the proportion of families that used their voucher, in this study) to estimate what the total effect would have been had the nonusing families actually used their vouchers.[41] However, the adjustment accounted for only those families that did not use the voucher at all, *not* for those that initially enrolled their children in private school but were unable to keep using the school because of excessive travel time; 11% of families that used a voucher in year 3 but dropped out said in a survey that they had done so because "it was too difficult to get the child to the private school each day."[41] Additionally and more important, although the Bloom adjustment method is mathematically sound, the IES researchers encountered major and complicated challenges in applying it in the OSP study because of the second problem, data collection dropout.

Study dropout and external validity in the OSP. The Bloom adjustment factor was estimated based on a 14% rate of nonuse, not the actual rate of nonuse of 25%, because the data analysis was based only on families that completed data collection efforts, and families that never used the OSP were understandably less likely to participate in several years of data collection than those choosing private school.[*] Additionally, although the IES researchers used incentives (e.g., small payments) to participate in data collection, the rate of data collection dropout was generally quite high *and* systematically related to study group assignment; 34% (468 of 1,387) in the voucher group and 46% (420 of 921) in the control group were *not* included in the student assessment testing in the program's third year. The IES investigators used intensive attempts to encourage participation in data collection, as well as complex multivariate systems of nonresponse weights so that students responding to data collection "represent not only students who responded … but also students who were like them in relevant ways but did not respond to outcome data collection."[41] However, even the highest-quality multivariate analyses cannot (and usually do not) guarantee absence of confounding effects.[26]

---

* To understand this point mathematically, consider a hypothetical sample of 100 voucher families in which 78% use the voucher and 22% do not. If the data collection dropout rates are 30% for the users and 45% for the nonusers, the numbers of cases available for analysis (i.e., 1 minus the percentage dropout) are 55 for users (70% of 78) and 12 for nonusers (55% of 22). Thus, although these hypothetical nonusing families are 22% of the sample overall, they are only 18% (12÷67) of families for which data are available.

Addressing external validity problems in the OSP. The high rates of voucher nonuse, data collection dropout, and the systematic relationship between the two perhaps could have been partially avoided with closer attention to the general principle of evidence quality that an intervention should be tested in a sample that is as similar as possible to the population in which it will be applied. For example, a drug that is going to be used for a condition that is common only in adults would not be tested in children, a drug that is going to be used to treat bacterial infections would not be tested in people with viral infections, and so on. Following the principle of eligibility to receive the intervention, perhaps the voucher trial analysis should have excluded *from both the intervention and control groups* children who, during the first program year, lived more than a reasonable distance from a voucher-accepting school that had space available and that charged no more than a reasonable amount in excess of the $7,500 tuition voucher for a family at 180% of FPL. Of course, under this approach, the decision rules for reasonable distance and cost would have to be established *a priori* to avoid introducing bias into the analysis, but the classification of families as eligible or ineligible for analysis could have been made at the time of data analysis based on the *a priori* decision rules. After making that exclusion, the analysis could have been performed using a standard intention-to-treat approach, following children through all remaining program years. For those who would argue that no exclusions should be made after randomization, it is notable that the IES investigators actually did just that when they excluded from both study groups those children who participated in the voucher lottery but were already attending private school, for the reason that the study was intended to assess the effect of new educational opportunities.

The question of avoiding data collection dropout is more difficult. Pre-screening for likely cooperation with data collection to determine eligibility for the voucher lottery, analogous to the JUPITER trial's placebo "run-in" period, would have been infeasible both from practical and public relations standpoints. A methodologically reasonable idea would be to charge families a nominal but salient fee, such as $50 or $100, for voucher lottery entry, promising them that the fee would be reimbursed after completion of the study in return for cooperation with data collection efforts. However, it is highly unlikely that the legislation that enabled the program gave the IES investigators the authority to charge any fees to applicant families. Still, it appears that the incentives offered by the IES for participation in data collection were simply not sufficient to motivate cooperation. Future evaluations might consider either larger cash incentives or a lottery, in which cooperation with each data collection phase entitles a family to a ticket in a lottery with a large cash prize. These design modifications would not be easy to execute but probably would have provided a better test of the voucher program than the well-done, but highly compromised, OSP evaluation.

Summing Up: What Have We Learned?

A summary of designs commonly used in health care research (Appendix 3A) highlights the **patterns suggested by study design controversies**, such as those surrounding JUPITER and OSP. **First,** there is no such thing as a perfect study. Instead, the most appropriate (but usually imperfect) research design for a given project depends in part on its purpose, on the groups in which it will be applied, and on practical and ethical constraints. **Second** and related, most research involves at least some amount of trade-off between internal and external validity. High-quality research designs balance the two as much as possible. Thus, there are times when observational research is critically important—for example, when an RCT has been performed but a large proportion of study subjects were excluded prior to randomization, or when the evidence available to guide a pressing, "real-life" treatment question is limited or nonexistent.

In considering a proposed observational research design, three **rules of thumb** are important. **First,** take time at the start of a project to identify ways to establish and/or test a reasonably plausible causal relationship, as Snow did in his seminal investigation of the Broad Street pump and cholera mortality rates for pure versus impure water sources. **Second,** avoid "overinterpreting" observational study findings, but do so without dismissing them out of hand. In other words, association does not definitively establish causation (no matter how much we want it to), but it just might lead to an important discovery that withstands the test of increasingly rigorous investigation or, as Grimes and Schulz express it, "the first scientific toe in the water in new areas of inquiry."[34] **Third,** because it is important to inform those who use study findings about the strengths and limitations of the research, one of the most important aspects of study quality is the transparency and clarity of the study report itself. The topic of good research reporting will be taken up in Chapter 10.

But first, in Chapter 4, we turn to a system that will enable an accurate and efficient literature review as a basis for sound project planning. We begin in the way that all great research projects begin—with an *idea*.

Helpful Resources

- Statistician Andrew Vickers has written an interesting and helpful tutorial on intention-to-treat analysis.[45]
- In their article on the use of claims databases for outcomes research, Motheral and Fairman include a discussion of various threats to validity.[46]
- The International Society for Pharmacoeconomics and Outcomes Research (ISPOR) guidance on nonrandomized comparative effectiveness research includes a discussion of various types of bias and confounding.[47]
- The GRACE (**G**ood **R**ese**A**rch for **C**omparative **E**ffectiveness OBSERVED) principles provide a clear explanation of hierarchy of evidence quality.[48]
- Grimes and Schulz provide a helpful overview of the strengths and limitations of descriptive evidence.[34]

References

1. Snow J. *On the Mode of Communication of Cholera.* London. December 11, 1854. Available at: http://www.deltaomega.org/snowfin.pdf.

2. Hughes S. The day after: experts puzzled over increased death rate in ACCORD (Action to Control Cardiovascular Risk in Diabetes). Theheart.org. February 7, 2008.

3. Miller JE. *The Chicago Guide to Writing about Numbers.* Chicago, IL: University of Chicago Press; 2004: quotation p. 35.

4. UCLA Department of Epidemiology, School of Public Health. Reaction and committee action. Available at: http://www.ph.ucla.edu/epi/snow/reactionandcommitteeaction.html.

5. Wakley T. The Public Health and Nuisances Removal Bill: Dr. Snow's evidence [editorial]. *The Lancet.* June 23, 1855;23:634-35. (Note: The entire volume of *The Lancet* for the year 1855 is available free of charge from Google books at books. google.com.)

6. UCLA Department of Epidemiology, School of Public Health. Snow's testimony. Available at: http://www.ph.ucla.edu/epi/snow/snows_testimony.html.

7. About The Lancet medical journal. TheLancet.com. Available at: http://www.thelancet.com/lancet-about.

8. UCLA Department of Epidemiology, School of Public Health. Competing theories of cholera. Available at: http://www.ph.ucla.edu/epi/snow/choleratheories.html. An interesting graphic depicting Farr's compelling—but misleading—analysis of the association between elevation above the Thames River level and cholera mortality in London (1849) is available here: http://www.ph.ucla.edu/epi/snow/farrgraph.html.

9. Cromwell J, McCall N, Burton J. Evaluation of Medicare Health Support chronic disease pilot program. *Health Care Financ Rev.* 2008;30(1):47-60.

10. Ullman K. Medicare dives into disease management: pilot program coordinates care of diabetes, other chronic illnesses. *DOC News.* 2006;3(9):1-8. Available at: http://docnews.diabetesjournals.org/content/3/9/1.2.full.

11. Curtiss FR, Fairman KA. Looking for the outcomes we love in all the wrong places: the questionable value of biomarkers and investments in chronic care disease management interventions. *J Manag Care Pharm.* 2008;14(6):563-70. Available at: http://www.amcp.org/data/jmcp/JMCPMaga_563-570.pdf.

12. Linden A. Estimating the effect of regression to the mean in health management programs. *Dis Manage Health Outcomes.* 2007;15(1):7-12.

13. McCall N, Cromwell J, Bernard S. Evaluation of Phase I of Medicare Health Support (formerly Voluntary Chronic Care Improvement) pilot program under traditional fee-for-service Medicare: report to Congress. June 2007. Available at: http://www.cms.gov/reports/downloads/McCall.pdf.

14. Stratton IM, Adler AI, Neil HA, et al. Association of glycaemia with macrovascular and microvascular complications of type 2 diabetes (UKPDS 35): prospective observational study. *BMJ*. 2000;321(7258):405-12. Available at: http://www.ncbi.nlm.nih.gov/pmc/articles/PMC27454/?tool=pubmed.

15. National Heart Lung and Blood Institute. Questions and answers: Action to Control Cardiovascular Risk in Diabetes (ACCORD) study. March 15, 2010. Available at: http://www.nhlbi.nih.gov/health/prof/heart/other/accord/q_a.htm.

16. Nainggolan L. Target HbA1c levels still the subject of much debate, but tailored therapy should be the aim. *Theheart.org*. October 9, 2009.

17. Gerstein HC, Riddle MC, Kendall DM, et al.; ACCORD Study Group. Glycemia treatment strategies in the Action to Control Cardiovascular Risk in Diabetes (ACCORD) trial. *Am J Cardiol*. 2007;99(12A):34i-43i.

18. Hughes S. Intensive-glycemic-control arm of ACCORD stopped. *Theheart.org*. February 6, 2008.

19. Hughes S. Latest results from ACCORD: mortality signal still there. *Theheart.org*. March 2, 2011.

20. Treatment guidelines included:

    - American Diabetes Association. Standards of medical care in diabetes—2010. *Diabetes Care*. 2010;33(Suppl 1):S11-S61. Available at: http://www.ncbi.nlm.nih.gov/pmc/articles/PMC2797382/pdf/zdcS11.pdf.

    - American Diabetes Association. Treatment of hypertension in adults with diabetes. *Diabetes Care*. 2002;25(1):199-201. Available at: http://care.diabetesjournals.org/content/25/1/199.full.pdf.

    - Chobanian AV, Bakris GL, Black HR, et al.; Joint National Committee on Prevention, Detection, Evaluation, and Treatment of High Blood Pressure. National Heart, Lung, and Blood Institute; National High Blood Pressure Education Program Coordinating Committee. Seventh report of the Joint National Committee on Prevention, Detection, Evaluation, and Treatment of High Blood Pressure. *Hypertension*. 2003;42(6):1206-52. Epub 2003 Dec 1. Available at: http://hyper.ahajournals.org/cgi/reprint/42/6/1206.

- Rosendorff C, Black HR, Cannon CP, et al.; American Heart Association Council for High Blood Pressure Research; American Heart Association Council on Clinical Cardiology; American Heart Association Council on Epidemiology and Prevention. Treatment of hypertension in the prevention and management of ischemic heart disease: a scientific statement from the American Heart Association Council for High Blood Pressure Research and the Councils on Clinical Cardiology and Epidemiology and Prevention. *Circulation.* 2007;115(21):2761-88. Available at: http://circ.ahajournals.org/cgi/reprint/115/21/2761.

21. ACCORD Study Group, Cushman WC, Evans GW, Byington RP, et al. Effects of intensive blood-pressure control in type 2 diabetes mellitus. *N Engl J Med.* 2010;362(17):1575-85. Epub 2010 Mar 14. Available at: http://www.nejm.org/doi/full/10.1056/NEJMoa1001286#t=articleTop.

22. Cook TD, Campbell DT. *Quasi-Experimentation: Design & Analysis Issues for Field Settings.* Boston, MA: Houghton Mifflin Company; 1979: quotations p. 37.

23. See:
- McAlister FA, van Diepen S, Padwal RS, Johnson JA, Majumdar SR. How evidence-based are the recommendations in evidence-based guidelines? *PLoS Med.* 2007;4(8):1325-32. Available at: http://www.plosmedicine.org/article/info%3Adoi%2F10.1371%2Fjournal.pmed.0040250.
- Grades of Recommendation, Assessment, Development, and Evaluation (GRADE) Working Group. Grading quality of evidence and strength of recommendations. *BMJ.* 2004;328:1490-94.

24. Fairman KA, Curtiss FR. Rethinking the 'whodunnit' approach to assessing the quality of health care research—a call to focus on the evidence in evidence-based practice. *J Manag Care Pharm.* 2008;14(7):661-74. Available at: http://www.amcp.org/data/jmcp/661-674_FairmanCurtiss-Final.pdf.

25. Guyatt GH, Oxman AD, Vist GE, et al; GRADE Working Group. GRADE: an emerging consensus on rating quality of evidence and strength of recommendations. *BMJ.* 2008;336(7650):924-26. Available at: http://www.bmj.com/content/336/7650/924.long..

26. Vandenbroucke JP, von Elm E, Altman DG, et al. Strengthening the Reporting of Observational Studies in Epidemiology (STROBE): explanation and elaboration. *PLoS Med.* 2007;4(10):e296. Available at: http://www.plosmedicine.org/article/info%3Adoi%2F10.1371%2Fjournal.pmed.0040297.

27. Dormuth CR, Patrick AR, Shrank WH, et al. Statin adherence and risk of accidents: a cautionary tale. *Circulation.* 2009;119(15):2051-57. Available at: http://circ.ahajournals.org/cgi/reprint/119/15/2051.

28. For example, see:
    - Simpson SH, Eurich DT, Majumdar SR, et al. A meta-analysis of the association between adherence to drug therapy and mortality. *BMJ.* 2006;333(7557):15. Epub 2006 Jun 21. Available at: http://www.ncbi.nlm.nih.gov/pmc/articles/PMC1488752/pdf/bmj33300015.pdf.
    - Curtis JR, Delzell E, Chen L, et al. The relationship between bisphosphonate adherence and fracture: Is it the behavior or the medication? Results from the placebo arm of the fracture intervention trial. *J Bone Miner Res.* 2011;26(4):683-88.

29. Fairman KA, Curtiss FR. Still looking for health outcomes in all the wrong places? Misinterpreted observational evidence, medication adherence promotion, and value-based insurance design. *J Manag Care Pharm.* 2009;15(6):501-07. Available at: http://www.amcp.org/data/jmcp/501-507.pdf.

30. Potischman N, Weed DL. Causal criteria in nutritional epidemiology. *Am J Clin Nutr.* 1999;69(6):1309S-1314S. Available at: http://www.ajcn.org/content/69/6/1309S.long.

31. Hill AB. The environment and disease: association or causation? *Proc R Soc Med.* 1965;58:295-300. Available at: http://www.ncbi.nlm.nih.gov/pmc/articles/PMC1898525/pdf/procrsmed00196-0010.pdf.

32. Burns WC. Spurious correlations. 1996, 1997. Available at: http://www.burns.com/wcbspurcorl.htm.

33. Ariely D. *Predictably Irrational: The Hidden Forces That Shape Our Decisions.* New York, NY: Harper Collins; 2008.

34. Grimes DA, Schulz KF. Descriptive studies: what they can and cannot do. *Lancet.* 2002;359(9310):145-49.

35. Kiviluoto T, Sirén J, Luukkonen P, Kivilaakso E. Randomised trial of laparoscopic versus open cholecystectomy for acute and gangrenous cholecystitis. *Lancet.* 1998;351(9099):321-25.

36. Psaty BM, Weiss NS. NSAID trials and the choice of comparators—questions of public health importance. *N Engl J Med.* 2007;356(4):328-30.

37. Psaty BM, Weiss NS, Furberg CD. Recent trials in hypertension: compelling science or commercial speech? *JAMA.* 2006;295(14):1704-06.

38. No author listed. Dabigatran for atrial fibrillation: why we can not rely on RE-LY. *Therapeutics Initiative*. January-March 2011.

39. Ridker PM, Danielson E, Fonseca FA, et al.; JUPITER Study Group. Rosuvastatin to prevent vascular events in men and women with elevated C-reactive protein. *N Engl J Med*. 2008;359(21):2195-207.

40. Curtiss FR, Fairman KA. Tough questions about the value of statin therapy for primary prevention: Did JUPITER miss the moon? *J Manag Care Pharm*. 2010;16(6):417-23. Available at: http://www.amcp.org/data/jmcp/417-423.pdf.

41. Wolf P, Gutmann B, Puma M, Kisida B, Rizzo L, Eissa N. Evaluation of the DC Opportunity Scholarship Program: impacts after three years. U.S. Department of Education, National Center for Education Evaluation and Regional Assistance. March 2009. Available at: http://ies.ed.gov/ncee/pubs/20094050/pdf/20094050.pdf.

42. What Works Clearinghouse. WWC quick review of the report "Evaluation of the DC Opportunity Scholarship Program: Final Report." March 2011. Available at: http://ies.ed.gov/ncee/wwc/pdf/quick_reviews/dc_final_030811.pdf.

43. Ladner M. What does the red pill do if I don't take it? Jay P. Greene blog. June 19, 2008. Available at: http://jaypgreene.com/2008/06/19/what-does-the-red-pill-do-if-i-dont-take-it/.

44. The 2008 HHS poverty guidelines. Available at: http://aspe.hhs.gov/poverty/08poverty.shtml.

45. Vickers AJ. Why Mr. Jones got surgery even if he didn't—intention-to-treat analysis. August 17, 2009. Available at: http://www.medscape.com/viewarticle/707140.

46. Motheral BR, Fairman KA. The use of claims databases for outcomes research: rationale, challenges, and strategies. *Clin Ther*. 1997;19(2):346-66.

47. Cox E, Martin BC, Van Staa T, Garbe E, Siebert U, Johnson ML. Good research practices for comparative effectiveness research: approaches to mitigate bias and confounding in the design of nonrandomized studies of treatment effects using secondary data sources: The International Society for Pharmacoeconomics and Outcomes Research Good Research Practices for Retrospective Database Analysis Task Force Report—Part II. *Value Health*. 2009;12(8):1053-61. Available at: http://www.ispor.org/taskforces/documents/RDPartII.pdf.

48. GRACE Initiative. GRACE principles. Good ReseArch for Comparative Effectiveness OBSERVED. April 10, 2010. Available at: https://pharmacoepi.org/resources/GRACE_Principles.pdf.

49. Hotopf M. The pragmatic randomised controlled trial. *Advances in Psychiatric Treatment.* 2002;8:326-33.
50. Mann CJ. Observational research methods. Research design II: cohort, cross sectional, and case-control studies. *Emerg Med J.* 2003;20(1):54-60.
51. Ostrom CW. *Time Series Analysis: Regression Techniques. Second Edition.* Newbury Park, CA: Sage Publications; 1990.

Appendix 3A
Commonly Used Designs in Health Care Research

Design and Description	Strengths	Weaknesses
Case-control "Cases" are selected based on having a particular outcome (e.g., a diagnosis of lung cancer) and their potential risk factors are compared with those of "controls" (e.g., those who do not have a diagnosis of lung cancer) to assess predictors.	• Useful for (1) rare outcomes that would require enormous sample sizes for adequate study and (2) relationships in which a long time elapses between exposure and outcome; either of these factors may make a cohort study infeasible.	• Surveillance bias (e.g., diagnosed cases may differ from those who have not yet been diagnosed). • Recall bias (e.g., depressed patients may be more likely than subjects without depression to recall childhood trauma). • Can examine only a single outcome.
Cohort Observation of a group of subjects over time for development of one or more study outcomes (e.g., incidence of lung cancer), often comparing subgroups with versus without an exposure (e.g., exposure versus no exposure to asbestos).	• Establishes temporal relationship—the hypothesized cause preceded the effect. • Often used when randomization is impossible or unethical (e.g., cannot randomize a group to asbestos exposure). • Can examine multiple outcomes (e.g., the Framingham Heart Study, which measured numerous cardiovascular biomarkers and outcomes over time).	• Confounding (e.g., those exposed to asbestos may differ from those unexposed in other relevant ways, such as health habits). • Expensive if performed prospectively, particularly for outcomes that occur a long time after exposure.
Cross-sectional Measurement of an outcome over a brief or single point in time, comparing two or more groups.	• Effective for measuring prevalence. • Inexpensive and easily performed.	• Weak internal validity; association does not establish causation.
Interrupted time series Analysis of repeated observations of a single measure, often assessing (1) the level of the series at the point of an intervention or change and (2) the trend (slope) in the pre- and post-change periods; may control for seasonality (e.g., analyses of influenza prevalence).	• Controls for changes over time that would have occurred without the intervention (e.g., maturation of study subjects, disease progression).	• Cannot distinguish between effects of two changes/interventions that take place simultaneously. • Difficult to interpret when interventions are implemented gradually rather than at a single point in time. • Results may be invalid when an insufficient number of time periods is available for analysis (e.g., only six months before and after an intervention). • Stronger when an equivalent comparison group is used; sometimes difficult to achieve.

Appendix 3A *(continued)*
Commonly Used Designs in Health Care Research

Design and Description	Strengths	Weaknesses
Pragmatic randomized trial Study subjects are selected using minimal exclusion criteria, randomly assigned to groups, and followed under conditions that closely approximate routine clinical practice (e.g., physicians can change initially assigned drug treatment at any time).	• Eliminates selection bias *if* randomization was performed properly. • Intended to combine the primary factor in determining internal validity (random assignment to study groups) with external validity for routine clinical practice.	• Relies on allocation concealment to prevent human intervention in the group assignment process. • Outcomes following assignment (e.g., dropouts or treatment refusal) can compromise internal validity. • Possible "Hawthorne Effect," in which knowledge that one is being observed affects behavior (e.g., compliance with study medication).
Pre-post Comparison of outcomes before versus after a change/intervention in a single group.	• Easy to perform as a start to more rigorous investigation.	• Weak design because of regression to the mean or other changes occurring naturally over time (e.g., disease progression).
Pre-post with comparison group Measure amount of change from pre-intervention to post-intervention and compare change amount for group with intervention versus group without.	• Comparison group change provides a benchmark against which to measure change in the intervention group.	• Requires a comparison group that is equivalent to intervention group on all factors except the intervention; sometimes difficult to achieve.
Randomized controlled trial Study subjects are assigned at random to study groups; outcomes often measured under tightly controlled experimental conditions.	• Eliminates selection bias *if* randomization was performed properly.	• Relies on allocation concealment to prevent human intervention in the group assignment process. • Stronger if all involved (i.e., subjects, investigators, assessors of study outcomes) are "blinded" to group assignment throughout the study, which is not always feasible. • External validity sometimes problematic if too many exclusions occur prior to randomization or if study setting is not representative of clinical practice (e.g., a study performed in a tertiary care center that will be applied in primary care). • Possible "Hawthorne Effect," in which knowledge that one is being observed affects behavior (e.g., compliance with study medication).

Sources:
Cook and Campbell. *Quasi-Experimentation: Design & Analysis Issues for Field Settings.*[22]
Hotopf. The pragmatic randomized controlled trial.[49]
Mann. Observational research methods.[50]
Ostrom. *Time Series Analysis.*[51]

CHAPTER 4

Accurate Literature Review and Project Planning Made Easier

"The problem is, human nature works against us ... [Most] of us embrace our first answer so strongly that we read less critically than we should. We easily spot data and arguments that confirm our claim, but we just as easily overlook or distort data that qualify or even contradict it. We don't do that deliberately; it's just human nature. ... You have to take notes more carefully than you think you need to."—Booth, Colomb, and Williams in *The Craft of Research*[1]

"I cannot give any scientist of any age better advice than this: the intensity of a conviction that a hypothesis is true has no bearing over whether it is true or not."— Zoologist Sir Peter B. Medawar, co-winner of the 1960 Nobel Prize in physiology or medicine and author of *Advice to a Young Scientist*[2]

"The scientific theory I like best is that the rings of Saturn are composed entirely of lost airline luggage."—Comedian Mark Russell[3]

What You Will Learn in Chapter 4

✓ Why *accurate literature review* is the foundation of a successful research project

✓ How to construct a *literature summary table* to guide you throughout the research process

✓ Which *three key parts of a research article* to read if you don't have time to read the entire report

✓ How to *calculate the sample size* that you need for informative statistical tests

✓ How to choose research topics and questions that your audience *really* cares about

---

Do you have an idea? Since you're reading this book, I assume that you probably do. It's something that you have always taken for granted but never actually had the opportunity to test. Or it's a pet theory. Or perhaps it's an assigned project, and you are not quite sure where to begin. Soon, you'll be investigating—good for you!

But first, you should take steps to make sure that your efforts are well spent. An investment of time in wise planning *before* you begin your research project can help you avoid backtracking, misusing resources (including your time, one of the most precious resources of all!), or finding out after you have disseminated the results of your hard work that you selected entirely the wrong research question or studied it using invalid methods. In other words, plan your project now to avoid disappointment later and ensure that your efforts will yield valuable information—or, in a rule known to every good woodworker, measure twice, cut once.

In this chapter, we'll look at how to conduct and interpret a literature review of previously published work on your topic to make good decisions about how your research will be performed. We'll look at how to formulate research questions and hypotheses, estimate the sample size needed, write an *a priori* analysis plan, and obtain critically important preliminary input about the study methods. We'll also briefly discuss how the important steps taken at this stage pave the way to an accurate and informative project report, the topic of Chapter 10. We begin with suboptimal examples to help illustrate better approaches.

Literature Review Inaccuracies:
The Case of the New Hampshire Medicaid Study

In 1991, a prominent research group reported the results of a study of a "cap" (limit) of three prescriptions per beneficiary per month, which had been implemented in the New Hampshire Medicaid program in September 1981 and replaced 11 months later with a $1 copayment for each prescription.[4] The study design was **quasi-experimental**. That is, the design was not **randomized,** meaning that the study subjects were not assigned to experimental conditions in a known probability (e.g., by using a random number generator); however, the authors used appropriate analytic techniques to control for **confounding**, the existence of factors other than the cap that could have influenced the outcomes. To do this, the authors used an **interrupted time series with comparison group**, a strong observational design in which trends in use of health care services before versus after an "interruption" (the implementation of the cap) were compared for New Hampshire versus New Jersey, a state that had no cap.

In both New Hampshire (n=411) and New Jersey (n=1,375), the study subjects were, as users of health care services go, distinct in a number of ways. They were all aged 60 years or older; they had filled a total of at least 36 prescriptions during the year prior to the cap implementation date; and they had "regular use" (at least eight claims per year) of at least one in five therapy classes indicating serious illness—for example, medications to treat heart disease, diabetes, and epilepsy. In other words, all study subjects were chronically ill, considerably older than most Medicaid beneficiaries, and—because all were enrolled in Medicaid—mostly low-income.[4]

The researchers found that prescription drug use in the New Hampshire sample declined from 2.8 to 1.9 "standardized monthly doses" after cap implementation, approximately 35% in the time series analysis.[*] In the 11-month period after cap implementation and prior to replacement of the cap with the $1 copayment, nursing home admission rates in the New Hampshire and New Jersey samples were significantly different at 10.6% and 6.6%, respectively ($P=0.006$).

However, the relationship between the cap and nursing home admission was not uniform throughout the sample; it held for only the sickest patients. That is, for a *subsample* of study patients (197 of 411 in New Hampshire and 756 of 1,375 in New Jersey) with at least eight claims per year for at least three of 26 chronic medication therapy classes for a wide variety of conditions (e.g., heart disease, mental illness, migraine, diabetes, ulcers, and many others), the risk of nursing home admission in New Hampshire was more than double that in New Jersey during the cap period (relative risk=2.2, 95% confidence interval=1.2-4.1). However, for those with less regular medication use (i.e., less than three chronic therapy classes or less than eight claims per year for each of the three therapy classes), the cap was not significantly associated with nursing home admission rates. Additionally, the cap was not significantly associated with hospitalization rates, either for the chronically ill sample overall or for the more chronically ill subsample.[4]

Partly because the effect of prescription drug benefit designs on enrollee health became a "hot topic" in the next decade and beyond, the New Hampshire study has been cited frequently—more than 300 times, according to a Web of Science search run in August 2011. Unfortunately, however, its results are often described incorrectly, as illustrated by the citations in Table 4A.

As shown in the table, an especially common and troubling error was the attribution of hospital stays to the cap, in contrast with the study finding that the cap was not significantly associated with hospitalization even among the sickest study subjects. Additional errors included describing the cap as a formulary (a list of preferred or covered medications),

---

[*] Subsequent research suggested the possibility that missing data may have substantially compromised the findings of the New Hampshire study; this research is discussed in detail in Chapter 7.

Table 4A
Inaccurate Descriptions of New Hampshire Prescription Drug Cap Study[a]

Study Year	Were Key Details About the Sample Reported?			Description of Findings	Problem(s) in Description
	Low-Income[b]	Elderly	Chronic Medication Use[c]		
1993	Yes	Yes	Yes	The cap "was associated with an increased nursing home admission rate and an increased mortality rate..."	• The authors did not measure mortality rate.
1993	No	No	No	Exogenous factors, such as reimbursement policies and formularies, "influence prescribing decisions."	• The authors did not study prescribing decisions.
1993	No	No	No	"...there have been few empirical studies which have provided strong evidence that federal payment policies can directly influence medical practice."	• The authors did not study medical practice or a federal policy.
1994	Yes	No	No	The cap "put Medicaid recipients at much higher risk of hospitalization (50% higher than the control group)."	• The relationship between the cap and hospitalization risk was not statistically significant. • The RR for hospitalization was 1.2, which would have indicated a 20% increase (not a 50% increase) if statistically significant.
1996	Yes	No	No	After the cap, New Hampshire's savings on prescription costs were "accompanied by a 20% increase in use of hospital services and a 220% increase in admissions to nursing homes."	• The relationship between the cap and hospitalization risk was not statistically significant. • A 220% increase would have been an RR of 3.2 (not 2.2).
1996	No	No	No	"Modification of physicians' practices carries the risk of causing patient harm while effecting change."	• The authors did not study physicians' practices.
1997	Yes	No	No	Limits on pharmacy reimbursements in Medicaid produce "generally a short-term savings from pharmacy charges, but over time, there have been increased expenditures from hospital services (i.e., emergency room) and other expenses, such as nursing homes and community care centers."	• The relationship between the cap and hospitalization was not statistically significant. • The authors did not study use of emergency rooms or community care centers.

Table 4A (continued)
Inaccurate Descriptions of New Hampshire Prescription Drug Cap Study[a]

Study Year	Were Key Details About the Sample Reported?			Description of Findings	Problem(s) in Description
	Low-Income[b]	Elderly	Chronic Medication Use[c]		
1997	No	No	No	Generic substitution and formulary use could mean that "expenditures for other resources, such as hospitalizations, emergency room visits, and inappropriate antibiotic use associated with acute asthma episodes" would increase.	• The authors did not study any of the outcomes described in the sentence except hospitalizations, and the relationship between the cap and hospitalization risk was not statistically significant.
1998	Yes	Yes	No	The cap "was associated with an increased risk of admission to nursing homes ... and hospitalization (RR = 1.2; 95% CI, 0.8-1.6)."	• As the CI around the RR shows, the relationship between the cap and hospitalization risk was not statistically significant.
2000	Yes	No	No	"Even among those covered by Medicaid, coverage limits and copayments reduce medication use and worsen clinical outcomes."	• The authors found that nursing home admission rates returned to pre-cap levels upon institution of a $1 copayment to replace the cap.
2000	No	No	No	"...formulary restrictions that reduce drug costs may be associated with increased hospitalizations and total health care costs if beneficial drugs are excluded."	• The New Hampshire cap was not a formulary. • The relationship between the cap and hospitalization risk was not statistically significant.
2005	Yes	Yes	Yes	After cap implementation, "the New Hampshire Medicaid patients ended up in nursing homes, hospitals, or cemeteries significantly more often than [comparison group patients], who retained full drug coverage."	• The relationship between the cap and hospitalization was not statistically significant. • The authors did not study mortality.

[a] Convenience sample of publications—that is, this is not a representative sample but was instead selected to illustrate specific problems.[5] Much of this table was previously presented in Fairman KA. Accuracy in pharmacoeconomic literature review: lessons learned from the Navajo Code Talkers.[6] It is reprinted here with permission.

[b] Includes explanations that the sample consisted of Medicaid enrollees.

[c] Full disclosure would include mention of the subsample criterion of at least eight claims for at least three chronic medication therapy classes. No publication shown in the table mentioned that specific criterion. A "Yes" in the table indicates mention of chronic disease.

CI = confidence interval; NA = not applicable; RR = relative risk.

although the New Hampshire cap was not limited to certain drugs, or as a copayment, although the study found that drug utilization returned to its pre-cap rates after it was replaced with a $1 copayment. Some literature reviews shown in the table cited outcomes that were not even studied in the New Hampshire research, including physician practice patterns, emergency room use, and mortality. Another common error, occurring both in the publications shown in Table 4A and in others too numerous to list here, was failing to report the highly selective characteristics of the subsample in which the elevated nursing home admission rate occurred.[6] This omission is important because this group represented less than 2% of Medicaid enrollees affected by the cap.[6]

Researchers citing the New Hampshire study were not alone in making errors when describing previous research. Content analyses of some of health care's most prestigious journals have documented numerous mistakes of this type, some of them serious. For example, Evans et al. (1990) used a random number generator to select a total of 50 citations from the August 1987 issues of three prominent surgical journals.[7] In addition to citation errors (e.g., mistakes in the names of the authors or of the cited journal) and other minor errors (i.e., "oversimplification or a generalization"), Evans et al. documented "major errors." These were defined as situations in which "the reference article failed to substantiate, was unrelated, or contradicted the authors' assertions," such as a study that was cited to document "an increased risk of esophageal cancer with alcohol consumption" although the study report was "about treatment and contains absolutely no mention of etiology."[7] Counting all three types of problems, the error rate overall was a troubling 48%, and major errors occurred in 25%.[7] Using a similar methodology, Eichorn and Yankauer (1987) identified major errors in about 15% of publications in three public health journals in May 1986, and either major or minor errors in 36% of articles with 29 to 53 references.[8] Commenting on these findings, Evans et al. concluded that they "support the hypothesis that authors do not check their references or may not even read them."[7]

A Better Way to Plan High-Quality Research Efficiently: The Literature Review Summary Table

It is clear that reporting information accurately is important, a topic that will be addressed in more detail in Chapter 10. But how does accurate literature review affect research project *planning*? The answer is that every study should be built on the foundation of previous work. *A researcher who begins with an accurate understanding of what is already known about a topic increases the likelihood of studying the right outcomes, sampling the right groups, asking the right research questions, recognizing and properly accounting for known confounding factors, and interpreting study findings correctly.* And, of course, the converse is true—an inaccurate literature review can lead to problems in study design and/or interpretation.

For example, in discussing a study of the relationship between preventable hospitalizations and socioeconomic status, Blustein et al. (1998) cited the New Hampshire cap study to suggest that barriers to securing medications could have caused an increased rate of preventable hospitalizations among lower-income beneficiaries in the Blustein et al. sample.[9] This misinterpretation of the New Hampshire study findings may have resulted in the loss of potentially important information in the research design. That is, the New Hampshire study findings suggested an *interaction effect* of the cap and extent of chronic drug use, in which the relationship between the cap and nursing home admission (not hospital admission) was significant only for those with intense use of chronic medications (not for all low-income beneficiaries). To build the study on the foundation of previously published work, Blustein et al. perhaps should have compared a subgroup of beneficiaries meeting medication use criteria similar to those in the New Hampshire study with a subgroup that had less intensive medication use.

An efficient way to synthesize the information gleaned from previously published work is a literature summary table, constructed during the planning phase of a research project. Although few researchers today have the time necessary to take copious notes on every article relevant to a given topic area, all should have the time to summarize key features, which can be obtained in a *targeted and abbreviated* reading of three key portions of the study report, as described in the next section of this chapter.

The literature summary table serves **four purposes**, the first three of which are discussed in detail below. **First,** it helps a researcher to identify the gaps in what is already known about a given topic. **Second,** it helps a researcher to maintain objectivity about the topic. **Third,** it helps the researcher to make sound methodological decisions, both early in the project and as questions arise throughout the research process. **Fourth,** it will be used to write an accurate and informative project report, the subject of Chapter 10.

Identifying and Reading Previously Published Studies *Efficiently*

Identifying previously published work on your research topic can seem like an overwhelming task, but the workload can be reduced considerably with a few **decision rules. First,** although it is common for authors of systematic (comprehensive) literature review articles to search multiple databases (e.g., MEDLINE, EMBASE, SciVerse Scopus), a MEDLINE

(PubMed) search is usually sufficient to identify peer-reviewed articles for *most* purposes in health care research. Of course, you will want to tailor your sources to fit your topic. For example, if your topic requires knowledge of clinical trials that have been completed but not yet published, you will want to search clinicaltrials.gov, a "registry" (database) that includes both ongoing and completed studies. Similarly, if your work involves economic research, you will want to search the "working publications and papers" database of the National Bureau of Economic Research. Influential journals in the field of study (e.g., *Diabetes Care* for a study of patients with diabetes) and clinical practice guidelines available at guidelines.gov are also good sources of information. At all these websites, advanced search functionality can typically help you find relevant articles reasonably quickly. Finally, asking knowledgeable colleagues or teachers/mentors is a great way to identify important sources of previously published work.

Second, it is often helpful to begin with systematic review articles—that is, systematic descriptions of all or most previously published work—and examine relevant cited references. A PubMed search can easily be narrowed to review articles using the "Limits" function available in the online interface. However, you don't want to stop there, especially if the review articles were not published recently, because important research could have been published after the date span covered by the review. Using the "published in the last …" (date span) limit option in PubMed can help with this problem. For example, if the most recent review article was published two years ago, you might want to limit your search for additional literature to the past three years, another easily invoked PubMed option.

One note of caution: it is *unwise* to use *nonsystematic* review articles, sometimes called "narrative reviews," which assess only a portion of the literature on a topic. These articles are often biased. You can usually distinguish a systematic from a nonsystematic review because the former contains *quantitative* information about the effect of each inclusion and exclusion criterion (e.g., 5 studies were excluded because they were published prior to 1990, 6 studies were excluded because they were not conducted in humans, etc.).

Third, strategic use of specific keywords in the search is also extremely helpful. For example, based on a PubMed search that I conducted for a hypothetical study in July 2011, a researcher who plans to study the effects of collaborative care by pharmacists and physicians for patients with chronic disease would identify an overwhelming list of 16,684 articles, most of which are irrelevant to the topic, by searching PubMed on "collaborative care." Adding the search term "pharmacist" narrows the scope to 360 articles. To that search, adding terms that represent common chronic diseases, such as "diabetes," "hypertension," and "dyslipidemia," produces manageable lists of 38, 18, and 8 articles, respectively, for additional screening. If you are having trouble with search terms, it often helps to ask an experienced colleague or teacher/mentor for assistance.

Fourth, if particular websites or organizations are influential in the field of study, it can be helpful to search these. However, use these sources with caution. An organization with an "axe to grind" is generally not a good source of information. For example, articles published on company websites may be thinly veiled advertisements for company products, and some organizations call themselves "nonpartisan" but are actually heavily slanted toward a particular political point of view.

Fifth, although it may seem a bit premature, it is wise to consult a research-reporting guideline appropriate for your study type (e.g., observational analysis, randomized trial, quality improvement assessment) at this stage or shortly thereafter. By explaining how you will be expected to report your methods and findings upon completion of the project, these guidelines can help you "stay on track" in collecting the necessary data. They are available at www.equator-network.org and are discussed in detail in Chapter 10.

What to read when you can't read the whole report. As the examples of the misreported New Hampshire study illustrate clearly, you should *never* rely solely on a second-hand account of the findings of any study. You should access and read the source material yourself. In an "ideal world," it is best to read the entire study report. *If you do not have time to read the full study report*—and many of us don't—the three most important parts of the article are (1) the Abstract, (2) the Methods section, and (3) the *data tables and figures* in the Results section. These usually contain all or nearly all of the information needed to construct an informative literature summary table. However, because questions may arise that require returning to the text of the article for clarification, it is a good idea to keep the entire article on hand throughout the research project.

How to Construct a Literature Summary Table

Although formats of literature summary tables may vary, the basic concept is to record key details of the study methods and findings for use throughout your project. (Note that only a small subset of these details will be included in your final published study report; the table is primarily for your reference.) Research methodologist Jane Miller calls these the "Ws"—who, what, when, and where.[10] More creatively and in a different context, the GRADE (Grading of Recommendations Assessment, Development and Evaluation) group,

Table 4B
Suggested Elements and Rationale for Literature Summary Table

Description and Example of Element	Rationale for Element
First author and year of publication	• Will be used for tracking purposes now and in the literature review section of your study report.
Where—the study setting (e.g., "clinic serving low-income elderly" or "academic teaching hospital")	• Findings that apply in one context might not apply in others; for example, a program might achieve great success in an academic teaching hospital but not in a small clinic in a remote rural area.
Who—key characteristics of study patients (e.g., "referred by physicians in 2007 because of A1c >8%" or "hospitalized at least once for diabetes during 2006"); number of cases in each study group or cohort	• Findings that apply to one group might not apply to others; for example, a disease management program might have one effect in a group of patients with severe diabetes and a different effect in patients with mild disease. • Sample size provides information about statistical power (probability of detecting a statistically significant difference).
What—specific intervention or change (e.g., "copayment increase from $10 to $20 for brand medication and decrease from $5 to $0 for generic medications")	• The effects of a policy often depend on the details; for example, the effects of a $5 copayment increase and a $25 copayment increase may differ.[a]
When—time periods for identification and follow-up of study subjects	• In health care (and in other fields) interventions and knowledge change over time; thus, knowing the year in which a study took place (not just when it was published) is important. • Knowing the length of the follow-up periods used in previous studies informs the methodological decisions to be made in your study.
Design—the overall structure of a study (e.g., "randomized controlled trial" or "pre-intervention versus post-intervention comparison")[b]	• Because trials in which subjects are randomized to an intervention usually have the best internal validity if carried out appropriately, topics not studied with at least one randomized trial should generally be considered understudied.[b]
Findings—be specific (e.g., "claims PMPM increased from 0.2 to 0.5 in the control group and decreased from 0.2 to 0.1 in the intervention group, $P < 0.001$")	• Both the direction and the amount (magnitude) of change are important. For example, a decline of 2.0 claims PMPM and 0.1 claims PMPM are both reductions but may have very different clinical implications. • You will use these details as examples in the literature review section of your study report.[c] • Noting statistical significance or nonsignificance in the table is important because nonsignificant findings should not be treated as if they were significant.
Other details relevant to the topic	• Depends on information that is important to those likely to use the results of your study.
Comments—any impressions of the study's quality or findings relative to those of other research	• This information helps you determine the gaps in available knowledge. • You will need this information for the study report literature review, and it is unlikely that you will remember it then—better to make notes now.

[a] For example, in commercially insured groups, typical copayment increases of up to $12 are not significantly associated with discontinuation of medications, but in one study, a copayment increase of $23 was associated with discontinuation of medication.[12]
[b] See Chapter 3.
[c] See Chapter 10.
A1c = hemoglobin A1c; PMPM = per member per month.

which promulgates systems for quality-of-evidence assessment in the development of clinical treatment guidelines, uses the acronym "PICO" (patient-intervention-comparator-outcome).[11] In Arizona, where I live, this term is easily remembered because pico de gallo is an especially delicious salsa! The point is to pick whatever acronym or system helps you identify key elements of a study's design and results. Depending on the study topic, your summary table might include the elements summarized in Table 4B.

A sample literature summary chart is in Table 4C. I wrote this unpublished chart initially in 2001, when I was working with a researcher who wanted information about studies of the clinical and economic effects of disease state management (DSM) programs for congestive heart failure (e.g., patient education, nurse "hotlines," assessments of medication use by pharmacists, and similar services). Because the researcher was especially interested in the administrative costs of these programs (e.g., costs of printing and mailing educational materials, salaries paid to nurses and pharmacists), I included information about that topic. To avoid delving here into details of specific studies, I have removed the "first author and year" column for illustration purposes only (citations available upon request).

Using the Literature Summary Chart to
Formulate Research Questions and Hypotheses

Having constructed a summary chart, a researcher is ready to describe two critically important aspects of his or her study—*what is already known* about the topic and *what the present study is intended to add*. In addition to providing vital information for planning, this information will be used later in writing up the study report so that the reader understands the present study in the context of previous work.

Identifying what is already known. To begin the process, look at your summary table. What patterns in methods, findings, and limitations do you see? In reviewing our congestive heart failure summary chart, the researcher and I noted the following patterns, which represented what was already known about DSM programs for congestive heart failure.

- Weakly designed studies, such as pre-post analyses without an adequate comparison group, uniformly found that DSM programs were effective. This pattern is common in this type of design and does not necessarily mean that the programs work, for reasons described in more detail in Chapter 3.
- *Randomized controlled trials* (RCTs) produced mixed results but generally suggested that DSM for congestive heart failure was ineffective.

- There was an important exception: RCTs of the highest-risk hospitalized inpatients suggested that post-discharge education and support reduced readmission rates, thereby improving both economic and humanistic outcomes.
- Some studies appeared to have insufficient **statistical power**; that is, the number of cases studied was so small that the probability of detecting a statistically significant effect was low, a topic that will be considered later in this chapter.
- In study abstracts, some authors described nonsignificant results as if they were significant.
- Complex and expensive interventions did not seem to work better than less intensive interventions; thus, there seemed to be an opportunity to study interventions of varying intensity levels to identify cost-effective approaches.

The researcher and I opted not to do a study of DSM programs. But had we done so, the literature summary table would have pointed the way both to an important unmet need and to a well-informed study hypothesis.

What was not known about the topic—identifying the unmet research need. At the time that we performed the literature review, all RCTs of DSM for congestive heart failure had been done in *inpatient* populations. The only information about the possible effects of these programs in *outpatients*—that is, patients in "ambulatory care" who receive most or all of their care in physician offices—came from weakly designed research, mostly pre-post designs with no comparison group or with an inadequate comparison group. This lack of rigorous evidence was especially problematic because outpatients constituted the vast majority of those served by DSM programs in the United States, at an estimated cost of $600 million in 2002.[13] Had we planned to proceed with a research project, we would have been able to articulate *what our study was intended to add*—rigorous (preferably RCT or quasi-experimental) information about the effects of DSM for outpatients with congestive heart failure, perhaps comparing higher-risk versus lower-risk patients and more-intensive versus less-intensive interventions.

An informed hypothesis. Because RCTs of DSM in inpatients had produced mixed findings with the best results for the *highest*-risk patient populations, it seemed unlikely that a study of DSM in outpatients—who are mostly *low* risk and therefore have fewer preventable medical events—would produce positive outcomes. Thus, the most informed **hypothesis**—a statement about what we expected to find based on what was already

Table 4C
Sample Literature Summary Chart for Studies of Disease
State Management Programs for Congestive Heart Failure

Who and Where? (Sample and Setting)	What (Intervention)	Design and Outcomes Reported	Comments
Members of a large Midwestern health plan; had one inpatient or two outpatient claims with HF diagnosis in 12 month period. 100% of members were enrolled unless they opted out (28% opted out); n=1,647 in baseline year (1999) and 1,973 in first program year (June 2000-May 2001).	Intensive, holistic program that coordinates all health needs, not just disease-related. Numerous physician services: cardiac care guidelines, visit(s) from service manager to discuss medication indications and dosing, multiple medication reminders and alerts, toll-free hotline, guideline compliance charts. Numerous patient interventions: multiple mailings, telephone calls made by nurses every 4-6 weeks, in-home electronic monitoring, toll-free hotline, website access.	• Simple pre/post without a comparison group. • Increase in LDL-C screening from 20% to 38%, in ACE-I use from 51% to 64%. Reductions of about 20%-25% in hospital use (from 1,410 to 1,149 admits per 1,000; from 1,240 to 935 ER visits per 1,000), but no statistical tests were reported. Medical cost reduction of 28% estimated by applying an assumed 18% inflationary factor to baseline expenditures before comparing to post-intervention period.	• Results probably represent regression to the mean.[a] • Costing method was nonstandard. • Administrative cost was not reported.
190 Swedish patients aged 65-84 years, hospitalized for HF between December 1991 and October 1993; patients with comorbidities were excluded; n=80 intervention, n=110 control.	Education program on HF, self-management of diuretics, and medication compliance; follow-up at clinic with nurse readily available.	• RCT, 1-year follow-up. • One-year survival 71.8% control versus 70.0% intervention (NS); mean time to readmission (days) 106 control versus 141 intervention ($P<0.05$); "trend" toward lower costs ($3,594 controls versus $2,294 intervention, $P=0.07$) and lower hospital days (8.2 control versus 4.2 intervention, $P=0.07$)	• Abstract's conclusion that program "reduces health care costs" was based on a P value of 0.07.

Table 4C (continued)
Sample Literature Summary Chart for Studies of Disease State Management Programs for Congestive Heart Failure

Who and Where? (Sample and Setting)	What (Intervention)	Design and Outcomes Reported	Comments
Patients with confirmed moderate to severe HF (class II or III), treated in a multispecialty medical group. Of 128 identified via claims, only 26 were enrolled because the rest did not have HF or because of physician or patient refusal. All other participants were volunteers (42 of 68 participants). Comparison group was patients in same medical group with ≥1 HF claim, matched on sex and 1995 claims. After matching, N was 43 program and 86 comparison.	Daily home monitoring via measurements taken and called in by patients; contacts to doctors for unacceptable values; weekly educational meetings and nurse telephone contact; offer of pager with medication reminders.	• Pre/post with comparison group; each period was 1 year. • No significant differences in baseline period between intervention and control in total claims, natural log of total claims, hospital admits or hospital days. In the post-intervention period, total all-cause medical costs decreased in the intervention group from $8,500 to $7,400 and increased in the comparison group from $9,200 to $18,800 ($P<0.05$). Not possible to assess HF-related utilization because of diagnostic inaccuracy.	• Study groups are not comparable because of high number of volunteers in intervention group. • All-cause medical cost was measured—not clear how much was disease-related.
287 patients hospitalized between July 1995 and April 2001 with HF diagnoses and/or clinical signs (LVD, pulmonary edema) in an academic medical center in Vermont that serves a mostly rural area; n=141 intervention and 146 control, of whom 122 and 112, respectively, completed the study.	Nurse case management: early discharge planning, care coordination, patient and family education, 12 weeks of phone follow-up, reminder letters to physicians about appropriate medications.	• RCT, 90-day follow-up. • Readmission rate 37% in both groups ($P>0.99$). All medication use measures NS (e.g. at 12 weeks, use of ACE-Is and ARBs was 84% intervention, 80% control, $P=0.40$). All differences in 90-day costs of care were NS, including mean readmission costs ($5,253 intervention vs. $5,163 control, $P=0.96$) and outpatient costs ($1,552 intervention vs. $1,307, $P=0.28$).	• Of 589 patients initially screened, 167 refused participation. • Abstract Results section indicated that the intervention reduced total cost and cost per readmission, but these results were NS ($P=0.14$ and 0.94).

Table 4C *(continued)*
Sample Literature Summary Chart for Studies of Disease State Management Programs for Congestive Heart Failure

Who and Where? (Sample and Setting)	What (Intervention)	Design and Outcomes Reported	Comments
443 veterans hospitalized with CHF in 1 of 9 VA hospitals.	An in-hospital visit with a nurse for education, a post-hospitalization nurse telephone call, and ongoing access to primary care nurse.	• RCT, 6-month follow-up. • Hospitalization rates per patient were *higher* in the intervention than control group (1.5 vs. 1.1, $P=0.02$). Of those clinically eligible for ACE-I, 75% in intervention group and 73% in control group received it ($P>0.02$).	• Of 3,209 patients eligible for randomization, 971 declined.
Hospitalized CHF patients aged 70 years or older with risk factors for readmission (e.g., at least four hospitalizations in the past five years), July 1990 to June 1994. Of 1,306 admissions in age range, 282 met study criteria; n=142 treatment and 140 control.	Intensive patient and family education by nurse, dietary assessment by dietician, social service consult, medication analysis by geriatric cardiologist, intensive home care (visits and phone calls).	• RCT, 90-day follow-up. • 90-day survival without readmission (primary outcome) 64.1% treatment and 53.6% control ($P=0.09$). RR for readmission 0.56, $P=0.02$. Net savings of $460/patient or $153 PPPM after accounting for administrative costs	• Well-done with promising results, but lacks external validity for outpatient populations because of very restrictive risk criteria for sample entry.
Hospitalized CHF patients. Of 1,145 patients, 573 met study criteria and 358 agreed to participate (n=130 intervention, 228 control).	Telephonic case management using proprietary software, targeting medication adherence, diet, signs and symptoms; mean of 17 phone calls per patient.	• RCT, 6-month follow-up, randomization at the physician level. • HF hospitalization rate 0.21 (intervention) versus 0.41 (control) at 6 months ($P=0.02$ after covariate adjustment); HF hospital days mean 1.1 intervention and 2.1 control at 6 months ($P=0.05$ after adjustment). No significant difference in many measures including HF readmissions, all-cause hospitalizations or readmissions, physician or ER visits. Net savings of ~$550/patient ($1,000 gross savings–$443 program cost).	• Although the program targeted medication compliance, drug costs were not included in the cost calculation. • Extent of exclusions prior to randomization is problematic.

Table 4C (continued)
Sample Literature Summary Chart for Studies of Disease State Management Programs for Congestive Heart Failure

Who and Where? (Sample and Setting)	What (Intervention)	Design and Outcomes Reported	Comments
27 male patients at one VA hospital with class II to class III-IV CHF and 3 month history of therapy with ACE-Is. Patients "with a history of non-adherence with physician appointments were excluded."	Mailed educational materials; digital BP machine, scale and pager; reminders to do self-care activities (e.g. weighing, BP, take meds); weekly phone contact with nurse; 24-hour nurse telephone access; doctor notified of problems.	• Simple pre/post pilot study, no comparison group; mean follow-up of 8.5 months. • CV hospitalizations declined from 0.6 PPPY to 0.2 PPPY but $P=0.09$. CV hospital days declined from 7.8 to 0.7 PPPY ($P<0.05$). High severity patients (two-thirds of participants) had greater reductions, as did patients who had a recent admission.	• Authors acknowledge weak design and inability to draw conclusions from results.
97 high-risk (high level of cardiac impairment) Australian patients hospitalized with CHF. High-risk patients were selected because they would be more likely to benefit from the intervention. n=49 intervention, 48 control.	One single home visit 1 week post discharge, by nurse/pharmacist team, to optimize meds, identify early problems, and educate caregivers.	• RCT, 18-month follow-up. • Rates for primary endpoint (composite of unplanned readmissions plus deaths) mean 1.4 intervention and 2.7 control ($P=0.03$). Mean hospital days 2.5 intervention and 4.5 control ($P=0.004$). Costs (Aus$) mean $5,100 intervention and $10,600 control ($P=0.02$).	• Strong design and follow-up time. • Highest risk patients only; may not be applicable to outpatients. • Probably low administrative costs.
117 hospitalized CHF patients meeting criteria for high risk (e.g., class III or IV, recent CHF hospitalization); enrolled July 1998 to April 1999; tertiary care center setting.	Multidisciplinary team, patient education manual, telephone and visit schedule based on severity stratification.	• Simple pre/post, no comparison group, 10-month follow-up, mean 4.7 months. • Beta-blocker use increased from pre- to post-intervention (52% vs. 76%, $P<0.01$). Hospitalization rate decreased (from mean 1.5 to 0 PPPY), and number of clinic visits increased (mean 4.3 to 9.8 PPPY), both $P<0.01$. Change in ACE-I use NS (78% vs. 79%).	• Results probably represent regression to the mean.[a] • Administrative costs of intervention not assessed.

[a] Regression to the mean is explained in Chapter 3 and discussed in detail in Chapter 5.
ACE-I=angiotensin-converting enzyme inhibitor; ARB=angiotensin-II receptor blocker; Aus=Australian; BP=blood pressure; CHF=congestive heart failure; CV=cardiovascular; ER=emergency room; HF=heart failure; LDL-C=low-density lipoprotein cholesterol; LVD=left ventricular dysfunction; NS=nonsignificant; PPPM=per patient per month; PPPY=per patient per year; RCT=randomized controlled trial; RR=risk ratio; VA=U.S. Department of Veterans Affairs.

known—would have been that DSM in outpatients with congestive heart failure would produce no significant improvements in clinical or economic outcomes.

Notably, this hypothesis—based on *specific* information about the available evidence—was in sharp contrast to prevailing wisdom at the time. Yet, as was discussed in more detail in Chapter 3, the Medicare Health Support experiment, an RCT conducted several years later, surprised advocates of DSM programs whose opinions had been based primarily on weakly designed studies, by producing the finding that DSM programs for congestive heart failure did not produce either meaningful clinical benefit or health care cost savings.[14]

Sound Knowledge, Sound Planning: Why Is Understanding Previous Research Critical to Effective Project Design?

Ask any student of history to cite a classic example of the importance of *knowledge* in developing a sound strategy, and chances are good that he or she will mention the Battle of Thermopylae, fought in 480 BC between the Persians and Greeks and considered pivotal in the ultimate termination of Persian efforts to invade Europe.[15,16] Although the sizes of the fighting forces are uncertain, it is clear that "the odds were overwhelmingly against the Greeks," as one account describes it, with the Persian fighting force numbering into possibly the millions.[17] Yet, because the Greeks had *knowledge* of the extremely narrow "mountain track" at Thermopylae, which controlled the only road into central Greece, they correctly surmised that it would represent the best vantage point for defense against the massive (and therefore cumbersome) Persian army. With what historian Herodotus described as only "a small force,"[17] the Greeks successfully defended the pass for three days before losing their lives, thereby giving the Athens government sufficient time to prepare its naval forces for warfare and ultimately defeat the Persians at the Battle of Plataea in 479 BC.[16]

Although engaging in hand-to-hand combat is obviously unlikely for most researchers—thankfully—the lessons learned from the battle apply nonetheless: *good strategic planning rests on a foundation of knowledge,* and *it is important to know the paths that others have walked before.*

For example, in considering a plan for research about DSM in congestive heart failure, **three critically important implications** of establishing *what was already known* (the "path" walked before) and *what our study was intended to add* are noteworthy. **First,** knowledge of the weak study designs used in research on outpatients revealed an important gap in current knowledge; an RCT was needed. **Second,** if we had limited our literature review to study abstracts, we would have been given a very misleading picture of the effectiveness of DSM because the abstracts were, unfortunately, sometimes inconsistent with the actual study findings. By requiring us to record specific details, the literature summary table prompted us to go beyond the sometimes vague statements in abstracts and obtain more useful and accurate information. **Third,** and perhaps most important, the literature summary table saved us from ourselves! As Booth, Colomb, and Williams (2008) observe in *The Craft of Research,* all researchers must find ways to guard against bias because human nature drives us to embrace information in support of our preconceptions and miss details that refute them.[1] A researcher who for any reason—philosophical, business, or professional—begins his or her project in support of a particular idea benefits greatly from the "reality check" provided by a literature summary table. That is, by prompting a researcher to examine *specific* findings, the literature summary chart "forces" objectivity on human beings, who are by nature less than objective.

Formulating a Preliminary Plan

Now that you have identified what is already known about your subject and what your study is intended to add, it is time to begin to flesh out details. That is, you will begin to *operationalize*—translate your study concepts into specific design rules. A checklist for the process is summarized in Table 4D and discussed in more detail below.

Design. Is a randomized design possible? If not, how will you control for **confounding** factors? Before making your choice, make sure that you understand **internal validity** (appropriateness of inference) and **external validity** (applicability), which were described in detail in Chapter 3. If a standard randomized test of the intervention is not possible for business reasons (e.g., a client who wants 100% of his or her enrollees to receive the intervention), consider a **staggered or phased randomized design**, in which the intervention is implemented first to one randomly selected subgroup, then to other randomly selected subgroup(s) at a later time. This type of design offers the researcher the opportunity to make several interesting comparisons. For example, assuming an intervention implemented to Group A in January 2009 and Group B six months later in July 2009, the researcher could compare: (1) Group A versus Group B from January 2009 through June 2009, when Group A had the intervention and Group B did not (measures initial intervention effect); (2) Group B from January 2009 through June 2009 (pre-

Table 4D
Summary Checklist of Study Planning Decisions

Check literature review summary table for:
➤ Gaps in what is already known about the subject.
➤ Methods used in previous research (e.g., design, sample inclusion and exclusion criteria, follow-up time).
➤ Diagnosis and procedure codes used in analyses of administrative claims (billing data), if applicable.

Pick the strongest possible research design, using the following steps:
➤ Consider a randomized controlled trial.
➤ If randomization of all cases is impossible, consider a staggered (phased-in) randomized implementation.
➤ If randomization is impossible, pick comparison group(s) that are as similar as possible to the intervention group.
➤ To draw conclusions about the effect of the intervention, avoid pre-post designs without a comparison group.
➤ To *describe* a relatively new intervention and explore possible research questions for future study, a pre-post design without a comparison group is appropriate.

Determine the necessary sample size by calculating statistical power, taking into account the effect sizes:
➤ That have been previously published.
➤ That you and/or others believe would represent a meaningful improvement.
➤ That you and/or others believe will result from the intervention.

Select sample inclusion and exclusion criteria based on:
➤ Previously published work.
➤ Consideration of internal validity (accuracy of inference) and external validity (applicability).

Select follow-up time for study based on:
➤ Previously published work.
➤ Specific features of the independent and dependent variables (e.g., the amount of time it takes for a drug or a program to take effect).
➤ Developments in the field of study taking place over time.

intervention) versus Group B from July 2009 through December 2009 (post-intervention); and (3) Group A versus Group B from July 2009 to December 2009, when Group A had six months of experience with the program and Group B was just starting the program (measures change in program effect over time).

Who. How, specifically, will study subjects be selected? At this stage, you will establish the *inclusion criteria* and the *exclusion criteria,* the specific requirements for entry into and omission from the sample. To make these decisions, look at your literature summary chart, consulting the original study reports if necessary for more details, to determine specific selection criteria used by others. For example, if you plan a study of patients who use antidepressant medications, you will find in examining previous work that some researchers limit their samples to those diagnosed with "major depressive disorder;" others include those with milder forms of depression; and some include patients with anxiety disorders, who often use antidepressant drugs. Some may choose to include patients with psychotic disorders, such as schizophrenia, because they are commonly treated with antidepressant drugs (along with other medications), whereas others may exclude those patients out of concern that the psychosis makes it impossible to draw valid conclusions about the relationships between antidepressants and the study outcomes.[18] In making your decisions, you will want to consider *both* which methods are most commonly used *and* which make the most sense to you given your research topic and objectives. It may also be appropriate to consider limitations in the data sources used in previous work; for example, a study based solely on pharmacy claims data cannot control for patient diagnosis. You will be verifying your understanding of all of these points later in this process; for now, the idea is to develop a preliminary plan.

If your study is nonrandomized but will compare two groups, you will select an **intervention group**, a group that receives the treatment or intervention of interest, and a **comparison group**, to which the intervention group's results will be compared. In addition to examining the literature summary chart for information about sample selection criteria used by other researchers, you should select for comparison a group that is as similar as possible to the intervention group except for the intervention itself. For example, if you are testing a DSM intervention in a group of blue-collar union members, the comparison group should not consist of white-collar computer programmers employed by a university. Similarly, if the intervention group patients pay a copayment of just $10 per month for Drug A, which costs $1,000 per month, the comparison group should not consist of patients who pay 100% of the cost of Drug A.

If you plan to use a database of administrative medical or pharmacy claims (billing data), you should check previous study reports on your topic for specific diagnosis and procedure codes used by other researchers. You should also check for **superbills**, preprinted billing forms used by physician offices, to determine the diagnosis codes that are most commonly used to bill for the medical condition of interest. These are available on the Internet using the search terms "superbill" plus the name of the specialty area (e.g., "superbill" plus "gastroenterology" or "superbill" plus "family practice").

You will also be making preliminary decisions about **sample size**, that is, the number of cases that you will study. This decision requires consideration of **statistical power**, a topic that will be discussed in the next section of this chapter.

When. What time period will you study? To make this decision requires consideration of **three major points**.

First, consider the specific features of your **independent variables** (variables that are intended to explain or predict the study outcomes) and **dependent variables** (the study outcomes). For example, if Drug A does not take effect in the body before 30 days of treatment, the outcomes of treatment with Drug A should be measured beginning at (and not before) 30 days. Similarly, in studying the effects of an educational program intended to improve the dietary habits of outpatients with congestive heart failure and possibly prevent hospitalizations, it would be unreasonable to study hospitalizations for just one month after program completion; one would expect so few hospitalizations in one month's time that no meaningful results could be produced.

Second, consider the time periods used in previous research and whether you are able to improve on them. For example, if no previous study has examined outcomes for more than six months of follow-up, and you have access to three years of longitudinal data, you have an opportunity to add to the literature by studying and reporting both the six-month and three-year outcomes.

Third, consider major developments that have taken place in the field of study over time. For example, any study of the cost of treating upper gastrointestinal disorders, such as ulcers and gastroesophageal reflux disease, would have to account for the major change to the field that occurred in 1992, when *Helicobacter pylori* infection was identified as the underlying cause of most peptic ulcer disease.[19] Similarly, a study of responses to medication cost changes would have to take into account dates on which any study drugs lost patent protection and were marketed as generics, which are available at a greatly reduced cost.

How Many Cases? Sample Size and Statistical Power

A key step in determining the number of cases to be selected for study is an assessment of **statistical power**. To understand the meaning and importance of power, a brief review of statistical testing principles is necessary.

A statistical test sets up a "what-if" or "straw man" scenario in which the relationships between or among the study variables are *not* as they were hypothesized (called the **null** *hypothesis*), and calculates the probability—called the **P value**—of obtaining the observed results *if* the null hypothesis (no relationship) were true. If that probability is low—that is, if it falls below a certain threshold, called the **alpha** or **critical P value,** which is usually set to 5% (0.05) or 1% (0.01)—the null hypothesis is rejected and the result is deemed statistically significant. The power of a statistical test is the probability that it will detect a statistically significant result when the hypothesized relationship exists (i.e., when the null hypothesis is false). The probability of **type 2 error** (sometimes called "false negative"), or failing to reject the null hypothesis when the null hypothesis is false, is 100% minus the power (e.g., if power is 80%, the probability of type 2 error is 20%). The primary cause of type 2 error is an **underpowered** study, a situation in which the number of cases studied is too small to reveal a statistically significant result even if the researcher's hypothesis is accurate. For this reason, power calculations should be considered at the planning phases of a study.[20]

Details of power calculations occupy entire textbooks, one of which is listed as a resource at the end of this chapter. Because many types of power calculations are now available free of charge online, detailed familiarity with the mathematics of these calculations is generally unnecessary for most purposes. However, knowledge of several **general principles** is helpful:

Limited benefit for large claims databases. Power analysis is seldom important in retrospective analyses of administrative health care claims (billing) data, for two reasons. **First**, most vendors and health plans today provide millions or even tens of millions of cases for analysis. Thus, unless the topic of the research is a rare health condition or the administrative claims database is unusually small (e.g., data from just one health plan), these analyses are seldom underpowered. **Second**, one of the key purposes of calculating statistical power is to ensure that resources are not expended on studying more cases than necessary to investigate the research question. This purpose is inapplicable in administrative claims data analysis because typically, it takes about the same level of effort to study 100,000 cases as 10,000,000 cases. So, if you are using a *large* administrative claims database to study a *common* health care condition, a power calculation is a good practice that doesn't take much time—and a journal peer reviewer may ask about it later—but it is unlikely to affect study planning.

The bigger the effect size, the greater the power. Calculating statistical power requires an estimate of the **effect size,** that is, the degree to which the independent variable affects or is associated with the dependent variable. The bigger the effect size, the greater the statistical power (all other things being equal), and the smaller the sample size needed. Or, put more simply, the bigger something is, the easier it is to see.

To understand this point in practical terms, think of political polls run before two elections. In the first, Candidate A has 49% support, and Candidate B has 51% support. In the second, Candidate C has 20% support, and Candidate D has 80% support. Which election is easier to "call?" Of course, the second election is; a small amount of sampling error in the poll for the first election could produce an error in its prediction of victory for Candidate B, but even with a great deal of sampling error, a victory for Candidate D is nearly certain.

For tests of differences in means, such as a t test, estimating the effect size for a power calculation will require knowledge not only of the expected mean difference, but also of the expected standard deviation, a statistical measure of dispersion (variability) in the data. Consider the commonly used "d" statistic, a standard indicator of effect size:[20]

$$d = \frac{MA - MB}{SD}$$

where MA=mean of group A, MB= mean of group B, and SD=standard deviation (assumed to be equal for the two groups, an assumption of the t test). The following two calculations reflect very different effect sizes, although both represent mean differences of 10:

$\frac{MA - MB^*}{SD} = \frac{280 - 270}{100}$ = effect size of 0.10, or one-tenth of a standard deviation

$\frac{MA - MB}{SD} = \frac{280 - 270}{20}$ = effect size of 0.50, or one-half of a standard deviation

Intuitively, the need to know about sample variability in estimating the necessary sample size makes sense. If the results for different study subjects are extremely diverse, the outcome of any statistical test is more difficult to "call;" therefore, more cases are

---

* Note that for two-tailed testing (i.e., nondirectional hypothesis testing, in which one tests for differences between the groups without specifying the expected direction of the difference), which constitutes the vast majority of statistical tests performed in health care research, the absolute value of the difference is calculated. Here, I show the larger mean first, for ease of explanation.

required to get a reliable answer. That is why variability (i.e., a bigger standard deviation) decreases the effect size, and the smaller effect size, in turn, increases the necessary sample size. For example, with 100 cases in each group and an alpha of 0.05 (i.e., a *P* value less than 0.05 will be deemed significant), a t test will have 11% power to detect an effect size of 0.10, compared with 94% power to detect an effect size of 0.50. To have 80% power to detect an effect size of 0.10 would require 1,570 cases in each group!

Expected means and standard deviations can often be determined from the literature review. Additionally, the effect sizes that are deemed meaningful should be determined as part of initial research planning meetings, described later in this chapter.

Power and binomials. A ***binomial*** (two-level variable, e.g., yes/no or Candidate A versus Candidate B) is a special case of a mean in which it is unnecessary to calculate a standard deviation to determine an effect size, because each variable has only two possible values. Cohen (1969) presents a formula that can be used to calculate the number of cases needed to test any combination of binomial results for two groups (e.g., 50% in Group A versus 30% in Group B, 50% in Group A versus 20% in Group B, etc.).[20] Inputting this formula into a spreadsheet takes just a few hours (using a copy and paste function for formula components) and provides a handy and easily used reference—a major timesaver.

Power and alpha. The critical *P* value (alpha) for a statistical test and the power of the test can be thought of as "first cousins" who don't always get along well. That is, the more stringent the alpha criterion, the lower the power, and the greater the number of cases required to get sufficient power. For example, with n=100 in each group and an effect size of 0.40, a t test has 81% power at an alpha=0.05 and only 60% power at an alpha=0.01. To get 81% power at alpha=0.01 requires 150 cases in each group.

Common sources of "power loss." Statistical power is decreased by random measurement error (e.g., keying mistakes, asking a survey question in a manner that is confusing and causes unreliable answers by respondents).[21] Additionally, although using a ***nonparametric test***—that is, a test that does not assume a particular data distribution (usually the normal distribution)—is appropriate if the assumptions for a parametric test (e.g., t test, analysis of variance) are not met, nonparametric testing diminishes statistical power if data are normally distributed and should be used only when necessary (e.g., when working with health care cost data, which are typically highly skewed).[21]

Discussing the Preliminary Study Plan

The next step is to write a preliminary study plan that will be used in planning discussions prior to beginning the project. An example is shown in Appendix 4A, a hypothetical plan for a study that I coauthored in 2001.[22] The idea is not to overwhelm everyone with detail, but rather to give those involved in the project—either as investigators or as eventual users of the study results—an opportunity to review the planned methods, make comments, and point out details or a need for information that might have been missed. It is helpful to include other knowledgeable researchers at these meetings as well. Disseminate your preliminary study plan prior to the meeting, if at all possible, to give those attending the meeting a chance to read and consider the details prior to discussing them.

At the planning meeting, "talk through" the background information—that is, what is already known about the subject, which eventually will become the introduction to your study report, and what your research is intended to add, which is the study objective. For example, in presenting the hypothetical study plan shown in Appendix 4A, you would briefly explain the findings of previous studies of copayments, explain that no studies of three-tier copayments have been performed, and say that the study would be the first to assess pharmacy and medical utilization outcomes associated with three-tier copayment implementation.

Explain the outcome measures, and ask those present if any important measures have been omitted. If you have worked hard on your plan and don't actually *want* to make changes, you might find it hard to ask this question—but if there is something that your information users need to know that you weren't planning to study, now is the time to find out so that you can make adjustments! Then explain, briefly, how you plan to operationalize the study measures into specific constructs. To facilitate understanding of the expected study output, the use of "table shells" (see Chapter 10, Appendix 10A for examples) is recommended.[23]

A good rule of thumb in your written document is that the study method should be explained in detail sufficient to enable a knowledgeable person to conduct the study using only the plan that you provide.[24] However, some details (e.g., numerous diagnosis or procedure codes) are best presented in writing rather than orally during the meeting. In the meeting, you can refer to this information briefly. For example, say something like "To control for comorbidities in our sample of patients with congestive heart failure, we selected all diagnosis codes representing diabetes, hypertension, or major depressive disorder in the six months prior to the first diagnosis of congestive heart failure. These are listed in Table 1." You don't need to name all the codes, but you should give your audience a sense of what they are, in terms that will be meaningful to the group (e.g., physicians will probably want more clinical detail than managed care account executives). When you present information at this level of detail, others may think of points that you missed, such as the importance of a particular comorbidity, the introduction of a new benefit design to the marketplace, or a practice pattern that changed during your study period because of an updated treatment guideline.

As part of the meeting, be sure to highlight the effect sizes that were assumed when you planned the study, because any discrepancies in these assumptions can have a profound impact on the number of cases needed for analysis. For example, say you assumed that a medication continuation rate difference of 80% in the comparison group versus 90% in the intervention group would be meaningful (clinically important)—but at the meeting, you learn that your information users would describe a much smaller difference, 80% in the comparison group and 85% in the intervention group, as meaningful and therefore worthy of measurement. At a critical P value of 0.05, the number of cases needed in each study group for 80% power to detect the minimum meaningful difference would change from 195 to 902! That does *not* mean that you should change the meaningful difference to "back into" the sample size you want—clinical meaning does not change just because of sample size requirements—but it does mean that you might need to adjust the therapy classes or time periods that are studied to have a sample that is both sufficiently powered and feasible.

Do I *Have* To? Why Planning Is So Important

Two common objections are sometimes made to this planning stage. The first objection is that it takes too much time. In reality, the information included in the preliminary plan translates nicely into a draft literature review and methods section for a research report after completion of the study. Hence, assuming that you want to write an accurate and informative report—which is a requirement of most journals—no extra time is spent to create the literature summary table and research plan. Actually, this step is often a time-saver because it prevents the unhappy situation in which the researcher completes a study only to find out that information users need to know about a different outcome or identify a major flaw in the methods. Removal of bias from the literature review, an important benefit of the literature summary table, also should ultimately save time in the peer review process; reviewers and editors are less likely to encounter errors in a manuscript that is based on a careful assessment of previous work.

The second objection is that the methods are too complex to explain to information users, who may (and often do) have less technical training in methods and statistics than the investigator. In reality, the investigator must be able to explain study methods clearly in order to write a publishable report after completion of the study analyses. Additionally, the act of "translating" statistical procedures into language that is understandable for those with less technical training sometimes reveals important flaws in the analytic technique. In other words, if you cannot explain the rationale underlying your procedures to somebody else, it may be that there is a flaw in the statistical analysis plan that has been missed. It is wise to uncover problems of this type at the planning stage.

Summing Up: What Have We Learned?

For those of us who are intellectually curious about our research results and "can't wait" to find out the answers to our questions, planning can be tough! It's just not as much fun to *plan* as it is to *do*. But laying the plans for a research project on a carefully developed foundation of what is already known about the study topic will yield huge returns relative to the investment of time spent: research questions that address what information users really need to know, valid methods, and appropriate interpretation of findings.

We now turn in Chapter 5 to the avoidance of common mathematical mistakes that can thwart effective and accurate calculation and presentation of study outcomes. We begin with a catastrophic launch into outer space.

Helpful Resources

- Booth, Colomb, and Williams. *The Craft of Research:* Chapter 3 "From Topics to Questions," Chapter 4 "From Questions to a Problem," Chapter 5 "From Problems to Sources," and Chapter 6 "Engaging Sources."[1] This book recommends a literature review method that is more lengthy and cumbersome than that presented in this chapter, but its sound underlying principles make these chapters excellent background material.

- Cohen. *Statistical Power Analysis for the Behavioral Sciences.* This book contains a classic explication of statistical power, underlying theory, and calculation methods. It is a good reference to keep on hand.[20]

- Statistician Russell Lenth has written a helpful, practical guide to sample size determination during project planning.[25]

- International Society for Pharmacoeconomics and Outcomes Research guidance on good research practices for comparative effectiveness research contains helpful information about research planning.[23]
- Remember to consult a reporting guideline prior to beginning your project! These are available at www.equator-network.org and discussed in detail in Chapter 10.

References

1. Booth WC, Colomb GG, Williams JM. *The Craft of Research. Third Edition.* Chicago, IL: University of Chicago Press; 2008: quotation p. 84.

2. Peter Medawar quotes. Goodquotes.com. Available at: http://www.goodquotes.com/ quote/peter-medawar/i-cannot-give-any-scientist-of-any-age.

3. Mark Russell quotes. Available at: http://www.brainyquote.com/quotes/quotes/m/ markrussel100093.html.

4. Soumerai SB, Ross-Degnan D, Avorn J, McLaughlin TJ, Choodnovskiy I. Effects of Medicaid drug-payment limits on admission to hospitals and nursing homes. *N Engl J Med.* 1991;325(15):1072-77. Available at: http://www.nejm.org/doi/full/10.1056/ NEJM199110103251505.

5. Sources for the table include:

   • Avorn J. *Powerful Medicines: The Benefits, Risks, and Costs of Prescription Drugs.* New York: Vintage Books; 2005.

   • Balkrishnan R. Predictors of medication adherence in the elderly. *Clin Ther.* 1998;20(4):764-71.

   • Bukstein DA. Incorporating quality of life data into managed care formulary decisions: A case study with salmeterol. *Am J Manag Care.* 1997;3:1701-06.

   • Elliott WJ. The costs of treating hypertension: What are the long-term realities of cost containment and pharmacoeconomics? *Postgrad Med.* 1996;99(4):241-52.

   • Fraser GL, Wennberg DE, Dickens JD Jr, Lambrew CT. Changing physician behavior in ordering digoxin assays. *Ann Pharmacother.* 1996;30(5):449-54.

   • Hennessey S. Potentially remediable features of the medication-use environment in the United States. *Am J Health Syst Pharm.* 2000;57(6):543-48.

   • Kountz DS. Cost containment for treating hypertension in African Americans: impact of a combined ACE inhibitor-calcium channel blocker. *J Natl Med Assoc.* 1997;89(7):457-60.

   • Lipton HL, Bird JA. Drug utilization review in ambulatory settings: state of the science and directions for outcomes research. *Med Care.* 1993;31(12):1069-82.

   • Lo B, Alpers A. Uses and abuses of prescription drug information in pharmacy benefits management programs. *JAMA.* 2000;283(6):801-06.

   • Powe NR, Griffiths RI, Anderson GF. Medicare payment policy and recombinant erythropoietin prescribing for dialysis patients. *Am J Kidney Dis.* 1993;22(4):557-67.

- Rosenberg GB. Opportunities for alliances between industry and pharmacy. *Am J Hosp Pharm.* 1994;51(24):3061-65.
- Sumner B, Lurie N. Financial payment systems and asthma care. *Med Care* 1993;31(3 Suppl):MS74-MS81.

6. Fairman KA. Accuracy in pharmacoeconomic literature review: lessons learned from the Navajo Code Talkers. *J Manag Care Pharm.* 2008;14(9):886-91. Available at: http://www.amcp.org/data/jmcp/886-891.pdf.

7. Evans JT, Nadjari HI, Burchell SA. Quotational and reference accuracy in surgical journals. A continuing peer review problem. *JAMA.* 1990;263(10):1353-54.

8. Eichorn P, Yankauer A. Do authors check their references? A survey of accuracy of references in three public health journals. *Am J Public Health.* 1987;77(8):1011-12.

9. Blustein J, Hanson K, Shea S. Preventable hospitalizations and socioeconomic status. *Health Aff (Millwood).* 1998;17(2):177-89.

10. Miller J. *The Chicago Guide to Writing about Numbers.* Chicago, IL: University of Chicago Press; 2004: quotation p. 11.

11. Guyatt GH, Oxman AD, Kunz R, et al. GRADE guidelines: 2. Framing the question and deciding on important outcomes. *J Clin Epidemiol.* 2011;64(4):395-400.

12. Fairman KA. The future of prescription drug cost-sharing: real progress or dropped opportunity? *J Manag Care Pharm.* 2008;14(1):70-82. Available at: http://www.amcp.org/data/jmcp/JMCPMaga_JanFeb%2008_070-082.pdf.

13. Foote SM. Population-based disease management under fee-for-service Medicare. *Health Aff (Millwood).* 2003; Suppl Web Exclusives:W3-342-56.

14. McCall N, Cromwell J, Bernard S. Evaluation of Phase I of Medicare Health Support (formerly Voluntary Chronic Care Improvement) pilot program under traditional fee-for-service Medicare: Report to Congress. June 2007. Available at: http://www.cms.gov/reports/downloads/McCall.pdf.

15. Gill NS. Persian Wars Battle at Thermopylae—480 BC. About.com. Available at: http://ancienthistory.about.com/cs/weaponswar/p/blpwtherm.htm.

16. Battle of Plataea, defeat of the Persians. Timeline index. Available at: http://www.timelineindex.com/content/view/2181.

17. Herodotus (Grene D, translator). *The History.* Chicago, IL: University of Chicago Press; 1987.

18. See, for example, Vlahiotis A, Devine ST, Eichholz J, Kautzner A. Discontinuation rates and health care costs in adult patients starting generic versus brand SSRI or SNRI

antidepressants in commercial health plans. *J Manag Care Pharm.* 2011;17(2):123-32. Available at: http://www.amcp.org/data/jmcp/123-132.pdf.

19. Marshall BJ. Helicobacter pylori: a primer for 1994. *Gastroenterologist.* 1993;1(4):241-47.

20. Cohen J. *Statistical Power Analysis for the Behavioral Sciences.* New York: Academic Press;1969.

21. Blalock HM. *Social Statistics.* New York: McGraw-Hill; 1972.

22. Motheral B, Fairman KA. Effect of a three-tier prescription copay on pharmaceutical and other medical utilization. *Med Care.* 2001;39(12):1293-304.

23. Berger ML, Mamdani M, Atkins D, Johnson ML. Good research practices for comparative effectiveness research: defining, reporting and interpreting nonrandomized studies of treatment effects using secondary data sources: the ISPOR Good Research Practices for Retrospective Database Analysis Task Force Report— Part I. *Value Health.* 2009;12(8):1044-52. Available at: http://www.ispor.org/taskforces/documents/RDPartl.pdf.

24. International Committee of Medical Journal Editors. Preparing a manuscript for submission to a biomedical journal. Available at: http://www.icmje.org/manuscript_1prepare.html

25. Lenth RV. Some practical guidelines for effective sample-size determination. March 1, 2001. Available at: http://www.stat.uiowa.edu/techrep/tr303.pdf.

Appendix 4A
Sample Study Planning Document

Note: This is a *hypothetical* document, which I constructed retrospectively based on a study that a coauthor and I published in 2001.[22]

Study Working Title: Effect of a Three-Tier Prescription Drug Copayment on Drug and Medical Utilization

Research Question(s) or Hypotheses:

Please note that there is relatively little information currently available on which to base a hypothesis; hence, we have mostly research questions at this point.

Research questions: Does the implementation of a three-tier prescription drug copayment affect (a) drug utilization and cost overall; (b) drug utilization and cost for third-tier drugs; (c) rates of continuation of chronic drug therapy; and (d) key measures of medical service use?

Hypothesis based on previous work: Implementation of a three-tier copayment design is associated with savings to payers in net drug costs (i.e., total drug cost minus copayments paid by members), mostly because of the cost offsets due to the copayment, with little effect on overall drug utilization.

Rationale/Relevance of the Project

Background. Three-tier copayment systems use member cost-sharing levels to provide incentives for members to use lower-cost and/or preferred brand drugs. Use of this design is increasingly rapidly. In 1998, only 36% of prescription drug plans offered a three-tier copayment; that proportion was 80% in 2000. (Managed Care Formulary Drug Audit, Scott-Levin. Newton, PA; 2000.) Yet, little is known about the effects of this benefit design, and some commentators have expressed concern that the structure will cause patients to stop using chronic drug therapy, leading to greater use of medical services. (Dalzell MD. Pharmacy copayments: A double-edged sword. *Manag Care.* 1999;8(8):26-31.)

What is already known: Several relevant studies of copayment increases (not three-tier plans) are summarized below:

- Motheral and Henderson used a quasi-experimental (pre-post with comparison group) design, comparing 6 months before versus 6 months after a copayment change. Generic/brand copayment change from $4/$10 to $5/$15 or from $5/$10 to $7/$15 (comparison group $5/$10) was associated with a total net plan drug cost decrease of $18 per member per month (PMPM) in the intervention group and increase of $31 PMPM in the comparison group; increase in generic fill rate of 1 percentage point in the intervention group and decrease of 6 percentage points in the comparison group; and no significant differences in continuation with chronic medications. (Motheral BR, Henderson R. The effect of a copay increase on pharmaceutical utilization, expenditures, and treatment continuation. *Am J Manag Care.* 1999;5:1383-94.)

- Harris et al. used a similar design to assess copayment changes from $0 to $1.50, then from $1.50 to $3.00 in an HMO. The $1.50 copayment was associated with a decline of 11% in the number of prescriptions filled, with the largest changes for "discretionary drugs." Utilization declined again by 11% when the copayment increased to $3. No measures of medical utilization or adherence to chronic drug utilization were performed. (Harris BL, Stergachis A, Ried LD. The effect of drug co-payments on utilization and cost of pharmaceuticals in a health maintenance organization. *Med Care.* 1990;28(10):907-17.)

- Johnson et al. conducted two studies of changes in copayments in elderly HMO members. Copayment changes in one group were from $1 to $3 and then to $5. Copayment changes in the other group were from 50% to 70% with maximums of $25 and $30, respectively. In the group subject to the larger copayment change, likelihood of use was less for antiasthmatics, diuretics, thyroid hormones, nonopioid analgesics, and topical anti-inflammatories. No significant changes in medical care utilization (office visits, emergency room visits, home health care, hospitalization) or total medical costs were found. It should be noted that these were Medicare groups and results may not have external validity (applicability) for commercially insured samples. (Johnson RE, Goodman MJ, Hornbrook MC, Eldredge MB. The effect of increased prescription drug cost-sharing on medical care utilization and expenses of elderly health maintenance organization members. *Med Care.* 1997;35(11):1119-31; *Health Serv Res.* 1997;32(1):103-22.)

What this study is intended to add. This will be the first study to examine medical and drug utilization and cost associated with a three-tier copayment system.

Methods
Design summary: Quasi-experimental: pre-post with comparison group.

Subjects: Preferred provider organization enrollees continuously enrolled from January 1997 through November 1999. Three-tier group will include enrollees whose employer changed from a two-tier to three-tier plan at any time from January 1998 through September 1998 and maintained the three-tier plan through November 1999. Comparison group will include enrollees whose employer retained a two-tier plan throughout the study period. Because these decisions were made by employers and not by enrollees, concerns about selection bias are minimal.

Copayment structures: The two-tier plan was generic $7 and $12 brand. The three-tier plan was $8 generic, $15 preferred brand, and $25 nonpreferred brand.

Inclusion/exclusion criteria: We will exclude any enrollees who were not continuously enrolled from 12 months before through 12 months after their employer's switch date to three-tier, or a comparable index date for the comparison group.

Study Variables
Dependent variables: These variables will be measured both pre-implementation and post-implementation of the three-tier copayment:
- Total drug utilization (claims PMPM)
- Drug utilization for nonpreferred drugs (match claims to nonpreferred drugs file; claims PMPM)
- Total cost (average wholesale price, inflation-adjusted)
- Rates of chronic medication continuation, defined for users with use in the last several months of the pre-intervention period (time period to be established based on preliminary analyses of sample size counts) and who used medications that cost more than the copayment amount in the pre-intervention period (to identify only those users likely to be affected by the change).
- Use of antibiotics (defined as GPI class 01, 02, 03, 08, and some combinations in GPI

- class 16—penicillins, cephalosporins, macrolides, sulfonamides) after an office visit for otitis media (ICD-9-CM code 381.XX)
- Numbers of office visits, emergency room visits, and inpatient hospital stays PMPM, overall and for those using drugs in the pre-intervention that were made three-tier in the post-intervention period

Independent variables:
- Gender
- Age
- Chronic disease score
- Two-tier versus three-tier plan

Statistical considerations

Sample size: For the analysis overall, there are no statistical power considerations. Preliminary analysis of the enrollment files indicates at least 5,000-10,000 cases in each group. For the analysis of continuation of chronic drug therapy, fewer cases are available. We will consider the meaningful effect size to be a difference of 90% versus 80% in continuation. At 80% power, and a one-tailed test at alpha=0.05, we need n=154 cases per group. We will measure continuation with therapy for all chronic drug therapy classes, measured using GPI at the 2-character level, that meet that criterion.

Data analysis: Multivariate techniques will be used if groups differ on important clinical or demographic factors. Otherwise, we plan to use bivariate analysis for most study questions.

Ethical considerations
De-identified dataset without any protected health information.

Budgetary Considerations
No special budgetary needs are anticipated.

Estimated completion date
Unknown at the present time because we have not yet received the data files. We expect to complete analysis no later than 3 months after files are received.

CHAPTER 5

To Be Accurate, Credible, and Interesting: Avoiding Common Mathematical Errors

"The essence of mathematics is not to make simple things complicated, but to make complicated things simple."—Mathematician Stanley Gudder[1]

"A general rule in science is: the more questions you ask, the more likely you are to get a silly answer to at least one of them."—Biostatistician Andrew Vickers, discussing cumulative type I error[2]

"Unfortunately it was a paper that received a lot of attention and had our director's name on it."—Dixie Snider, Chief of Science at the Centers for Disease Control and Prevention, commenting on the retraction of a study report because of simple mathematical errors[3]

O n December 11, 1998, a Delta II 7425 rocket was launched from Cape Canaveral carrying the spacecraft "Mars Climate Orbiter," sophisticated radiometry and color imaging equipment, and the hopes of National Aeronautics and Space Administration (NASA) scientists that the $327.6 million, six-year project would allow them to "witness the atmospheric conditions on Mars through each of its seasons, and from this data, perhaps understand the past and future weather conditions on Mars."[4,5] Just nine months later, the Orbiter was destroyed in an unexpected crash landing. Investigation revealed a surprising cause for the mishap: the

---

> **What You Will Learn in Chapter 5**
>
> In this chapter, you will learn about five common mathematical problems and how to prevent them from damaging the validity of your study results:
>
> ✓ Regression to the mean
> ✓ Confusing statistical significance with practical significance
> ✓ "Unit of analysis" discrepancies
> ✓ Percentages calculated incorrectly—simple math errors, wrong denominator, and denominator-text mismatch
> ✓ Extended "fishing trips"— cumulative type I error

subcontractor that helped build the Orbiter had used English (Imperial) mathematical units, whereas NASA scientists had used metric units, causing a miscalculation and catastrophic navigational error upon entry into the Mars atmosphere.[6]

About one month after the Orbiter launch, a team of scientists at the Centers for Disease Control and Prevention (CDC) announced the retraction of a report that natural disasters prompt suicides, which they had published in the prestigious *New England Journal of Medicine* in February 1998.[7] Because of an "error in computer programming," deaths in 1990 had inadvertently been counted twice. Corrected data showed no significant relationship between natural disasters and suicide.[7] More than five years later, another embarrassed CDC team admitted that a "widely reported" study of the effects of obesity on mortality in the United States, which had been published in the *Journal of the American Medical Association* eight months previously, would have to be retracted. The problem, which caused an overestimate of approximately 80,000 deaths, was "simple mathematical errors, such as including total deaths from the wrong year."[3]

These three cases, although distinctive by notoriety, illustrate a phenomenon common to much less widely publicized projects. Frequently, when research projects fail, the cause is *not* subtly nuanced, technologically sophisticated, or complicated. Instead, catastrophic failures are often attributable to simple and avoidable technical flaws. In this chapter, we'll explore five basic mathematical errors that thwart the intentions of even the best researchers. We'll review "tricks of the trade" to help you avoid these shortcomings and produce work that readers, teachers/mentors, and information users will find compelling and credible.

#1: Regression to the Mean

Does intensive multidisciplinary (e.g., physician, pharmacist, and nurse) "team care" of patients with diabetes improve patient outcomes? This question was addressed in a retrospective analysis by Domurat (1999), who studied patients enrolled in a diabetes care management (DCM) program from 1995 to 1997.[8] In addition to routine office visits with an endocrinologist, the program provided "intensive one-on-one case management evaluation," screening appointments (e.g., eye and foot examinations, blood tests), and education either in group sessions or by telephone. The program was targeted to a minority (about 30%) of patients who were especially high-risk. Criteria for DCM enrollment included "multiple hospital, emergency department, or urgent clinic admissions or visits," complications of diabetes, comorbidities (e.g., uncontrolled hypertension or "general debility"), or other risk factors including "poor understanding of disease self-care."[8]

Domurat found that compared with lower-risk patients ("usual care"), the high-risk patients enrolled in the DCM program had better (higher) routine screening rates—for example, 75% compliance with lipid screening in the DCM group versus 49% in usual care. But on the important question of *change* in outcomes over time, Domurat documented an interesting pattern in most analyses. Among DCM patients who had *favorable* measures at baseline (e.g., hemoglobin A1c within goal, blood pressure within goal) outcomes *worsened* significantly over time, although on average patients remained within goal (e.g., mean A1c changed from 7.0% to 7.5%). In contrast, among patients with *unfavorable* measures at baseline, outcomes significantly *improved* (e.g., mean A1c changed from 10.7% to 9.4%). Similar patterns were observed in the usual care group—on average, patients with good baseline values got worse, and patients with poor baseline values got better. However, blood pressure decreased slightly but significantly more for DCM than usual care patients.

To what can we attribute these results? Are the study outcomes attributable solely to the DCM program? Domurat appropriately explored alternative explanations, including **confounding** factors, in discussing his results. Those who have read Chapter 3 will notice the potentially important effect that **selection bias** could have had on the findings. That is, as Domurat pointed out, patients who were more motivated to improve their health could have been more likely to receive a physician referral to DCM or to remain consistently enrolled in the DCM program. Yet, an equally important threat to the validity of the study findings is a crucial but seldom-discussed mathematical phenomenon, **regression to the mean** (RTM).

What is RTM? To understand RTM, think about anything that you do well—writing, athletics, or a hobby. You probably do not perform the activity *equally* well *every* time; instead, you have good days and bad days. In technical terms, your performance displays "within-subject variability."[9] This variability lies at the heart of the RTM phenomenon, which is that "when observing repeated measurements in the same subject, relatively high (or relatively low) observations are likely to be followed by less extreme [values] nearer the subject's true mean."[10] That is, if one performs especially well (at anything) on a given occasion, one is likely to perform less well on the next occasion, and vice versa. An amusing example of RTM was provided in a 2007 commentary by biostatistician Andrew Vickers, who described "the curse of *Sports Illustrated*," a phenomenon in which "athletes making the cover of *Sports Illustrated* typically have a rapid decline in performance, or get injured, shortly after being featured." The reason for the decline is RTM: "Now of course the reason why athletes get picked [for] the cover is that they have done something spectacular … and at any randomly picked subsequent time [they] are likely to be just average."[11]

Domurat's results, in which subjects with good baseline results tended to deteriorate and subjects with poor baseline results tended to improve, displayed classic signs of RTM. DCM patients who were selected for the program specifically because they were experiencing unfavorable outcomes (e.g., hospitalizations or diabetic complications) at a given point in time would mathematically be expected to show improvement, on average, *with or without intervention*. Linden (2007) demonstrated the same phenomenon in an analysis of health care cost data for health plan members with coronary artery disease (CAD) in 2001 and 2002.[9] Without any health care management intervention at all, mean annual costs for those in the highest cost quintile in 2001 declined sharply from nearly $30,000 to approximately $5,000 in 2002, whereas mean annual costs for those in the bottom four quintiles rose by approximately $920 (after accounting for inflation in both groups).[9] "Had a [disease management] program targeting CAD existed during this period," Linden concluded, "an evaluation of the impact on costs would have wrongly concluded that this outcome was a program effect."[9] This is *not* to say that Domurat's program had no impact; instead, the effects of the program are unknown until measured with a design and/or analytic technique that account for RTM.

And, in failing to mention that RTM had likely been partially responsible for his results, Domurat was not alone. Reviews of the literature performed by scientists familiar with RTM have spotlighted examples of misinterpretations in a wide variety of applications, including analyses of standardized educational tests, immunizations, birthweights, laboratory test values, and health care costs.[9,10,12] In a review and commentary on RTM, Smith and Smith (2005) describe the experience of witnessing an interview for a tenure-track academic job with a candidate whose specialty was educational testing. When asked "how she would interpret data showing that a student who had scored 1.0 standard deviation above the mean on a test administered at the start of the school year scored 0.8 standard deviations above the mean on a similar test administered at the end of the year," the candidate's answer was that "the school had failed this student."[12]

Avoiding or Mitigating the Effects of RTM

The best way to prevent RTM from affecting the validity of research findings is to design the study in a way that takes RTM into account. A highly effective approach is a randomized trial, such as the Medicare Health Support experiment described in Chapter 3, in which subjects who meet study entry criteria are randomly allocated to treatment and control groups.[9,10] In a design of this type, *both* the **intervention** (treatment) and **control** groups experience RTM, and the key focus of the analysis is determining whether the intervention group experienced greater improvement than did the control. For example, a widely cited randomized trial by Rich et al. (1995) assessed the effects of nurse-directed multidisciplinary care on patients aged 70 years or older who were hospitalized for congestive heart failure.[13] By sampling design, study patients were at high risk for hospital readmission because of medical history. *Both* treatment and control group patients experienced improvements in the study's quality-of-life (QOL) measure, the Chronic Heart Failure Questionnaire, during the 90-day follow-up. However, the treatment group's average questionnaire score improvement was approximately double that of the control group, suggesting that the program had positive effects on QOL even after accounting for RTM.

Another design approach to mitigate the effects of RTM is to select study subjects based on two or more measurements, instead of just one, in an attempt to obtain a baseline value that is closer to each subject's true mean than a single measurement would indicate.[9,10] An additional option is to use a formula that calculates the estimated effect of RTM using known or estimated summary statistics for the population distribution, and subtract that result from the observed change to provide an RTM-adjusted estimate.[9,10] Finally, some researchers favor "regression discontinuity" designs, in which study subjects are assigned to treatment or comparison groups based on a pre-specified cutoff point for a baseline measure (e.g., baseline health care cost or educational testing score); separate linear regression lines are estimated for each group; and the intervention effect is measured as the difference ("discontinuity") between the regression lines at the cutoff point.[9,14]

Key Points: RTM

❖ A natural mathematical phenomenon resulting from "within-subject variability."

❖ An important reason why pre-post designs without an adequate comparison group often produce inaccurate results.

❖ There are several appropriate ways to deal with it—but don't ignore it!

#2: Confusing Statistical Significance with Practical Significance

If you are like many researchers today, you work with a personal computer that has a hard drive size of 300-500 gigabytes, 4-8 gigabytes of RAM, and a nearly instantaneous response time. With the push of a computer key, you can access a dataset containing information about thousands of people, such as General Social Survey data available from the National Opinion Research Center,[15] nationwide Medicaid drug claims data available from the Centers for Medicare & Medicaid Services,[16] or even health care claims (billing) data for tens of millions of people, which are available for purchase from a number of vendors. It's quite a change from 20 or 30 years ago, when researchers wanting to analyze a large number of cases needed to use a university mainframe, if they were fortunate enough to have access to such a large dataset at all.

This embarrassment of riches has created a challenge of interpretation. In studies with sample sizes of several thousand to tens of thousands of cases, nearly every result is statistically significant. For example, in a study of two cohorts comprising 40,000 cases each (not uncommon in published health care studies today), a difference of 14.5% versus 15.0% is statistically significant ($P=0.046$) using a two-tailed Pearson chi-square test and an alpha threshold of 0.05. Even with a much smaller sample size, 2,500 in each group and again using a Pearson chi-square test, a difference of 14.0% versus 16.0% is significant ($P=0.048$). Do these miniscule differences have any substantive meaning? It depends on the research question, but in most studies, probably not. Thus, problems arise when researchers confuse *statistical significance* with *practical significance*.[17]

A study by Chernew et al. (2008), a retrospective observational comparison of the employees and dependents of two employers, provides a widely publicized example.[18] The first employer (intervention group) had made sharp reductions in drug copayments in selected medication classes for its 37,867 members in January 2005, from $5 to $0 for generic drugs, $25 to $12.50 for preferred brand drugs, and $45 to $22.50 for nonpreferred brand drugs. The other employer (comparison group), which had 70,259 members in 2005, had left copayments unchanged from 2004 through 2005, averaging $16.22 for generic and $29.72 for brand drugs in 2004. The investigators measured change from 2004 to 2005 in the medication possession ratio (MPR), a commonly used measure of medication adherence that represents the proportion of days during which drug is available to the patient (e.g., a patient who fills prescriptions totaling 60 dispensed days of medication during a 120-day time period has an MPR of 50%).

Chernew et al. found that the increase in MPR from 2004 to 2005 was significantly greater in the intervention group than in the comparison group for four of the five drug classes studied: blood pressure medications, beta blockers, antidiabetic drugs, and cholesterol-lowering drugs. Because "clinical evidence supports adherence to these medications," the investigators noted in their study report, "we expect health improvements, although we do not quantify them in this study." Extending this line of thinking, the investigators noted that they expected "some savings in nondrug spending associated with improved adherence," adding that "there might be gains in worker productivity or reduced absenteeism or disability."[18] Popular press coverage of the study report was enthusiastic, not surprisingly because a press release by the sponsoring university confidently predicted that "just by cutting a few dollars off the co-pay … employers could increase the chances that employees with chronic illnesses will take certain preventive medicines. And that could pay off in the long run, in the form of fewer hospitalizations or emergency room visits for employees with diabetes, high blood pressure, asthma and other conditions."[19,20] Just a "few dollars" for such a big health benefit—who could resist?

The problem with this exuberance over the report by Chernew et al., lost in the popular press coverage, is evident with a close examination of the study findings. As a colleague and I pointed out in a critique of the study,[21] the between-group differences in MPR (i.e., the effect sizes for the intervention, expressed in percentage points) ranged from 2.59 for blood pressure medications to 4.02 for antidiabetic drugs—in other words, averages of approximately 9 to 15 additional *days* of therapy per *year* (e.g., $0.0402 \times 365 = 14.7$), surely not enough to achieve any therapeutic benefit, let alone decreases in hospitalizations or absenteeism. In other words, the findings were statistically significant because of the powerful statistical technique and large sample size, but clinically meaningless.[22]

How *should* a researcher interpret statistical significance? The key is to remember its technical meaning. A statistically significant result is one that is unlikely to be attributable to random sampling error—the effects of "chance" in drawing the sample (see detailed explanation in Chapter 4).[23] If the number of cases is very large, the likelihood that a finding is attributable solely to chance is small, and the result will be deemed statistically significant. However, the fact that a finding is unlikely to be attributable to chance does not itself indicate anything at all about the finding's importance.

How to Report Statistical Significance and Practical Significance Appropriately

To interpret statistically significant results, especially those obtained using large sample sizes, consider not just the *P* value but also the results in absolute terms (e.g., for Group A the rate was X%, for Group B it was Y%) and, most importantly, *express what those results mean using concepts that are of practical importance to your audience.* A commonly used metric in health care is the **number needed to treat** (NNT), calculated as the mathematical reciprocal of the estimated benefit of the treatment. For example, if a treatment reduces a negative outcome by two percentage points, the NNT is $1 \div 0.02 = 50$, meaning that 50 patients have to be treated to prevent a single additional negative outcome. Kaul and Diamond (2010) provide a helpful review of additional mathematical approaches to interpretation.[17]

Research methodologist Jane Miller offers a cogent example of practical interpretation in her indispensable guide to reporting quantitative information, *The Chicago Guide to Writing about Numbers.*[24] Suppose, she says, you were considering a change in the mathematics curriculum for fourth grade students. In a nationwide comparison of the old versus new curricula, "a difference of even half a point in average test scores might be statistically significant because the sample size was so large." Thus, the real question is not whether the result was statistically significant but "is it worth incurring the cost of producing and distributing the new materials and training many teachers in the new curriculum for such a small improvement?"[24] To address this question, the researcher should put the findings "in perspective by providing evidence about how that half-point improvement translates into mastery of specific skills, the chances of being promoted to the next grade level, or some other real-world outcome to evaluate whether that change is worthwhile."[24]

Statistician Russell Lenth (2001) observed in a helpful tutorial on sample size determination that it is wise to identify these meaningful effect sizes at a study's planning stage rather than after findings are obtained.[25] In addition to helping researchers calculate an appropriate sample size for the planned project (Chapter 4), establishing meaningful effect sizes *a priori* greatly reduces the temptation to "over-interpret" statistically significant but meaningless results upon project completion.

An especially commendable way to plan for statistical interpretation is to use published information about the meaning of the effect sizes *to the population that is represented by the sample of research subjects.* For example, in a study of a rheumatoid arthritis disease therapy management

> ## Key Points: Statistical Versus Practical Significance
> - Statistical significance—refers to small likelihood that a finding is due to sampling error.
> - A statistically significant finding is not necessarily important.
> - Interpret results in practical terms that have meaning for the audience of information users—e.g., NNT, MCID.

program, Stockl et al. (2010) found a statistically significant improvement of 0.08 on the Health Assessment Questionnaire-Disability Index (HAQ-DI) score, a commonly used functional measure.[26] Instead of limiting their interpretation to statistical significance alone, the authors took the additional, important step of comparing the observed HAQ-DI improvement with the "minimally clinically important difference (MCID), which is defined as the threshold of improvement that is perceptible and considered clinically meaningful to an individual patient," identified as 0.09 in a previous study.[26] Information of this type, if available at the design stage, is worth its weight in gold to avoid interpretation problems during analysis and write-up.

#3: What Does a "Mean Mean" Mean?
"Unit of Analysis" Discrepancies in Basic Mathematical Calculations

For baseball fans, 1941 was a year to remember. In what would be the final season before the bombing of Pearl Harbor and the entry of the United States into World War II, an America weary of increasingly frightening news from Europe thrilled to the exploits of players who today are remembered as some of the greatest in the history of the game. New York Yankee "Joltin' Joe" DiMaggio achieved a 56-game hitting streak and took the American League's most valuable player (MVP) award.[27] Stan Musial, who would go on to play an astonishing 22 years for the Cardinals and later be described by broadcaster Vin Scully as "good enough to take your breath away," made his major league debut in St. Louis.[28] Boston Red Sox outfielder Ted "Splendid Splinter" Williams refused to leave the final game of the season early to protect a historic batting average of 0.39955 (which would have been rounded to a record-setting 0.400) and instead continued to play, batting 6 for 8 and finishing the season with an average of 0.406—a record unmatched by any player since.[29] And 1941 was a good year for the Red Sox in general—the team boasted a batting average of 0.283 (1,517 hits in 5,359 at-bats), just besting the 0.269 average (1,464 hits in 5,444 at-bats) achieved by their ubiquitous archrivals, the New York Yankees.

In the more than 70 years since that timeless 1941 Major League Baseball (MLB) season, the method of calculating a batting average has not changed. But what if MLB *did* make a change to its method? What if it calculated the *team* batting averages by averaging *each player's* batting average—that is, calculating a mean of the mean, or simple average of the batting averages (summed batting averages divided by total number of players)? The result is shown in Table 5A.

Table 5A
Batting Averages 1941 Season: Boston Red Sox and New York Yankees

NEW YORK YANKEES				BOSTON RED SOX			
Player	At-Bats	Hits	Batting Average	Player	At-Bats	Hits	Batting Average
Dickey	348	99	0.284	Pytlak	336	91	0.271
Sturm	524	125	0.239	Foxx	487	146	0.300
Gordon	588	162	0.276	Doerr	500	141	0.282
Rizzuto	515	158	0.307	Cronin	518	161	0.311
Rolfe	561	148	0.264	Tabor	498	139	0.279
J. Dimaggio	541	193	0.357	Williams	456	185	0.406
Keller	507	151	0.298	Finney	497	143	0.288
Henrich	538	149	0.277	D. Dimaggio	584	165	0.283
Rosar	209	60	0.287	Fox	268	81	0.302
Selkirk	164	36	0.220	Peacock	261	74	0.284
Priddy	174	37	0.213	Newsome	227	51	0.225
Crosetti	148	33	0.223	Spence	203	47	0.232
Bordagaray	73	19	0.260	Flair	30	6	0.200
Silvestri	40	10	0.250	Hale	24	5	0.208
Lindell	1	0	0.000	Carey	21	4	0.190
Ruffing	89	27	0.303	D. Newsome	78	19	0.244
Russo	78	18	0.231	Harris	55	6	0.109
Gomez	59	9	0.153	Wagner	63	10	0.159
Chandler	60	11	0.183	Grove	45	5	0.111
Donald	62	5	0.081	Dobson	47	7	0.149
Bonham	50	8	0.160	Wilson	44	7	0.159
Breur	46	4	0.087	Ryba	37	8	0.216
Peek	28	1	0.036	Johnson	34	10	0.294
Murphy	18	1	0.056	Hughson	17	1	0.059
Stanceu	12	0	0.000	Dickman	11	1	0.091
Branch	10	0	0.000	Fleming	9	2	0.222
Washburn	1	0	0.000	Judd	4	2	0.500
				Potter	3	0	0.000
				Hash	2	0	0.000
Sums	5,444	1,464	5.042	Sums	5,359	1,517	6.372
Player count			27	Player count			29
Unweighted (simple) average of players' averages			0.187	Unweighted (simple) average of players' averages			0.220
Actual (correct) batting average			0.269	Actual (correct) batting average			0.283

Source: www.mlb.com.

Using this alternative method, the team batting averages are dramatically different. The Red Sox maintain their superiority over the Yankees, but this time by a much wider margin—0.220 versus 0.187, respectively. While such a drubbing for the Yankees would have thrilled Red Sox fans in 1941 (something else about the game that hasn't changed in 70 years), this result is mathematically wrong. What happened?

The problem is that the "mean mean" (the simple average of percentages) is unweighted; that is, it gives equal weight to players who saw action in nearly every game, such as Dom DiMaggio (0.283 in 584 at-bats), and players who came to the plate only a few times, such as "Lefty" Grove (0.111 in just 45 at-bats) and Herb Hash (no hits in 2 at-bats). Thus, the unweighted average "drags down" the average for the whole team by "overweighting" results for the players who saw little time at home plate and "underweighting" results for the better hitters. In other words, each team's *actual* batting average was far better than the simple player average would suggest because each team, wisely, sent its better players to the plate more often.

But why did the *comparison* of the teams change when we calculated the erroneous simple average? Why was the Yankees' average deflated so much more than that of the Red Sox? The answer is clear from the Pearson correlations between number of at-bats and batting average (not shown in the table)—0.704 for the Yankees, 0.537 for the Sox—indicating that the relationship between performance at the plate (batting average) and playing time (at-bats) was much stronger for the Yankees. Thus, when we calculated the "mean mean" (the simple average of the batting averages for all players), thereby erroneously "underweighting" the results for the better hitters with more playing time, the average for the Yankees was deflated disproportionately.

This example illustrates **three basic principles** that apply in multiple contexts:

1. The results of simple (unweighted) mathematical calculations may be distorted when the "unit of analysis" (i.e., the entity of interest, number of *team* at-bats in this example) does not match the structure of the dataset (*individual player* batting data in this example).
2. This problem is exacerbated when there is a systematic relationship between the outcome of interest (e.g., batting average) and the unit of analysis (e.g., number of at-bats), as it was in this example (i.e., better batters went to the plate more often).
3. The problem can be avoided by weighting the results to prevent underweighting

and overweighting (e.g., instead of "counting" each player as representing a single unit, treat each player's data as if the player represented his number of at-bats).

We shall return to these principles again, but first we review two research applications. In other words, we look at why this problem is important in health care research.

Unit of analysis discrepancies in calculating percentage share of cost. The problem of knowledge gaps about unit of analysis in health care became clear to me some years ago. A young employee whom I had been supervising informed me that he had, as requested, calculated the overall percentage of drug costs paid by patients versus payers (health insurance plans) in our "book of business" and had found that, on average, patients were paying 65%. Knowing that the actual average share of drug cost paid by consumers in the United States has been less than 30% since 2000 (in 2008 it was 21%),[30] I recall staring at him, open-mouthed, for what I hope was no more than a few seconds—until I realized that, using a method similar to the erroneous hypothetical team batting average calculation described above, he had probably calculated each patient's cost-sharing percentage, then calculated a simple (unweighted) average of all the percentage shares.

The problem with calculating an average of the percentages in this instance is that healthy people typically use inexpensive drugs—for example, generic ampicillin to treat a strep throat. These patients often pay 100% or nearly 100% of the low cost of the medication. For example, a patient who paid the average copayment for a generic drug in an employer-sponsored health plan in 2009, $10,[30] paid 100% of the cost of ampicillin, which costs approximately $10.[31] In contrast, patients with chronic illnesses, who fill prescriptions more often, also typically use more expensive drugs. For example, a 30-day supply of a brand-name oral antidiabetic drug (e.g., Actos or Januvia) costs about $200; thus, a patient with a typical "preferred brand drug" copayment of $27[30] pays about 14% of its cost. In a simple example of just two patients in a year, one with a single case of strep throat and the other with 12 prescriptions for an oral antidiabetic drug, the simple average erroneously estimates the patient share of cost as 57% ([100%+14%] ÷ 2), whereas the actual share of cost paid by the two patients is 14% ($334 patient share ÷ $2,410 total cost).*

---

* Patient share=(12×$27)+$10; total cost=(12×$200)+$10. Note that a percentage is just a special case of averaging because it is calculated as the average amount per 100; for example, a patient who paid $400 of a total bill of $1,200 paid an average of approximately $33 per $100, or 33%.

Unit of analysis discrepancies in calculating cost per month or per year. A common variation of the "mean mean" problem arises when study subjects are followed for varying lengths of time and the researcher calculates a simple average (per study subject) of an outcome that has been measured per unit of time. For example, to calculate monthly health care cost for a group of patients, researchers sometimes first calculate each patient's mean cost per month (the patient's total cost divided by the patient's total months of follow-up) and then calculate a simple per patient average of the monthly means. A common variation on this approach is to "annualize" costs, that is, calculate each patient's cost per month of follow-up, multiply those monthly costs by 12, then calculate the simple per patient average of those annualized numbers. This technique is intended to provide a familiar metric (annual costs) while adjusting outcomes for time spent under observation; for example, a patient with only 2 months of follow-up would be expected to incur lower health care costs than a patient followed for 6 months, all other things being equal.

The problem with these cost calculation techniques is that often all other things are *not* equal. Specifically, the calculation distorts the results if the reason for **loss to follow-up** is systematically related to the study outcome. For example, health care resource utilization at end-of-life is typically intense, resulting in high costs during the final few months of health care.[32] The one-month cost of a health plan member at end-of-life, if multiplied by 12, will usually *greatly* overstate the cost that would have been incurred by a living person over 12 months' time. As a very simplified example, a patient who is hospitalized with a cardiovascular event but dies after just one day of inpatient care at a cost of $25,000 certainly would not have incurred total health care costs of $9.125 million during the subsequent year had he or she lived; however, an annualized cost calculation would multiply $25,000 for a single day times 365 days and produce that very improbable (and meaningless) result.

For this reason, researchers sometimes require that patients be enrolled for a specific minimum amount of time (e.g., two months)[33] to be included in a calculation of annualized cost. However, even after making this adjustment, the "mean mean" (i.e., the per member average of the monthly average cost) may grossly overstate actual cost, as shown in the hypothetical example in Table 5B:

Table 5B
Monthly Cost Calculation Example

Member	Months Enrolled	Total Cost	Monthly Cost
A	12	$600	$50
B	8	$700	$88
C	10	$1,500	$150
D	12	$300	$25
E	2	$30,000	$15,000
Totals	44	$33,100	
Simple per member average of monthly costs (mean mean)			$3,063
Actual (correct) cost PMPM (total cost ÷ total months)			$752

PMPM=per member per month, a standard measure used in health economics research and health care finance.

Note that because the result obtained using a "mean mean" method is *not* mathematically equivalent to a per member per month (PMPM) or per member per year (PMPY) cost, it should *never* be described as a PMPM or PMPY in the text of a research report.

How to Handle Unit of Analysis Discrepancies

Although unit of analysis problems are usually (not always) addressed in peer review so that they seldom make it into published work, they are among the most common errors we see in manuscripts submitted to *JMCP*. Steps to determine if a study has a unit of analysis problem and, if it does, to address the issue appropriately, are described below.

First, determine if you have a problem. Think of your analysis in terms of its research question (talk this question through with a knowledgeable friend or colleague if you are unsure).

- What is the team's batting average, defined as the number of hits as a proportion *of* at bats?
- What is the average share *of* total cost that is paid by patients?

The "of" variable is a good clue about the unit of analysis—team at bats in the first example, total dollars in the second. *If the format of your data does not match your unit of analysis—for example, if you have individual player data when you want a team batting average, or patient-level data when you want to know share of dollars paid by patients overall, simple per unit calculations using your data in its present format, such as a simple average, may produce distorted results.*

In considering this question, give preference to methods that are standard for your area of study. For example, A1c is a percentage measure—the proportion of glucose that is bound to hemoglobin in red blood cells. In a study of patients with diabetes, calculating a simple per patient mean of the A1c percentage is common and acceptable, because A1c has a specific clinical meaning.[34] However, if you want to analyze health care costs and have patient-level data, it is important to be aware that PMPM cost calculations are the "coin of the realm" in the health insurance industry. If you are conducting a project for health care executives, you should present cost analyses in PMPM form, using the standard PMPM definition, total dollars divided by total months, with both values summed across the entire sample. (Note that the weighting method described below will permit you to calculate the mathematical equivalent of a PMPM using the data that you already have.)

Second, verify your initial impressions. If you are not sure whether you have an important unit of analysis discrepancy, run study results using more than one method. If the answers are different, think about why they are different and whether the difference is important for your research question. For example, in a study of total drug costs for 548 health plans, Liberman and Roebuck (2010) calculated *both* the member cost share as a percentage of total dollars (i.e., dollars spent by members divided by total dollars spent, with both figures summed across all members in all 548 plans) *and* mean per plan member cost-sharing percentage (i.e., a simple average of member cost-sharing percentages, in which the numerator was the sum of the member cost-sharing percentages for the 548 plans and the denominator was 548).[35] Notably, the percentage of total dollars was approximately 1 percentage point lower than the simple average of the percentage shares, suggesting that health plans with greater total drug expenditures, which were underweighted using the simple averaging method, had lower member cost-sharing requirements.

Third, consider the kind of output that you need. If you determine that you have a unit of analysis discrepancy but do not need to perform statistical tests on your data, the solution is easy—just use sums that *do* represent your unit of analysis. For example, if the dataset contains data measured at the patient level, and the outcome measure is percentage of total cost paid by patients: (1) sum the total dollars paid by patients; (2) sum the total dollars paid by all sources; and then divide (1) by (2). When this approach is taken, "bootstrapping" (repeated sampling from the same dataset used to simulate a sampling distribution) can be used to generate confidence intervals and/or standard deviations for study reports.[36]

However, in many studies, a measure of statistical significance using the original unit of analysis (e.g., health plan members) is needed. Researchers need a way to use the data that they have but produce results equivalent to the summed method. The solution is to calculate and apply a set of weights to the data.[37]

Fourth, if needed, calculate weights. The basic logic underlying the calculation of weights to address unit of analysis discrepancies is to think of the dataset as displaying "disproportionate stratification," a term used in sampling theory.[38] In disproportionate stratification, study subjects in different groups have unequal probabilities of selection into the sample (e.g., the researcher samples 1% of patients who took Drug A and 10% of patients who took Drug B). Thus, a study subject in one group ("stratum") of the sample represents a different number of people than does a study subject in another group.

To account for stratified samples, each case is weighted by the reciprocal (multiplicative inverse) of its selection probability—that is, n people in the sample represent N people in the population, the selection probability is $n \div N$, and the resulting weight is a function of $1 \div (n \div N)$, which simplifies to $N \div n$.[38,39] For example, if 500 users of Drug A in the sample represent 50,000 users of Drug A in the health plan, the selection probability is 1% and the reciprocal is 100 for all members of the Drug A stratum. (In practice, each weight is often multiplied by a constant to avoid inflating sample size, for reasons explained below.) If we treat the cost analysis situation as a stratified sampling problem, a single unit (n=1 person) represents a variable number of months of care, dollars, or whatever the unit of analysis is (u). Because n=1, $u \div n = u$; thus, the weight simplifies to u—the number of months of follow-up in the PMPM cost example or total dollars in the percentage cost example.

How to apply this weight depends on the statistical package. Returning to the example shown in Table 5B, calculating a simple average of the monthly costs per patient produced an inflated cost result, $3,063. As shown in the SPSS output below, weighting each health plan member by his or her number of enrollment months produces the correct result of $752

PMPM (i.e., the answer equivalent to summed cost ÷ summed months) but inflates the sample size and distorts the results of statistical tests because the "inflationary weights fool SPSS," as SPSS documentation describes it.[37] In other words, because of the weighting, SPSS "thinks" that the sample size is 44, the total number of months for all members in the sample.

COMPUTE monthly_cost=cost/months.
WEIGHT BY months.
FREQ monthly_cost/format=notable/statistics=mean.

Statistics
monthly cost

N	Valid	44
	Missing	0
Mean		752.3

To avoid this inflation, each weight (number of months) may be multiplied by a constant, N÷U, where N is the sample size and U=$\sum u$, the total number of units of analysis (enrollment months in this example), or 5÷44 = 0.1136. The result is shown in Table 5C:

Table 5C
Monthly Cost Calculation Example and Weights

Member	Months Enrolled	Total Cost	Monthly Cost	Constant	Weight (Months × Constant)
A	12	$600	$50	0.1136	1.36
B	8	$700	$88	0.1136	0.91
C	10	$1,500	$150	0.1136	1.14
D	12	$300	$25	0.1136	1.36
E	2	$30,000	$15,000	0.1136	0.23
Totals	44	$33,100			
Simple per member average of monthly costs			$3,063		
Actual cost PMPM (total cost ÷ total months)			$752		

PMPM=per member per month.

Applying the new weight yields the following result:

COMPUTE adj_weight=months*(5/44).
WEIGHT by adj_weight.
FREQ monthly_cost/format=notable/statistics=mean.

Statistics
monthly_cost

N	Valid	5
	Missing	0
Mean		752.3

Thus, use of the new weight produces the correct PMPM, this time with the correct sample n. This calculation is actually more straightforward than it may seem because $u \times (N \div U) = (u \div U) \times N$. In other words, the weight for a case equals its percentage share of the total units of analysis for the sample ($u \div U$, e.g., $12 \div 44$ for Member A above), multiplied by the constant N (the sample size), or $12 \div 44 \times 5 = 1.36$ for Member A.

Because the method of "invoking" (using) weights depends on the statistical package, and as a general check for error, it is a good idea to calculate one or two results using *both* the summed method *and* the weighted method. The results should be equal using both methods, and the total number of cases should remain the same after weighting. If either of these two conditions is not met, the weights or statistical program should be rechecked.

Finally, whatever method you use should be explained specifically in your research report (with citations to references documenting the method, of course) for two reasons. **First**, as will be discussed in more detail in Chapter 10, good research-reporting practices require that mathematical methods be transparent. **Second**, in a pool of three or four reviewers, chances are good that at least one will notice and question any unusual methodology, and it is better strategically to address those questions "up front" rather than "playing catch up" later on in the process.

#4: Percentages Calculated Incorrectly

It is perhaps surprising that erroneously calculated or improperly presented percentages are by far the most common mistakes we see in manuscripts submitted to *JMCP*. Generally, the mistakes fall into one of three categories: (1) simple math errors, including rounding mistakes; (2) use of the wrong denominator; and (3) denominator-text mismatch, meaning that the denominator is correct but does not match to the description in the text.

The effects of problems (1) and (3) can range from mild to severe. At the "mild" end of the spectrum, editors get cranky about having to correct numerous math errors, and we generally prefer papers that are completely "clean" and therefore easier to copy-edit and produce. More serious problems can arise for an author when a peer reviewer interprets mathematical errors as a sign that the author lacks skill and rejects the paper on that basis. This does not happen often (and never happens for just one or two mistakes), but it does happen, and you do not want it to happen to you.

Avoiding Errors in Calculating and Presenting Percentages

Avoiding problem (1) is simple. If you are not using a statistical package (e.g., SPSS, SAS, SYSTAT) to obtain the output that will be used in the study report, enter the numerator and denominator for *every* percentage into a spreadsheet package (e.g., Microsoft Excel). Although it is tempting to calculate percentages manually on a calculator "to save time," this method is error-prone. If you plan to submit your paper to a journal, check the journal's style (e.g., online instructions or a sample article) to identify its preferred reporting method. For example, *JMCP* uses the format XX.X% (one decimal). Then, use the statistical package or spreadsheet to calculate your percentages using that format, so that you do not have to perform rounding by hand. Of course, it should be assumed that your calculations will be checked by an internal peer reviewer as part of the work product review (Chapter 2).

To avoid problems (2) and (3), the key is to use the *purpose* of the calculation as the indicator of which denominator to use and of the denominator "key word," which indicates

> ## Key Points: Unit of Analysis Discrepancy
>
> ❖ Will distort results if there is a systematic relationship between the outcome measure (e.g., health care cost, share of drug cost) and unit of analysis (e.g., number of months of follow-up, total drug cost).
>
> ❖ If unsure whether there is a unit of analysis problem, test outcome using summed values (e.g., a true PMPM, total sample costs divided by total sample months) versus simple averaging (e.g., per member average of monthly cost).
>
> ❖ If necessary, weight calculations using options in your statistical package.
>
> ❖ Explain the method clearly in your study report.

Table 5D
Identifying the Correct Denominator and Using Denominator "Key Words"

Purpose #1: Predictor or causal—you hypothesize that factor X (predictor or independent variable) predicts or causes outcome Y (predicted or dependent variable).
Example A: You believe that age is a predictor of attitudes toward Jane Smith, a political candidate who is running against Joe Jones.
Example B: You believe that age is a predictor of whether a patient will discontinue use of Drug A before 30 days of use.
Denominator groups: The predictor (independent) variable groups
Denominator key word: "of"
Calculation method: For each category of the independent variable, calculate $C_o \div C$, where C_o is the total number in the category with the outcome of interest and C is the total number in the category.
Calculation method example A: For each age group, divide the total number of Smith supporters in that age group by the total number of people in that age group.
Calculation method example B: For each age group, divide the total number in that age group who discontinued their medication by the total number of people in that age group.
Example A using denominator key word: Of likely voters aged 55 years or older, 57% expressed support for Jane Smith. In contrast, only 25% **of** those aged 34 years or younger and 35% **of** those aged 35 to 54 years said that Smith would be their choice.
Example B using denominator key word: Only 10% **of** patients aged 34 years or younger, compared with 20% **of** patients aged 35 to 54 years and 30% **of** patients aged 55 years or older, discontinued Drug A before 30 days.
Purpose #2: Profiling—you want to describe a group.
Example of purpose A: You are writing an article about the candidacies of Jane Smith and Joe Jones and are creating a data table to show characteristics of each candidate's supporters.
Example of purpose B: You are writing an article about factors predicting medication adherence and are creating the first table in the article, a quantitative description of the study sample. The sample includes two cohorts (subgroups): users of antidepressant drugs and users of antihypertensive drugs.
Denominator groups: The groups that are being profiled
Denominator key word: "of"
Calculation method: For each group being profiled, calculate $O_c \div O$, where O_c is the total number in the group with the characteristic of interest and O is the total number in the group.
Calculation method example A: Divide the total number of Smith supporters aged 55 years or older by the total number of Smith supporters, the total number of Smith supporters aged 35 to 54 years by the total number of Smith supporters, etc., for all age groups. Repeat for Jones supporters.
Calculation method example B: Divide the total number of antidepressant users aged 55 years or older by the total number of antidepressant users, the total number of antidepressant users aged 35 to 54 years by the total number of antidepressant users, etc., for all age groups. Repeat for antihypertensive users.

Table 5D (continued)
Identifying the Correct Denominator and Using Denominator "Key Words"

Example A using denominator key word: This congressional district encompasses Tangerine City, a retirement community that requires homeowners to be older than 54 years of age. Thus, 83% **of** all Smith supporters, 63% **of** all Jones supporters, and 73% **of** survey participants overall were aged 55 years or older. Just 9% **of** the sample overall was younger than age 35 years.
Example B using denominator key word: As expected, antidepressant drug users were younger than patients using antihypertensive drugs. Only 25% **of** antidepressant drug users, compared with 60% **of** antihypertensive drug users, were older than 54 years of age.
Purpose #3: Comparing two groups—you want to compare one group with another group.
Example of purpose: You are comparing patients in Hospital A, which has an intense educational program for patients with heart disease, with patients in Hospital B, which has no educational program.
Denominator group: Depends on the context, but usually is the comparison group—that is, the group to which your group of interest is being compared.
Denominator key words: "than" or "compared with"
Calculation method using comparison group as a denominator: Calculate $(I-C) \div C$, where I is the outcome for the intervention group and C is the outcome for the comparison group.
Calculation method example: Calculate the result for Hospital A (intervention, has program) minus the result for Hospital B (comparison, no program). Then divide that number by the result for Hospital B.
Examples using denominator key word "than": Patients in Hospital A experienced a survival rate of 95%, that is, 18.8% higher **than** the 80% survival rate in Hospital B.
Example using denominator key word "compared with": **Compared with** the 80% survival rate for Hospital B's patients, the survival rate for Hospital A's patients was 18.8% higher at 95%.
Alternative example using the intervention group as the denominator: For patients in Hospital B, which did not use the educational program, the rate of survival was 80%, 15.8% lower **than** the 95% survival rate for Hospital A.[a]
Purpose #4: Comparing two time periods—you want to assess change over time.
Example of purpose: Because of medical advances, treatment of Disease X improved greatly from 2000 to 2009, resulting in fewer disease exacerbations requiring inpatient care. You are using national hospitalization data to assess the proportion of U.S. citizens hospitalized for Disease X in 2000 versus 2009. The population of the United States was 281,421,906 in 2000 and 307,006,550 in 2009. For 2000 and 2009, respectively, the rates of Disease X hospitalizations per 1,000 population were 8.88 (0.89%) and 7.79 (0.78%).
Denominator: Depends on the context, but usually is the *earlier* time period.
Denominator key words: "from" or "compared with"
Calculation method: Calculate $(L-E) \div E$, where L is the rate for the later time period and E is the rate for the earlier time period.
Calculation method example: $(7.79 - 8.88) \div 8.88 = -12.3\%$, or a 12.3% decline.
Example using denominator key word "from": In 2000, 2,498,309 adults were hospitalized for Disease X. **From** 2000 to 2009, that number declined to 2,392,875. Measured as hospitalization rate per 1,000 population, the decline **from** 2000 to 2009 was a remarkable 12.3%, that is, a rate of 8.88 in 2000 versus 7.79 in 2009.

[a] Note that because the denominator changed from Hospital B's rate of 80% to Hospital A's rate of 95%, the percentage difference changed. Hospital A's survival rate is 18.8% higher than Hospital B's, but Hospital B's survival rate is 15.8% lower than Hospital A's.

how the calculation will be described in the text. The **four most common purposes** for calculating percentages are:

1. *Predictor or causal*—you hypothesize that factor X (a predictor or *independent variable*) predicts or causes outcome Y (a predicted or *dependent variable*).
2. *Profiling*—you want to describe a group.
3. *Comparing groups*—you want to compare one group with another group.
4. *Comparing time periods*—you want to measure change over time.

> ### Key Points: Avoiding Percentage Calculation Errors
>
> ❖ Use statistical or spreadsheet software to calculate percentages—avoid calculating manually.
> ❖ Calculations and text should be checked as part of internal work product review (Chapter 2).
> ❖ Use the purpose of the calculation to guide the selection of the denominator and the denominator key word.

Methods and denominator key words for each of these calculations are shown in Table 5D.

#5: Extended "Fishing" Trips: Cumulative Type 1 Error

In an entertaining 2006 commentary on the approaches to statistical analysis that have become unfortunately common among clinicians-turned-researchers, Andrew Vickers described a conversation that he overheard between a statistician and a surgeon:[40]

> Statistician: "Oh, so you have already calculated the P value?"
> Surgeon: "Yes, I used multinomial logistic regression."
> Statistician: "Really? How did you come up with that?"
> Surgeon: "Well, I tried each analysis on the SPSS drop-down menus, and that was the one that gave the smallest P value."

In a later commentary, Vickers described a similar phenomenon, "waterboarding and Wilcoxon," that is, torturing a data set until it confesses to anything.[2] Like Vickers, most research analysts and methodologists have at least one story of a research study in which they were asked by a supervisor or principal investigator who did not like or agree with the initial study results to repeat the analyses using new methods—"fishing" for answers—until the desired results were obtained.[41] Decision makers can, and sometimes do, ask for changes in primary endpoint outcomes, duration of follow-up observation, sample selection criteria, statistical adjustment methods, or in Vickers' words recalling one of these incidents, "probably some other stuff that I have forgotten, but by now I am so depressed living through it again that I don't even want to look at our 20-page project file detailing every new analysis that was requested."[2]

In retrospective analyses of administrative data sources, such as health care claims, national survey data, or educational testing data, the opportunities for repeating analyses are even greater because the data are easily accessible. In health care studies, one might retrospectively revise the sample identification period, the number of diagnoses or drug claims used to indicate a medical condition, the "washout" time to identify new users, or type of diagnosis (e.g., primary, secondary, etc.), to name just a few options.[41] A variation on this theme is the use of multiple analyses of study subgroups (e.g., men and women, older and younger, patients with certain comorbidities versus those without)—sometimes planned *a priori*, sometimes performed after initially planned analyses do not produce the desired result.[42]

It is important to note that there *are* times when one legitimately has no choice but to change an *a priori* analytic protocol. In a 2010 commentary, Vickers described the situation in which he found himself when he wrote a statistical analysis plan for a study of what he thought would be three endpoint outcomes. After completion of the trial, he discovered that there are a number of different ways of measuring each outcome and "the laboratory had done them all. As a result, I had to develop a different way of analyzing data on the fly, without reference to the protocol."[43]

I encountered a similar situation as principal investigator of a study assessing the relationship between use of a new injectable therapy and disease outcomes. In my initial analyses of health care claims data, I realized that use prevalence for the therapy was much lower than expected given known clinical prevalence of the disorder. Investigation revealed that because the therapy was new during my study period, insurance companies used makeshift coding methods while awaiting the promulgation of a billing code. I researched billing memoranda from numerous health plans to providers, redid the analyses using the new and expanded coding list, and completed the study.

Whether legitimate or illegitimate, *post hoc* changes to study protocols and subgroup analyses subject a research study to a common threat to validity, "cumulative type I error." To understand this problem, recall that a statistically significant result is one that is unlikely to be attributable to sampling error (chance) alone. In a *single* statistical test with an alpha (*P* value threshold) set to the typical value of 0.05, the probability of type I or "false positive" error—that is, concluding that there is an effect when actually the result was attributable to chance—is 5%. However, as the number of statistical tests increases, the *cumulative* probability of obtaining at least one false positive result increases. The formula for calculating the cumulative type I error probability in K trials is $CP=1-(1-a)^K$, where CP=the cumulative type I error probability and a=the alpha (usually 0.05).[17] For example, after ten trials with alpha=0.05, the cumulative probability that at least one of the ten trials will produce a false positive answer is 40%. Double the number of trials to 20, and the cumulative type I error probability jumps to a whopping 64%.

Avoiding or Mitigating the Effects of Cumulative Type I Error: Don't "Go Fish"

First, if you followed the guidance in Chapter 4, you have established an *a priori* analysis plan, including subgroups of interest (e.g., men versus women, high-risk versus low-risk) in the planning stages of a research study. You have also had an initial planning meeting at which your information users had the opportunity to provide input into the plan. There is no substitute for obtaining this type of input early in the project to help reduce the likelihood of "what if we did it this way instead of that way" questions later on.

Second, when beginning an analysis, include a data exploration phase, in which you run a few basic frequencies and crosstabulations to determine if the data appear to be reasonable. (The data exploration phase of a research project is discussed in more detail in Chapter 7.) For example, if the estimated prevalence of the disease state being studied is 10%, and in a dataset of 1 million people you identify only 2,000 cases (i.e., prevalence of 0.2%), you have identified a problem that should be addressed *before running any analyses of the study outcome according to the a priori plan.* Performing this step in a systematic way before beginning analyses of the study research questions will help you (and supervisors or other members of the research team) avoid the temptation to stop analyzing the data when the desired result is reached (e.g., we like the answer with the subset of 2,000 cases; why look for the missing 98,000). Additionally, establishing that the dataset is reasonable *before* analyzing the data will help prevent "fishing expeditions" later on. In other words, in an ideal scenario, you will reach agreement that the data are reasonable, then move on to analyze the data, and the answer to the research question is whatever it is.

Third, if it is necessary to run a number of *a priori* or *post hoc* analyses, an adjustment to the *P* value threshold is recommended.[17,42] A commonly used approach is the "Bonferroni correction," in which the threshold is adjusted to a÷K (the single-test alpha divided by the number of tests performed).[17,44] For example, if ten tests are performed, the adjusted alpha is 0.05÷10=0.005, and the cumulative type 1 error probability is 4.9%, approximately equal to that of the typical 0.05 threshold.[17] The Bonferroni correction has been criticized because it reduces statistical power (the probability of rejecting the null hypothesis when the null hypothesis is false); it has been suggested that

> **Key Points: Cumulative Type 1 Error**
>
> ❖ Increases with number of statistical tests performed.
> ❖ Formula in K trials is $1-(1-a)^K$.
> ❖ Avoid by having an *a priori* analysis plan and using data exploration.
> ❖ Consider *P* value adjustment for multiple trials.
> ❖ Describe number of analyses and changes to *a priori* plan transparently in study report.

researchers should instead use standardized effect size calculations, such as the Cohen's d statistic, or focus primarily on practical significance rather than statistical significance.[44] However, when analyzing datasets containing tens of thousands of cases, a typical scenario today, power is not as much of a concern as is type 1 error.

Fourth, no matter how the data are analyzed, be transparent in describing procedures in the research report. State how many analyses were performed, which were *a priori* and which *post hoc*, and describe any changes to the *a priori* analysis plan that were made and the reasons for making them.[45] As the examples in Chapter 3 illustrated, no study is perfect; the key is to describe procedures clearly so that readers can understand the study's potential imperfections when they interpret its findings.

Finally, take the problem of cumulative type 1 error seriously. Thoughtful observers have noted that ignoring type 1 error in medical research has led to erroneous findings or even to suboptimal patient care.[17,42] High-speed computing capability certainly enables researchers to repeat analyses, sometimes over and over, until a desired outcome is reached. But the fact that a researcher *can* "go fish" does not make it right. Fishing expeditions produce bad information, and to disseminate "fishy" information that is "caught" knowingly, without making appropriate *P* value adjustments or other changes to interpretation, is unethical.

Summing Up: What Have We Learned?

The five shortcomings described in this chapter, although mathematically distinct, share a few common solutions. Be *aware* of phenomena that affect your work, like RTM and cumulative type 1 error. Be *systematic* in checking and analyzing data. And be *careful* about accuracy, using the tools described both here and in Chapter 2.

In Chapter 6, we focus on the use of multivariate and decision analytic modeling in common health care research applications, continuing to emphasize that most errors are caused by simple and basic, rather than complicated and nuanced, problems. If you have ever thought—or been taught—that complex statistical methods obviate the need for good basic design or attention to practical and clinical significance, read on.

Helpful Resources

- Booth, Colomb, and Williams. *The Craft of Research*. Chapters 8 ("Making Claims"), 9 ("Assembling Reasons and Evidence"), and 15 ("Communicating Evidence Visually").[46]
- Miller. *The Chicago Guide to Writing about Numbers*. This entire book is an invaluable resource to which the editors of *JMCP* frequently refer authors. See especially Chapters 2 ("Seven Basic Principles"), 3 ("Causality, Statistical Significance, and Substantive Significance"), 4 ("Technical but Important: Five More Basic Principles"), 6 ("Creating Effective Tables"), and 7 ("Creating Effective Charts").[24]
- Maletta's tutorial on sample weighting is an easily understood and informative guide to the rationale, calculation, and application of this helpful tool.[37]
- Kalton. *Introduction to Survey Sampling*. The discussion of weighting in this chapter is intended to address only the simplest and most frequently encountered weighting problems. More complicated weighting problems and mathematical considerations are addressed in Kalton's book.[38]

References

1. Quotations by Stanley Gudder. Available at: http://strangewondrous.net/browse/author/g/gudder+stanley.

2. Vickers AJ. Waterboarding and Wilcoxon: what medical researchers might learn about statistics from the CIA. February 18, 2009. Available at: http://www.medscape.com/viewarticle/588146.

3. Yee D. Obesity deaths inflated by math error. *Associated Press.* November 24, 2004. Available at: http://seattletimes.nwsource.com/html/nationworld/2002099269_obese24.html.

4. Mars Climate Orbiter fact sheet. Available at: http://science.ksc.nasa.gov/mars/msp98/orbiter/fact.html.

5. Mars Climate Orbiter: mission overview. Available at: http://science.ksc.nasa.gov/mars/msp98/orbiter/mission.html.

6. No authors listed. Metric mishap caused loss of NASA orbiter. September 30, 1999. Available at: http://articles.cnn.com/1999-09-30/tech/9909_30_mars.metric.02_1_climate-orbiter-spacecraft-team-metric-system?_s=PM:TECH.

7. Krug EG, Kresnow MJ, Peddicord JP, et al. Retraction: suicide after natural disasters. *N Engl J Med.* 1999;340(2):148-49. Available at: http://www.nejm.org/doi/pdf/10.1056/NEJM199901143400213.

8. Domurat ES. Diabetes managed care and clinical outcomes: The Harbor City, California Kaiser Permanente diabetes care system. *Am J Manag Care.* 1999;5(10):1299-307.

9. Linden A. Estimating the effect of regression to the mean in health management programs. *Dis Manage Health Outcomes.* 2007;15(1):7-12.

10. Barnett AG, van der Pols JC, Dobson AJ. Regression to the mean: what it is and how to deal with it. *Int J Epidemiol.* 2005;34(1):215-20. Available at: http://ije.oxfordjournals.org/content/34/1/215.full.pdf+html.

11. Vickers AJ. Regression to the Mike: a statistical explanation of why an eligible friend of mine is still single (and some implications for medical research). August 7, 2007. Available at: http://www.medscape.com/viewarticle/560205.

12. Smith G, Smith J. Regression to the mean in average test scores. *Educational Assessment.* 2005;10(4):377-99. Available at: http://economics-files.pomona.edu/GarySmith/aveTestScores.pdf.

13. Rich MW, Beckham V, Wittenberg C, Leven CL, Freedland KE, Carney RM. A multidisciplinary intervention to prevent the readmission of elderly patients with

congestive heart failure. *N Engl J Med.* 1995;333(18):1190-95. Available at: http://www.nejm.org/doi/pdf/10.1056/NEJM199511023331806.

14. Trochim WMK. The regression-discontinuity design. *Research Methods Knowledge Base.* 2006. Available at: http://www.socialresearchmethods.net/kb/quasird.htm and http://www.socialresearchmethods.net/kb/statrd.php.

15. GSS General Social Survey. Available at: http://www.norc.org/GSS+Website/.

16. Centers for Medicare & Medicaid Services. State drug utilization data. Available at http://www.cms.gov/MedicaidDrugRebateProgram/SDUD/list.asp.

17. Kaul S, Diamond GA. Trial and error. How to avoid commonly encountered limitations of published clinical trials. *J Am Coll Cardiol.* 2010;55(5):415-27.

18. Chernew ME, Shah MR, Wegh A, et al. Impact of decreasing copayments on medication adherence within a disease management environment. *Health Aff (Millwood).* 2008;27(1):103-12.

19. University of Michigan Health System, Department of Public Relations and Marketing Communications. The co-pay connection: lowering drug co-pays for chronic disease patients increases use of important preventive medicines, rigorous study shows. January 8, 2008. Available at: http://www.med.umich.edu/opm/newspage/2008/drugcopay.htm.

20. Reuters. New study indicates decreasing prescription copayments results in increased adherence for patients with chronic diseases. *Reuters.* January 8, 2008.

21. Fairman KA, Curtiss FR. Making the world safe for evidence-based policy: let's slay the biases in research on value-based insurance design. *J Manag Care Pharm.* 2008;14(2):198-202. Available at: http://www.amcp.org/data/jmcp/JMCPMaga_March%2008_198-204.pdf.

22. Fairman KA, Curtiss FR. What do we really know about VBID? Quality of the evidence and ethical considerations for plan sponsors. *J Manag Care Pharm.* 2011;17(2):156-74. Available at: http://www.amcp.org/data/jmcp/156-174.pdf.

23. Griffee DT. Research in practice: understanding significance testing program evaluation. *Journal of Developmental Education.* 2004;27(3):28-34.

24. Miller JE. *The Chicago Guide to Writing about Numbers.* Chicago, IL: University of Chicago Press; 2004:quotation p. 49.

25. Lenth RV. Some practical guidelines for effective sample-size determination. March 1, 2001. Available at: http://www.stat.uiowa.edu/techrep/tr303.pdf.

26. Stockl KM, Shin JS, Lew HC, et al. Outcomes of a rheumatoid arthritis disease therapy management program focusing on medication adherence. *J Manag Care Pharm.*

2010;16(8):593-604. Available at: http://www.amcp.org/data/jmcp/593-604.pdf. For another good example of this approach, see Flynn KE, Lin L, Ellis SJ, et al. Outcomes, health policy, and managed care: relationships between patient-reported outcome measures and clinical measures in outpatients with heart failure. *Am Heart J.* 2009;158(4 Suppl):S64-71.

27. Biography.com. Joe DiMaggio biography. Available at: http://www.biography.com/articles/Joe-DiMaggio-9274899.

28. Stan Musial quotes. Available at: http://www.baseball-almanac.com/quotes/quomusl.shtml.

29. Whitley D. Pure hitter: Ted Williams. Available at: http://espn.go.com/classic/000706tedwilliams.html.

30. Kaiser Family Foundation. Prescription drug trends. May 2010. Available at: http://www.kff.org/rxdrugs/upload/3057-08.pdf.

31. All drug prices were obtained from a health plan pricing tool that reflects the actual average cost of the medication. Available at: http://www.regencerx.com/learn/rxPriceGuide/index.html.

32. Hanchate A, Kronman AC, Young-Xu Y, Ash AS, Emanuel E. Racial and ethnic differences in end-of-life costs: why do minorities cost more than whites? *Arch Intern Med.* 2009;169(5):493-501.

33. Laliberté F, Bookhart BK, Vekeman F, et al. Direct all-cause health care costs associated with chronic kidney disease in patients with diabetes and hypertension: a managed care perspective. *J Manag Care Pharm.* 2009;15(4):312-22. Available at: http://www.amcp.org/data/jmcp/312-322.pdf.

34. See for example, Gilmer TP, O'Connor PJ, Rush WA, et al. Predictors of health care costs in adults with diabetes. *Diabetes Care.* 2005;28(1):59-64. Gilmer et al. calculated a mean HbA1c at baseline (study start date) for adult patients with diabetes and followed them for the subsequent 3 years to measure the relationship between baseline HbA1c and total subsequent health care costs.

35. Liberman JN, Roebuck MC. Prescription drug costs and the generic dispensing ratio. *J Manag Care Pharm.* 2010;16(7):502-06. Available at: http://www.amcp.org/data/jmcp/502-506.pdf.

36. See, for example:
   - McAdam-Marx C, McGarry LJ, Hane CA, Biskupiak J, Deniz B, Brixner DI. All-cause and incremental per patient per year cost associated with chronic hepatitis

C virus and associated liver complications in the United States: a managed care perspective. *J Manag Care Pharm.* 2011;17(7):531-46. Available at: http://www.amcp.org/WorkArea/DownloadAsset.aspx?id=10710.

- Campbell, Torgerson DJ. Bootstrapping: estimating confidence intervals for cost-effectiveness ratios. *QJM.* 1999;92(3):177-82.

37. Maletta H. Weighting. March 12, 2007. Available at: http://www.spsstools.net/Tutorials/WEIGHTING.pdf: 2,10.

38. Kalton G. *Introduction to Survey Sampling.* Thousand Oaks, CA: Sage Publications; 1983.

39. Wooldridge JM. *Econometric Analysis of Cross Section and Panel Data.* Cambridge, MA: The MIT Press; 2002:593.

40. Vickers AJ. Shoot first and ask questions later: how to approach statistics like a real clinician. July 26, 2006. Available at: http://www.medscape.com/viewarticle/540898.

41. Fairman KA. Differentiating effective data mining from fishing, trapping, and cruelty to numbers. *J Manag Care Pharm.* 2007;13(6):517-27. Available at: http://www.amcp.org/data/jmcp/pages%20517-27.pdf.

42. Lagakos SW. The challenge of subgroup analyses—reporting without distorting. *N Engl J Med.* 2006;354(16):1667-69.

43. Vickers AJ. Math as mass hypnosis: on mortgage-backed securities, maritime warfare, and medical research. January 11, 2010. Available at: http://www.medscape.com/viewarticle/714772.

44. Nakagawa S. A farewell to Bonferroni: the problems of low statistical power and publication bias. *Behavioral Ecology.* 2004;15(6):1044-45. Available at: http://beheco.oxfordjournals.org/content/15/6/1044.full.pdf+html.

45. Vandenbroucke JP, von Elm E, Altman DG, et al. Strengthening the reporting of observational studies in epidemiology (STROBE): Explanation and elaboration. *Ann Intern Med.* 2007;147:W-163-W-194. Available at: http://www.annals.org/cgi/reprint/147/8/W-163.pdf.

46. Booth WC, Colomb GG, Williams JM. *The Craft of Research. Third Edition.* Chicago, IL: University of Chicago Press; 2008.

CHAPTER 6

Multivariate, Not Magical:
Six Rules of Thumb for
Advanced Statistical Analysis

"Naturally, there is a strong desire to substitute intellectual capital for labor. That is why investigators often try to base causal inference on statistical models."—Statistician David Freedman on the role of multivariate statistics in the long-standing debate over association versus causation[1]

"I do not know of a complicated model in any area of science that performs well in explanation and prediction and have challenged many audiences to give me examples. So far, I have not heard about a single one."—Arnold Zellner, econometrician and co-founder of the *Journal of Econometrics* and the International Society for Bayesian Analysis[2]

"The statistics on sanity are that one out of every four Americans is suffering from some form of mental illness. Think of your three best friends. If they're okay, then it's you."—American writer Rita Mae Brown[3]

What You Will Learn in Chapter 6

✓ Characteristics of a *sensible* data analysis, and why they are important for information users and readers

✓ How *confounding* can affect even high-quality multivariate work

✓ Why *you* (and your literature review)—*not* your statistical model—should be in charge of your analysis

✓ Why exploratory data analysis and diagnostic tools should be used *prior* to finalizing an advanced statistical analysis

✓ What we can *learn from validation* of even the best statistical model

---

A number of years ago, while working on my first large-scale health care research project, I had the opportunity to work with a highly skilled expert panel that included several clinicians, a psychologist, and an internationally known statistician. At our first meeting, I was to present our study analysis plan. Bursting with knowledge gained in my coursework on advanced multivariate statistics, I was eager to apply the "very latest" techniques to the study of our research questions. Today, I am embarrassed—and a little amused—to recall that instead of clearly connecting our research questions to the planned data analysis, one of the first sentences of my presentation was "We will first examine log-minus-log survival plots," referring to the commonly used technique to ensure compliance with a key assumption of Cox proportional hazards analysis.

The statistician listened politely as I explained my "plan," which, as I remember, involved throwing an arsenal of every multivariate method that I had learned in graduate school at the data. Finally, when I had finished, the statistician gently asked a few questions. Where was my plan to calculate and assess basic frequencies and crosstabulations? What about examining the data distributions for normality or skewness? Why was it necessary to conduct multivariate analyses? Had I considered the possibility that simple bivariate statistics, such as t tests and Pearson chi-square tests, would answer my research questions effectively without introducing unnecessary complexity into the analysis and presentation of the research findings?

Although a little embarrassed by the encounter, I learned a valuable lesson. Ultimately, although a few of our research questions *did* require use of multivariate techniques, most were more clearly presented to our audience using simple bivariate statistical analyses that most undergraduate students learn as part of any college course of study. In the years since then, I have come to understand the limitations of what I more recently dubbed "The Enchanted Forest of Statistics" analytic strategy—an answer emerges from within, but readers cannot determine how it was derived or what, exactly, it means.[4] With this understanding, I now know why that statistician—and others knowledgeable in the field—believe that the most important attribute of a data analysis is not whether it uses the *latest* techniques, but whether it uses the *most appropriate* techniques. In other words, is the analysis *sensible*?

This chapter is devoted to the art and science of being *sensible* in the use of advanced statistical analysis, including both **multivariate analysis** and **decision analytic modeling**. Because an excellent, step-by-step guide to the calculation and presentation of multivariate analysis is available in Jane Miller's reference, *The Chicago Guide to Writing about Multivariate Analysis*,[5] some of my discussion of multivariate modeling summarizes and refers to her work. I focus in this chapter on commonly used health care applications and highlight key points that often present challenges to health care researchers. I assume basic knowledge of multivariate methods but provide brief definitions of terms throughout, as well as in this book's Glossary.

What Is a "Sensible" Analysis?

A sensible analysis has several interrelated features. These are summarized in Table 6A, described briefly below, and discussed in more detail throughout this chapter.

Table 6A
"Sensible Analysis" Checklist

➢ Demonstrates a clear and logical connection between study research questions or hypotheses, analytic output, and explanation of results
➢ Reflects knowledge of basic research principles (e.g., rules of causal inference)
➢ Reflects understanding that a sophisticated technique is an often useful but never perfect substitute for a strong basic research design
➢ Describes results in quantitative terms that have practical meaning for the information user or reader
➢ Consistent with a plausible causal process
➢ Validated

First and foremost, a sensible analysis is characterized by a clear and logical connection between the study research questions, the analytic output (data tables and graphs), and the explanation of results. If a reasonably knowledgeable reader is unable to understand the rationale for the analytic method, cannot determine how the quantitative results inform the study research questions, or does not understand the findings, the analysis is probably either not clearly described or not well conceived.

Second, a sensible analysis reflects knowledge of the basic research principles that were discussed in Chapters 3 and 5, such as association versus causation, general principles of causal inference for epidemiological data, confounding, the problem of cumulative type I error, and the difference between statistical significance and practical significance. For example, repeated multivariate analyses carry a mathematically predictable risk of cumulative type I error, just as repeated bivariate analyses do.

A particularly important point is that a sensible analysis reflects a **plausible causal process**. For example, we saw in Chapter 3 that, after accounting for measured confounding factors using standard multivariate analytic techniques, Dormuth et al. (2009) found an association between adherence to statin (cholesterol-lowering) medication and reduced rates of many negative outcomes, including burns, falls, and other accidents.[6] However, as Dormuth et al. pointed out, a conclusion that increasing statin adherence would reduce accident rates would be obviously inappropriate because there is no plausible biological relationship between cholesterol levels and burns, falls, or accidents. Similarly, for A to be a plausible cause of B, A must precede B— that is, if A occurred after B, then A cannot possibly have caused B.

Third, a sensible analysis produces results in quantitative and practical terms that are meaningful to those who will use the research information. For example, it is uninformative to report only that the raw coefficient in a logistic regression analysis was 0.30. Instead, it is more informative to calculate the ***odds ratio*** (i.e., exponentiate the raw coefficient) and report that the odds were multiplied by a factor of 1.35, or increased by 35% ($e^{0.30}$=an odds ratio of 1.35).

Fourth, a sensible analysis has been validated using whatever means are available to the researcher. This validation process helps the researcher to comply with standard methodological guidance that alternative explanations for study findings, rather than just the researcher's preferred or hypothesized explanation, should be considered in interpreting study results.[5,7] A common example in health care is the association between a ***disease-specific*** independent variable and an ***all-cause*** dependent variable. In a simplified example, consider a researcher who uses a multivariate analysis to assess the relationship between voluntary participation in a disease state management (DSM) program for diabetes and all-cause hospitalizations (i.e., inpatient stays for *any* diagnosis). Say, hypothetically, that after statistical adjustment for a variety of factors, the researcher finds a predicted (adjusted) average of 50 all-cause hospitalizations in the DSM group and 100 all-cause hospitalizations in the comparison group, measured per 1,000 patients per year. However, in the DSM group, all hospitalizations were for diabetes. The comparison group had adjusted averages of 50 hospitalizations for diabetes and 50 hospitalizations for cancer. The finding of equal adjusted rates of diabetes-related hospitalizations in each group suggests that the DSM program was not responsible for the reduction in all-cause hospitalizations. Instead, the relationship might be spurious—that is, a diagnosis of cancer might have affected both the key independent variable (decision to participate in the DSM program, with patients who had cancer less likely to choose DSM participation) and the dependent variable (all-cause hospitalization).

Why Perform an Advanced Statistical Analysis?

Although this chapter assumes some coursework and/or experience with advanced statistical analysis, a brief review of typical applications is helpful to an understanding of sensible approaches. Typical applications are summarized in Table 6B, and detailed descriptions and examples are provided following the table.

Table 6B
Summary of Common Applications for Advanced Statistical Techniques in Health Care Research

Technique	Example(s) of Uses in Health Care
Ordinary least squares multiple regression	Dependent variable is *normally distributed or* has been *log-transformed* (e.g., natural logarithm) to meet assumption of normally distributed dependent variable. Examples: • Medication possession ratio • Patient-reported scales (e.g., pain rated on a scale of 0 to 100) • Disease-related or all-cause health care costs
Logistic regression analysis (binomial)[a]	Dependent variable is a *binary or dichotomous event*, and measuring time-to-event is *not* important. Examples: • Occurrence of an ER visit for a drug side effect at least once during the first month of treatment • Occurrence of a hospitalization at least once during a one-year follow-up in a study designed to explain annual health care utilization and cost • Receipt of a particular recommended test or screening at least once annually (e.g., retinal examination in patients with diabetes)
Cox proportional hazards analysis	• Dependent variable is a *binary or dichotomous event*, and measuring time-to-event *is* important (e.g., length of progression-free survival in a patient with cancer). • Observations may be *censored* (i.e., the study period for some subjects ends prior to observation of the outcome event). • Especially helpful when one or more independent variables are *time-dependent* (e.g., cumulative effect of compliance with osteoporosis medication on incidence of fractures).[b]
Generalized estimating equations that assume pre-specified exponential distributions	Dependent variable: • Is an outcome with a non-normal distribution, especially when "retransformation" of coefficients is desired so that the information user can easily see the effect of the independent variable in practical terms (e.g., "each additional day was associated with an additional average cost of $100") • May consist of repeated measures on the same subject Model specification depends on purpose; commonly: • Gamma distribution with log link for cost data[c] • Poisson distribution for count data (e.g., counts of hospitalizations or ER visits) that are not "overdispersed"[d] • Negative binomial regression for count data that are "overdispersed"[d]
Time series analysis; interrupted time series analysis	• Compares a *pre-intervention* or pre-change period with a *post-intervention* or post-change period. • Assesses change in *trend* over time, as well as change in *level* (i.e., immediate change in trend line at the point of the intervention). • Often used with a comparison group—that is, the analysis compares time series for a group that experienced the intervention or change versus time series for a group that experienced no intervention or change. • Commonly adjusted for *seasonality* if applicable (e.g., outcome is use of medications for asthma or allergies).

Table 6B (continued)
Summary of Common Applications for Advanced Statistical Techniques in Health Care Research

Technique	Example(s) of Uses in Health Care
Decision analytic modeling; pharmacoeconomic modeling	Dependent variable is *not directly measurable* because it has not yet occurred, for example: • Anticipated effects of recently approved drugs or treatments on future health outcomes • Anticipated effects of a change in treatment algorithm on total health care expenditure (budgetary impact analysis)
Propensity scoring—the calculation of an algorithm to predict the propensity (likelihood) of membership in the study group of interest, based on a logistic regression analysis in which group membership is the dependent variable	• Often used in nonrandomized studies that are "confounded by indication" (e.g., health status affects *both* the likelihood of getting the treatment of interest *and* the study outcomes). • Score can be used for matching, sample stratification, or as a single covariate in a multivariate equation. • Does *not* adjust for unmeasured confounders.
Instrumental variable analysis—the use of an "instrument" (a carefully selected covariate) intended to adjust for *unmeasured* confounders	• Commonly used to adjust for confounding by indication • Feasible only when an instrumental variable can be identified that has (1) no systematic relationship with *measured or unmeasured* confounders; (2) a strong systematic relationship with the treatment or independent variable of interest (exposure); and (3) no association with the outcome except through the exposure (i.e., no direct effect on the outcome).
Bootstrapping—the selection of multiple "samples" from within a sample; intended to represent a sampling distribution	• Estimating confidence intervals and/or standard deviation when data are non-normally distributed or in any situation in which direct measurement of variance is infeasible. • Relies on the assumption that the sample adequately represents the population (e.g., bootstrapping a sample of families with annual incomes of >$100,000 does not produce a sampling distribution that represents families with annual incomes <$30,000).

[a] Multinomial logistic regression analysis is also available for dependent variables with more than two levels (e.g., no hospital utilization, ER visit only, inpatient hospital stay).

[b] See, for example, an analysis of the relationship between bisphosphonate adherence and fracture risk, with a time-dependent measure of bisphosphonate adherence as the key predictor, reported by Halpern et al. (2011).[8]

[c] The choice of the link function depends both on the distribution of the dependent variable and on how the researcher wants to interpret the coefficients; log link is commonly used for cost data, with results expressed as the average dollar amount of change associated with a one-unit change in the independent variable.[9]

[d] The definition of overdispersion is that the variance exceeds the mean. The choice between Poisson and negative binomial regression can often be made based on goodness-of-fit testing.[9]

Sources:
Ballinger. Using generalized estimating equations for longitudinal data analysis.[9]
Bosco et al. A most stubborn bias.[10]
Campbell and Torgerson. Bootstrapping: estimating confidence intervals for cost-effectiveness ratios.[11]
Dunteman and Ho. *An Introduction to Generalized Linear Models.*[12]
Glynn and Schneeweiss. Indications for propensity scores.[13]
Pedhazur. *Multiple Regression in Behavioral Research.*[14]
Wooldridge JM. *Introductory Econometrics.*[15]
ER = emergency room.

Most commonly, multivariate analysis is used in health care research to correct for **confounding**, the association of one or more factors known to affect health care outcomes—such as age, gender, and common comorbidities (e.g., hypertension, diabetes)—with *both* the **exposure** (the treatment or intervention of interest) and the outcome, as was discussed in detail in Chapter 3. In these circumstances, multivariate analysis is used to estimate the **marginal effect**, that is, the association of the exposure with the outcome *after* controlling for—taking into account—the effects of the confounding factors.[5]

The specific techniques used to address confounding depend primarily on three factors. **First** is the **distribution** of the dependent variable, as discussed in more detail under "technical requirements" below. For example, ordinary least squares (linear) regression is used for normally distributed dependent variables, whereas different techniques are necessary for non-normally distributed dependent variables (e.g., logistic regression for binary variables, generalized linear modeling using an assumed exponential distribution for skewed data). **Second** is whether the study design created **censoring**, the situation in which the outcomes for some subjects were not observed by the researcher because they did not occur prior to the end of the study period. For example, in a five-year study of survival time following Surgery A, subjects who died prior to the end of the five-year follow-up are *uncensored* because their outcome (death) was observed, whereas subjects who lived longer than five years after Surgery A are *censored*, meaning that their date of death was not observed. When some observations are censored, Kaplan-Meier analysis is commonly used if there is no need to control for confounders, and Cox proportional hazards regression is used when it is necessary to control for confounding factors.

The **third** factor is among the most difficult problems in health care research—the situation in which the researcher hypothesizes, based on the literature review conducted at the start of the project, that some confounding factors are not measurable. For example, assume a retrospective observational (nonrandomized) study of whether Surgery A, compared with drug treatment only, was associated with better outcomes for Disease B. In choosing whether to use Surgery A or drug treatment for a particular patient, a physician might consider (1) the patient's recent medical history (e.g., comorbidities); (2) the adequacy of the patient's social supports for the surgical recovery period (e.g., availability of adult children who get along well with the patient and are willing to engage in care activities); and (3) the patient's severity of Disease B. All three factors clearly affect both treatment choice and outcome; thus, all are confounders. As such, all would be controlled in an ideal multivariate analysis—but only the first set of confounders is measurable; the second is almost certainly not measurable; and the third might or might not be measurable, depending on the data source. As discussed in more detail later in this chapter, the presence of unmeasured confounders greatly complicates the selection of an appropriate analytic technique.[16]

Multivariate analysis is also necessary for time series and forecasting analyses, in which past trends are used either to predict future trends or to provide a quantitative assessment of the difference between trends *prior to* an intervention (e.g., a benefit design change) compared with *after* the intervention (e.g., an **interrupted time series**, sometimes including a comparison group that does not receive the intervention to make a stronger research design). Another commonly used technique is **decision analytic modeling**, which allows the researcher to forecast outcomes based on assumptions that are often complex and numerous. This technique is most appropriate when there is little "real-world" experience with an innovation, such as a new drug treatment, making it necessary to perform assessments based on hypothetical assumptions.

Finally, advanced statistical analyses are sometimes performed for nontechnical reasons. For example, a particular technique might be standard for the journal to which the researcher wants to submit an article. Similarly, a supervisor or journal peer reviewer may request that a particular analytic approach be undertaken. The topic of tailoring a data presentation to the target journal is discussed in detail in Chapter 10.

A complete presentation of the rationale and appropriate use for all advanced statistical techniques used in health care is beyond the scope of this chapter. However, regardless of specific technique, sensible application can be achieved with attention to six basic approaches, or "rules of thumb." Each of these is discussed in detail below.

> ### Key Points: Choosing a Technique to Adjust for Confounding
>
> ❖ Distribution of dependent variable.
> ❖ Censoring.
> ❖ Measurable versus unmeasurable confounding factors.

Rule of Thumb #1: The usual laws apply.

Used properly and in accordance with the specific purposes for which they were designed, advanced statistical techniques are highly effective tools—but they do not magically transform a weak design into a strong one, negate the usual principles of cause-and-effect, or alter the basic rationale of statistical significance testing. Like any good tools, sophisticated analytic tools are most effective when the user understands what they are—and are not—capable of doing. This observation should perhaps go without saying, but is nonetheless sometimes overlooked.

Association versus causation and residual confounding. In a typical example, the literature review of one research report, describing the results of a previous study, said that "doubling patient copayments [for prescription drugs] resulted in a 34 percent reduction in the use of lipid-lowering agents and a 26 percent reduction in use of antihypertensives."[17] In reality, the cited study, performed by Goldman et al. (2004), had not measured *change* in drug copayments at all. Instead, it used a **cross-sectional** design in which the unit of analysis was the person-year (e.g., a person who was included in the analysis for three years contributed three observations) and measured the *association* between copayments and utilization.[18] A two-part model was used to calculate the predicted impact of a doubling of the copayment in each drug class. First, probit regression estimated the probability of having at least one pharmacy claim in the class; then, for those with at least one claim, a generalized linear model predicted total drug spending, controlling for numerous measured factors. The results suggested large copayment effects; the authors reported that the doubling of copayments was associated with utilization declines of 25%-45% depending on the therapy class.[18]

However, previous research suggests a problem in attributing causality to the cross-sectional association between copayment and drug utilization. Studies in which the investigators *directly* measured response to price *change* (e.g., comparing a group that experienced a copayment increase with a group that experienced no increase, measuring change in utilization from pre-increase to post-increase) have suggested that prescription drug purchasing behavior displays little price sensitivity in response to typical copayment increases (i.e., approximately $10-$15) except for special populations (e.g., disabled, low-income) or drugs for which over-the-counter alternatives are available (e.g., pain or heartburn relievers).[19,20] Thus, although Goldman et al. used appropriate analytic techniques, their findings might have been affected by **residual confounding**, that is, confounding that remains after multivariate statistical adjustment, often because of factors that the authors were unable to measure and therefore unable to statistically adjust.

Examples of possible residual confounders in analyses of the association between copayment and drug utilization include employment sector and organizational culture. For example, employer groups of hotel workers and computer programmers may have different copayment structures *and* may also exhibit systematically different drug purchasing behaviors because of their occupational characteristics. Similarly, an organization with higher copayments may be likely to have other cost-saving or quality-improvement measures in place, such as an educational program that has been ongoing for a decade to encourage patients and physicians to try nonpharmacologic interventions (e.g., diet and exercise) prior to drug therapy for some chronic conditions.

Stukel et al. (2007) encountered residual confounding when they analyzed the association between the receipt of cardiac catheterization following a heart attack and long-term survival.[21] For **two reasons**, analyses of this type are often *confounded by indication*—that is, selection of the treatment is a function of factors that directly affect the outcome, making it difficult to determine the degree to which the treatment caused the outcome.[16] **First**, in order to have surgery, patients must survive until the surgery date; thus, an association between surgery and survival is nearly inevitable (and does not necessarily indicate a surgical benefit). **Second**, many of the factors taken into account in making these decisions, such as the patient's attitude toward surgery, can affect the outcome but are not easily measurable (or, in some situations, may not be measurable at all).

To assess the merits of various approaches to adjusting for confounding by indication, Stukel et al. compared the performance of four standard statistical methods. These included:

1. Cox proportional hazards regression;
2. *Propensity score* risk-adjustment, in which the propensity for (likelihood of) being treated with catheterization was calculated as a function of numerous predictor variables using logistic regression analysis, and the resulting score (in deciles) was entered as a covariate into a Cox proportional hazards regression model;
3. Propensity score matching, in which catheterized and noncatheterized patients were matched as closely as possible on the propensity score; and
4. *Instrumental variable analysis*, an econometric technique intended to remove the bias associated with unmeasured variables. In instrumental variable analysis, the researcher identifies a variable that has (a) *no* systematic relationship with measured or unmeasured confounding factors; (b) a *strong* systematic relationship with the exposure (surgery in this example); and (c) *no* association with the outcome except through the exposure (i.e., no direct effect on the outcome).[10,22]

The instrumental variable is then used as covariate in one or more multivariate equations in an attempt to adjust for the unmeasured factor(s) associated with treatment selection.[10,22] The instrumental variable used by Stukel et al. was the regional cardiac catheterization rate (i.e., a measure of geographic variation in use of cardiac catheterization).

Stukel et al. found that in contrast with the mortality benefit (i.e., reduction in mortality) measured in clinical trials—approximately 8%-21%—analyses performed using the first three statistical methods predicted a mortality benefit of about 50% from cardiac catheterization.[21] Stukel et al. pointed to residual confounding, a problem that could not be eliminated "even controlling for complete information on patients' admission severity," as the likely culprit in the inaccurate predictions. Instrumental variable analysis performed much better than did the other three statistical techniques, predicting a mortality benefit of 16%. However, the authors noted an important caveat about the instrumental variable analysis; "high cardiac catheterization rate regions had more high-volume hospitals with specialized staff and equipment, and coronary care units" that likely affected the study outcome. Thus, Stukel et al. concluded that an instrumental variable analysis based on geographic variation might be better suited to addressing regional policy questions, such as whether to invest in additional catheterization equipment, than to making predictions about treatment outcomes for individual patients.[21]

Bosco et al. (2010) faced similar challenges when they assessed breast cancer recurrence rates in women aged 65 years or older who were treated with chemotherapy versus those who did not receive chemotherapy. They compared standard multivariate regression, several propensity-score adjustment methods, and an instrumental variable analysis in which "each patient's surgeon's chronologically preceding patient's receipt of adjuvant chemotherapy" was the instrument.[10] In other words, for each patient, the treatment choice made for the surgeon's chronologically previous patient was the instrumental variable.

Like Stukel et al., Bosco et al. found that none of the methods produced results consistent with the chemotherapy benefits that had been suggested by previous research. The instrumental variable analysis suggested that chemotherapy was beneficial, but standard tests of the assumptions for instrumental variable analysis* suggested "imbalance"

---

* These included comparisons of measurable patient characteristics—including tumor size, node positivity, and histology—across levels of the instrumental variable. The rationale for these comparisons is that nonsignificant differences (i.e., "balance") in *measured* confounding factors across levels of the instrumental variable provide reassurance that *unmeasured* confounding factors are not systematically associated with the instrumental variable (i.e., a key assumption of the statistical technique).[10]

across levels of the instrumental variable, which indicated residual confounding by indication. In other words, the instrumental variable had not fully adjusted for unmeasured confounding factors. Bosco et al. concluded that although nonrandomized studies "will remain important contributions to our scientific knowledge base," these studies would "remain susceptible to confounding by indication, despite advancing methods to control this seemingly intractable bias."[10]

The results of the studies by Stukel et al. and Bosco et al. highlight the obstacles often faced by researchers who attempt to adjust for confounding, especially unmeasured (and sometimes unmeasurable) confounding. Propensity score adjustment, propensity score matching, and standard multivariate analysis adjusting for measured covariates all performed equally well (or, more accurately, equally poorly)—not a surprising result because all techniques used the same inadequate set of *measured* confounding factors.[10,21] Even instrumental variable analysis, which generally performed better than the other adjustment techniques, proved to be inadequate because of difficulties in identifying and interpreting appropriate instrumental variables—a common problem with this technique.[10,21,22]

Difficulties in controlling for intent. Even with the best multivariate analysis, it may be difficult or impossible to control for the *intent* of study subjects (or the intent of their health care providers). For example, a retrospective observational study of patients with hypertension, conducted by Hess et al. (2008), assessed fixed-dose combination (FDC) therapy (two antihypertensive drugs in a single pill) versus "free combination" (FC) therapy (two antihypertensive drugs taken separately).[23] The study compared patients who were switched from FDC to FC and had at least two pharmacy claims for each of the FC drugs (FC group) with patients who were treated continuously with FDC (FDC group). The two study groups were matched on a propensity score derived from demographic characteristics and medical comorbidities measured in the six months prior to the date of switching from FDC to FC (FC group) or a comparable assigned date (FDC group) and were followed for 12 subsequent months.

Logistic regression analyses assessed persistence with treatment, defined in a standard way using the fill date and "days supply" field in pharmacy claims data. Specifically, persistence was defined as having a supply of medication for all drugs in the treatment regimen (i.e., one drug for an FDC patient and both drugs for an FC patient) throughout the follow-up period with no more than a 30-day gap between refills for any one drug.

Generalized linear modeling assessed compliance, measured in a similar way as persistence but on a continuous scale—that is, number of days during the year on which the patient had a supply of medication for one drug (FDC) or both drugs (FC), divided by 365 days. Multivariate techniques were also used to assess between-group differences in use of other medical services during the follow-up period.

After controlling for demographics, comorbidities, and health care expenditures in the six months prior to the observation period, Hess et al. found a strong association between regimen choice and the study outcomes. Comparing FDC with FC patients, the rate of persistence was 43 percentage points higher; the rate of compliance was 23 percentage points higher; and medical service use rates were lower (e.g., hypertension-related office visit rates of 59% for FDC versus 66% for FC). The results certainly seemed to reflect a "win" for FDC, and the authors reported that their findings supported "the hypothesis that simplifying antihypertensive drug regimens may improve persistence and compliance."[23]

But there was a problem with this interpretation. Prescribers could have made the switch from FDC to FC with the *intent* of making *subsequent* changes to the drug regimen, possibly because the patient's hypertension was not sufficiently controlled by the medications and/or dosages in the FDC. Notably, the measures of persistence and compliance assessed only compliance with the *study* drugs, not with any other antihypertensive drugs. Thus, drug switches made by the physician would have reduced "persistence" and "compliance" as defined by the investigators. Similarly, one would expect that patients who are switched from one drug regimen to another because of poorly controlled hypertension would use more medical services than those who are maintained on a single regimen that is working well for them. Thus, despite the soundness of the statistical techniques used by Hess et al., their study may provide an example of residual confounding that cannot be overcome with any multivariate technique.

> ## Key Points: Limitations of Multivariate Analysis
>
> ❖ Even with advanced statistical techniques, some residual confounding is likely with a nonrandomized design.
>
> ❖ All techniques that adjust for the same measured confounders will produce similar results.
>
> ❖ Instrumental variable analysis can be helpful in addressing unmeasured confounders but is difficult to execute.
>
> ❖ Controlling for subject intent may be impossible.

Rule of Thumb #2: Rely primarily on foundational theory rather than "data mining."

One of the most important rules of thumb in advanced statistical analysis is that the technique is not in charge—*you* are in charge. More specifically, choices of the analytic method and covariates should be based primarily on specific theoretical constructs (hypotheses or research questions) that should, in turn, be derived from the literature review that was performed and summarized at the start of the research project (Chapter 4).

In planning the analysis, it may be helpful to depict the theory in graphic form. For example, as we saw in the discussion of the Medicare Health Support experiment in Chapter 3, patients who opt to engage actively in DSM services may be, on average, healthier and less costly at baseline than those who opt not to participate.[24] Thus, better health status may predict *both* a choice to participate in DSM programs *and* better health outcomes. Figure 6A shows the structure of a model to analyze a DSM program given this knowledge.

Figure 6A
Model Structure for Hypothetical Study of Disease Management Program

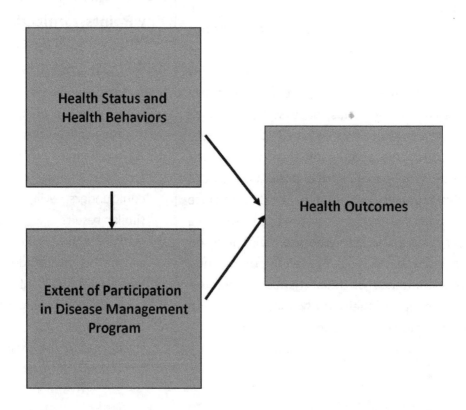

Depicting the theoretical construct in this way helps the researcher to avoid *specification error*, that is, the situation in which the model structure and/or assumptions are inconsistent with the data, often resulting in erroneous findings.[14] Examples of specification error in health care research include erroneous assumptions about the *form of a relationship* (e.g., assuming that the relationship between A and B is linear when it is actually loglinear); erroneous specification of *direction* of causation (e.g., assuming that treatment nonadherence causes poor health, when for some patients, poor health may cause treatment nonadherence); exclusion of important *covariates* (e.g., controlling only for age and sex in an analysis of health care cost); and misspecification of the *distribution of the independent or dependent variables* (e.g., using linear regression for counts of hospital stays, for which nearly all of the values are zero because most subjects are not hospitalized).

Of course, the literature review is not the only source of information about proper model specification. The development of a good multivariate model should be informed by exploratory bivariate analyses and, sometimes, by "stepwise" multivariate techniques that select predictor variables based on specific quantitative criteria. Patterns observed in the bivariate or preliminary multivariate analyses may prompt a researcher to "rethink" the model. Additionally, "data mining"—that is, exploratory data analysis of multiple relationships among study variables—is sometimes appropriate when little is known about the study topic, as *one part of* the process of constructing hypotheses and research questions. However, these choices should *always* be made with an eye toward plausible causal relationships, as discussed in Chapter 3, and the theoretical constructs derived from previously published work, as discussed in Chapter 4. An example of how *not* to construct a theory may help to illustrate the point.

Pedhazur's "Philadelphia Story." A sound approach in which model construction is built on a foundation of previous work can be contrasted with "theory building," in which the researcher uses stepwise analysis and/or tests of every possible interaction among independent variables as the sole source of information to determine a theory. In an example that might be amusing if it hadn't been so serious, statistician Elazar Pedhazur (1982) recounted the story of the "Philadelphia School District Studies," a two-report examination of factors affecting student reading achievement, published and circulated in the 1970s.[14,25,26] The studies became so influential that they were summarized in an educational resource booklet provided free of charge to the public, highlighted in the *New York Times*, and featured in a publication of the American Education Research Association.[14]

Yet, their authors candidly acknowledged that they were based on no theory at all. Instead, they were based *solely* on

> "... *many regressions ... The data have been mined, of course. One starts with so few hypotheses convincingly turned up by theory that classical hypothesis testing is in this application sterile. The data are there to be looked at for what they can reveal.*"[26]

In the report of the second study, for which the authors described running more than *500* multiple regression equations, the authors indicated that "the final equation was regarded as The Theory—the hypothesized relationship between growth in reading achievement ... and many inputs."[14]

Pedhazur pointed out that the authors' haphazard analytic approach resulted in errors, such as including interaction effect terms without main effect terms in one of the key published multivariate models. Additionally, and more important from a public policy perspective, the analyses produced contradictory findings that made little common sense. For example, the interaction terms from one analysis indicated that elementary students whose performance was below grade level (e.g., a third-grader with first-grade reading skills) did better in class sizes less than 28; other students could be placed in class sizes of up to 33 children without negative academic consequences; and class sizes of 34 or more children were harmful "for all elementary students in the sample."[25] However, a subsequent analysis found that "students do better in larger classes."[14] The authors explained the first finding by saying that "it is possible that the negative relationship may arise from a teacher's hostile reaction to a class size larger than mandated by the union contract, rather than from largeness itself"[25] and the second by saying that "it is a finding which emerges when many other variables are controlled,"[14] although both contradictory findings were based on similar multivariate analyses.

The authors apparently found themselves in an awkward spot when describing one finding in particular: "What is one to say about the finding that, for students who are at or below grade level, more [disruptive incidents] ... are associated with greater achievement growth?" After suggesting several explanations, the authors concluded that "it would seem a bit premature to engage in a policy of encouraging disruptive incidents to increase learning!"[26] Pedhazur's pointed assessment of the Philadelphia studies' internally inconsistent results was that "there are, of course, many other alternative explanations [for the inconsistencies], the simplest and most plausible being that the model reflected by the [final] regression equation has little or nothing to do with a theory of the process of achievement in reading."[14]

It is to be hoped that no researcher in health care—especially one reading this book!—would consider running *500* multivariate equations with no supporting theory or hypotheses at all, since the hazards of doing so should be immediately apparent (even putting aside the enormous cumulative type I error rate, as described in Chapter 5). In health care—as in education and many other fields—a myriad of factors are *associated* without being causally related at all. And, as Pedhazur has observed, the data for any given study may be consistent with numerous very different model structures. For example, if A causes B, a regression analysis in which B is used to predict A will likely produce a significant coefficient for B—but that result does not alone indicate that B actually causes A. Thus, "theory building" invites the "building" of nonsensical theoretical constructs.[14] Pedhazur notes in his excellent discussion of causal attribution in multivariate research that "controlling variables without regard to the theoretical considerations about the pattern of relations among them may amount to a distortion of reality and result in misleading or meaningless results."[14]

So if you do choose to engage in exploratory "data-mining," do so with caution, knowing that it is possible to produce meaningless results *if* you fail to consider causal plausibility, based on a foundation of previous research, in interpreting the data. "Data-mining" as a part of theory development should be used only in the early stages of a research project and only in conjunction with literature review and sound project planning (Chapter 4). Finally, hypotheses generated using one dataset should be tested with a different dataset, rather than retrospectively "fitting" the hypotheses to match the data and reporting the results as if the hypotheses had been derived from the literature review.

Rule of Thumb #3: Construct primary data tables *prior to* multivariate analyses.

A literary legend, perhaps apocryphal, tells of an exchange between Nobel Prize-winning novelist Ernest Hemingway and a group of friends. Known for his sparse and characteristically understated writing style,[27] Hemingway bet his companions that he could write an entire short story in just six words. When his friends agreed to the challenge, Hemingway thought a few moments, then reached for a napkin and wrote a poignant series of two-word phrases: "For sale. Baby shoes. Never worn."[28] He won the bet.

As in short stories or any other form of communication, when trying to convey research information—to say nothing of understanding it yourself—the simplest presentation necessary to meet the study objective is generally the best presentation. As methodologist Jane Miller describes the choices to be made:

> *"Writing about statistical results is equivalent to the evidence portion of a legal trial. Before you launch into a detailed description of your findings, provide justification for the methods of analysis. ... Explain why a simpler method won't suffice to answer your research question with the data at hand. In statistical terms, 'if a bivariate test will do, why estimate a multivariate model?'"*[5]

There are good reasons why knowledgeable statisticians recommend undertaking multivariate analysis only after carefully considering bivariate results.[5] **First**, from the perspective of the information user—whose needs should be paramount in the decisions made at every stage of the research process—bivariate analyses are easily understood. For this reason, as discussed in more detail in Chapter 10, bivariate results should be included in research reports, even those that also present multivariate results. **Second**, after the important first step of establishing study hypotheses, bivariate analyses provide a critical second step; they begin to reveal to the researcher both the direction and the magnitude of the associations between the independent and dependent variables. **Third**, a bivariate analysis of the relationships *among* the independent variables, such as a table of Pearson correlations, takes little time to produce and helps the researcher to determine the nature and extent of variance shared by the independent variables; this step can provide important information for selection of the final multivariate model.

Rule of Thumb #4: Pay attention to technical requirements and the specific meaning of coefficients.

In the rush to obtain the answers to research questions, it can be tempting to skip the seemingly uninteresting step of verifying that the multivariate technique and model structure are consistent with the data—but it is important to remember that technical details matter. As statistician Marija Norušis has said succinctly:

> *"Cranking out regressions without considering possible violations of the necessary assumptions can lead to results that are difficult to interpret and apply. Significance levels, confidence intervals, and other results are sensitive to certain types of violations and cannot be interpreted in the usual fashion if serious violations exist."*[29]

ОПЫТЪ СИСТЕМЫ ЭЛЕМЕНТОВЪ.

ОСНОВАННОЙ НА ИХЪ АТОМНОМЪ ВѢСѢ И ХИМИЧЕСКОМЪ СХОДСТВѢ.

Ti = 50	Zr = 90	? = 180.
V = 51	Nb = 94	Ta = 182.
Cr = 52	Mo = 96	W = 186.
Mn = 55	Rh = 104,4	Pt = 197,1.
Fe = 56	Ru = 104,4	Ir = 198.
Ni = Co = 59	Pl = 106,6	O· = 199.
Cu = 63,4	Ag = 108	Hg = 200.

H = 1

Be = 9,4	Mg = 24	Zn = 65,2	Cd = 112
B = 11	Al = 27,4	? = 68	Ur = 116	Au = 197?
C = 12	Si = 28	? = 70	Sn = 118
N = 14	P = 31	As = 75	Sb = 122	Bi = 210?
O = 16	S = 32	Se = 79,4	Te = 128?
F = 19	Cl = 35,6	Br = 80	I = 127

Li = 7 Na = 23

K = 39	Rb = 85,4	Cs = 133	Tl = 204.
Ca = 40	Sr = 87,6	Ba = 137	Pb = 207.
? = 45	Ce = 92
?Er = 56	La = 94
?Yt = 60	Di = 95
?In = 75,6	Th = 118?

Д. Менделѣевъ

Early drawing of the Periodic Table of the Elements by chemist and inventor Dmitri Ivanovich Mendeleev (1872). A compelling example of the scientific value of powerful foundational theory, the table grouped elements by patterns of electron arrangement, which in turn produce patterns of common actions and reactions. The system was so elegant that Mendeleev was able to predict the existence of four elements that had not yet been discovered, simply by observing the gaps in table cells. Source: Zumdahl SS, Zumdahl SA. *Chemistry*. Boston, MA: Houghton Mifflin; 2007. Public domain image from Wikimedia Commons.

Inconsistencies between data and technical requirements can occur in a number of ways, depending on the technique. To cite a few common examples encountered by health care researchers, a variable measured on a three-level ordinal scale, such as an opinion question measured as "agree strongly, agree somewhat, disagree," should not be treated as a linear predictor in a multivariate regression. Skewed data, such as counts for which 90% of the values are zero, should not be treated as linear.[9,29] Strong correlations among independent variables, such as total number of physician office visits and total number of drugs taken during a one-year period of time, can produce *multicollinearity*, a situation in which coefficients may be unstable because the predictor variables share so much variance that it is difficult or impossible to determine their independent (marginal) effects on the dependent variable.[14] And, in a time series analysis in which the outcomes display a seasonal pattern, failure to account for seasonality will produce inaccurate results.

Generalized estimating equation (GEE) modeling, an increasingly used feature of major statistical packages, is a special case in point because of its flexibility. Like any powerful tool, GEE requires attention to detail to produce useful results.[9] For example, a normal distribution and identity (nontransformed) link should be assumed only for normally distributed data, and exponential distributions should be assumed for dependent variables that are non-normally distributed. Poisson or negative binomial distributions are commonly assumed for count data; binomial distributions are assumed for binary (two-level) variables; and a gamma distribution is commonly assumed for cost data, typically with a "log link" function that is used to "retransform" the coefficients from a nonintuitive form (e.g., expected change in the natural logarithm of the mean of cost associated with one month of therapy) into more intuitively meaningful quantitative associations (e.g., each additional month of therapy was associated with an average cost increase of $100).[9]

Three main points are important in ensuring that multivariate analyses are consistent with technical requirements. **First**, nothing beats an exploratory data analysis, including frequencies, crosstabulations, summary statistics (e.g., mean, standard deviation, median, and range), and histograms, to help a researcher identify problems that are likely to compromise multivariate results. Issues identified at this stage might include a higher-than expected number of missing values, extreme values, skewness, an unexpectedly bimodal distribution (i.e., one-half of the sample values cluster around one outcome, whereas the other one-half cluster around a different outcome), and higher-than-expected variance. Scatterplots of the dependent variable with key independent variables should also be examined to check for unexpected relationships (e.g., you hypothesized a linear relationship, but a scatterplot shows that the relationship appears to be curvilinear). "Outlier" values detected in exploratory data analysis and/or plotting may represent either errors (e.g., a days supply of 900 on a pharmacy claim) or challenges to interpretation (e.g., a subject with a $200,000 hospital stay because of an automobile accident in a study of health care costs for 100 patients with cancer).

Second, major statistical packages generally include diagnostic tools specific to each technique. These tools are intended to help the researcher ensure compliance with important assumptions and should be used *early in the analytic process* to ensure that final analytic results are not based on a technique that was inappropriate for the data. For example, linear regression analysis procedures commonly include multicollinearity diagnostics, such as tolerance and variance inflation factor; the Durbin-Watson statistic for "autocorrelation," used to test for violation of the assumption that "residuals" (also known as error, the difference between predicted and actual values) are not inter-correlated; tests for influential cases, including Cook's distance; and partial regression plots, which help the researcher to identify influential cases and nonlinearity.[29] In Cox proportional hazards regression, the model calculates hazard "ratios" for various groups and covariates, assuming that for two cases, "the ratio of their hazards will be a constant for all time points."[30] If the survival functions for the groups of interest cross—that is, their hazards are not proportional—using the technique is problematic. To test for proportional hazards, log-minus-log (LML) survival plotting of the hazards functions for the groups can be used; if the LML plot suggests nonproportional hazards, an interaction term for group × time can be added to the equation.[30]

Additional technical requirements apply for weighting in the context of regression analysis, for example, if a stratified sampling technique was employed. Statistical packages include various commands and subcommands for weighting in these circumstances. If the sampling weights are "solely a function of independent variables included in the model" (e.g., the researcher selected 100% of cases with Disease A and 5% of cases without Disease A, and the model adjusts for presence of Disease A), weighting may be unnecessary or inadvisable, depending on the statistical package.[31] However, in more common applications in health care, weighting may be necessary, as discussed in Chapter 5. (Weighting for complex survey sampling designs is discussed briefly in Chapter 8.)

Third, in interpreting multivariate findings, it is important to remember the specific technical meanings of the coefficients. Typical examples are shown in Table 6C.

Table 6C
Coefficient Interpretations for Commonly Used Multivariate Techniques

Coefficient and Analysis Type	Interpretation[a]
OLS unstandardized (raw) coefficient, nontransformed dependent variable, nontransformed independent variable	Change in the dependent variable associated with a one-unit change in the independent variable
OLS *standardized* coefficient, nontransformed dependent variable	Number of SD units of change in the dependent variable associated with a one-SD change in the independent variable (permits comparisons of magnitude of coefficients in the same equation)
OLS unstandardized (raw) coefficient, log-transformed dependent variable, nontransformed independent variable	Percentage change in the dependent variable associated with a one-unit change in the independent variable
OLS unstandardized (raw) coefficient, nontransformed dependent variable, log-transformed independent variable	Change in the dependent variable associated with a 1% change in the independent variable
Logistic regression analysis, odds ratio	Exponentiated raw coefficient.[b] The amount by which the *odds* (*not* the probability)[c] of an event (e.g., a hospital stay, an emergency room visit) are multiplied for each one-unit change in the independent variable
Cox proportional hazards analysis, hazard ratio	Exponentiated raw coefficient.[b] The amount by which the hazard of an event is multiplied for each one-unit change in the independent variable
Generalized linear modeling, exponential distribution with link function	Change in average response associated with a one-unit change in the independent variable

[a] For all interpretations, the effects represent marginal effects. For dummy variables, the coefficient for the characteristic coded as 1 represents the effect of having that characteristic (e.g., if 0=male and 1=female, the coefficient represents the effect of female sex).

[b] Exponentiation refers to calculating the "antilog" of numbers that are expressed in log terms. For example, a logistic regression coefficient represents the change in "log odds" associated with a one-unit change in the independent variable. The odds ratio is calculated as $e^{\log \text{odds}}$.

[c] The odds of an event are $p \div (1-p)$, and odds should *not* be equated to probability. For example, if the probability of an event for males is 25% and the probability for females is 75%, the odds for males are $0.25 \div (1-0.25)=0.33$, the odds for females are $0.75 \div (1-0.75)=3.00$, the odds ratio for males relative to females is $0.33 \div 3.00=0.11$, and the odds ratio for females relative to males is $3.00 \div 0.33=9.09$. Note that the *odds* for females are 9.09 times those for males, but the *probability* for females is only 3 times as high.

Sources:
Ballinger. Using generalized estimating equations for longitudinal data analysis.[9]
Miller. *The Chicago Guide to Writing about Multivariate Analysis.*[5]
Norušis. *SPSS Advanced Statistics.*[30]
OLS=ordinary least squares; SD=standard deviation.

One note about interpreting dummy variable coefficients is particularly important. A sometimes forgotten point is that these variables represent the effects of a characteristic *relative to the reference* (omitted) category. For example, according to popular press reports in January 2010, a study by Yeh et al. found that in a sample of community residents aged 45 to 64 years, smokers who quit smoking "ironically" increased their risk of diabetes.[32] No doubt, the finding had popular appeal because of the common experience of weight gain among many ex-smokers who find themselves substituting food in the place of cigarettes. In reality, though, the popular press

> ### Key Points: Multivariate Analytic Assumptions
>
> ❖ Conduct exploratory and bivariate data analyses prior to running multivariate analyses.
>
> ❖ Use diagnostic tools available in statistical software prior to finalizing choice of technique.
>
> ❖ Remember the specific meaning of regression coefficients when interpreting results.

interpretation reflected a misunderstanding about the meaning of hazard ratios. The analysis by Yeh et al. was a Cox regression in which the reference group was adults *who had never smoked*. The hazard ratio of incident type 2 diabetes for adults who quit smoking was 1.73 (95% confidence interval [CI]=1.19-2.53), and the hazard ratio for those who continued to smoke was 1.31 (95% CI=1.04-1.65).[33] Thus, the findings indicated only that *compared with those who had never smoked*, those who quit smoking had a higher risk of type 2 diabetes. Those who continued to smoke also had a higher risk *compared with those who had never smoked*.[33] These findings did *not* address the question of whether those who quit smoking had a higher risk than those who continued to smoke—contrary to the popular press reports.

Rule of Thumb #5: Validate analytic results.

The spring of 1942 was an especially dangerous time for American forces battling the Japanese in the Pacific—and a critical juncture for Navy Admiral Chester Nimitz.[34] A series of Japanese victories had left the Pacific fleet "in ruins," according to an account by the U.S. National Security Agency. In pathetic contrast to the extensive and relatively unscathed Japanese fleet, the U.S. force consisted of only 3 aircraft carriers, 45 small warships, and 25 submarines. Nimitz turned to Commander Joseph Rochefort's team of cryptographers, who had worked for many months to break the remarkably complex Japanese message transmission code:

"It consisted of approximately 45,000 five-digit numbers, each number representing a word or phrase. For transmission, the five-digit numbers were super-enciphered using an additive table. Breaking the code meant using mathematical analysis to strip off the additive, then analyzing usage patterns over time, determining the meaning of the five-digit numbers. ... Rochefort and his staff were able to make progress because the system called for the repetitive use of the additive tables. This increased the code's vulnerability. Even so, the work was painfully slow."[34]

By June 1942, Rochefort and his staff had deciphered enough of the code that they could "make educated guesses regarding the Japanese Navy's crucial next move." Based on a series of transmissions referring to "a pending operation," they believed that the most likely location for the next attack would be Midway Island. But, with his entire meager fleet at stake, Nimitz needed to be sure. So, in mid-May he ordered the commanding officer of the Midway installation to send a message indicating that the island's water distillation (desalination) plant had suffered serious damage. Shortly thereafter, Nimitz had the confirmation that he needed: a Japanese transmission regarding the upcoming battle—the troops, the message said, would need a supply of fresh water.[34]

The careful verification step taken by Admiral Nimitz holds important lessons for researchers today. Although the cryptographers had done their complex and difficult work diligently and well, it was nonetheless important to validate their conclusions prior to making consequential decisions. In health care, *even carefully performed, high-quality statistical analyses require validation*, especially when they are to be used to make decisions that affect policy or patient care.

A good example of the potential value of validating multivariate analytic results in health care can be found in close examination of a study by Roebuck et al. (2011), who assessed the association between adherence to chronic medication therapy (e.g., antihypertensives for high blood pressure, cholesterol-lowering drugs for dyslipidemia) and total medical expenditures.[35] (It should be noted here that one reason why this study provides such a good example is the commendable transparency and clarity of its report.) Roebuck et al. used "fixed-effects" modeling, which statistically controls for the effects of unmeasured subject characteristics that do not vary over time, to adjust for the "healthy adherer" effect. This effect, which was discussed in detail in Chapter 3, is a confounding relationship in which healthy behaviors (e.g., eating right, exercising) affect both adherence to medical treatment and health outcomes, causing an association between adherence and positive outcomes that is partially spurious.

After adjusting for a number of measured factors including age, sex, and Charlson Comorbidity Index,[36,37] Roebuck et al. found strong associations between increased medication adherence and lower medical costs. For example, patients with dyslipidemia whose medication possession ratio (MPR) for cholesterol-lowering medications exceeded 80% had annual medical expenditures that were, on average, $1,860 lower than those of patients with lower MPRs, mostly due to avoided hospitalizations. (Adherent patients also had higher prescription drug costs, but for the sake of simplicity, we won't consider those in this example.)[35]

The results sound like a "big win" for medication adherence, but a simple validation test suggests a problem in ascribing causality to the association between adherence and lower medical costs. Assume 5,000 nonadherent patients with dyslipidemia who become newly adherent. If adherence (compared with nonadherence) *caused* the medical expenditure reduction estimated by Roebuck et al., one would expect this change from nonadherence to adherence to yield an annual medical cost savings of $9.3 million (5,000 patients × $1,860 per patient). Now, assume that a reasonable "ballpark" cost estimate for a cardiovascular hospitalization and follow-up care is approximately $70,000—based on three factors: (1) in 2006, *inpatient charges* per hospital stay billed to private insurance were $44,733 for coronary artery disease, $54,697 for heart attack, and $44,239 for stroke;[38] (2) billed charges typically far exceed actual cost (i.e., payments); and (3) one should assume some additional cost for outpatient follow-up care and for health care inflation. (Note that although the $70,000 estimate is a "ballpark" figure, results of this simple validation will be similar even if somewhat higher or lower costs are assumed.)

Using the assumed cost of $70,000 per cardiac event, to achieve the $9.3 million annual savings suggested by the study findings would require avoiding approximately 133 hospitalizations ($9.3 million ÷ $70,000) annually among the 5,000 newly adherent patients, *solely* due to the change from nonadherence to adherence. The problem is that the calculated effect of greater *adherence* to the drugs would far exceed the expected effects of the drugs themselves, based on clinical trials comparing statin-treated patients with those receiving *placebo*—no drug at all (Table 6D). In other words, if treatment with statins avoids about 25-50 cardiac events per year in a group of 5,000 patients, it is not reasonable to believe that better adherence to antihyperlipidemic medication avoids 133 events per year in the same group. Thus, the study's estimate that greater adherence saved $1,860 in annual medical cost per patient seems implausible. What happened?

Table 6D
Effectiveness of Statin Treatment in Preventing Major Cardiovascular Events in a Hypothetical Group of 5,000 Patients[a]

Trial and Events Avoided	Per-Subject Rate of ≥1 Avoided Event	Length of Follow-Up (Years)	Annual Probability of Event Avoidance[b]	Annual Number with ≥1 Avoided Event[c]
LIPID trial, secondary prevention[d] Events (death, heart attack, stroke) were avoided in 48 patients for every 1,000 treated.	0.048	6.1	0.0080	40
Meta-analysis, secondary prevention[d] Major vascular events were avoided in 48 patients per 1,000 treated.	0.048	5.0	0.0098	49
Meta-analysis, primary prevention[d] Major vascular events were avoided in 25 patients per 1,000 treated.	0.025	5.0	0.0051	25
JUPITER, primary prevention[d] 0.59 events per 100 person-years[e]	NA	NA	0.0059	30[e]

[a] Much of the material in this table was previously reported in Fairman KA, Curtiss FR. What do we really know about VBID?[39] It is reprinted here with permission. Trial report sources: JUPITER, LIPID, and a meta-analysis by Baigent et al.[40]

[b] Annual rate is derived algebraically from the cumulative probability formula: $C = 1-(1-a)^n$, where C=cumulative probability, a=annual probability, and n=number of years[41]—that is, $a = 1-(1-C)^{1/n}$.

[c] Assumed hypothetical cohort of 5,000 treated patients × annual avoided event rate, for example, using the LIPID trial data, 5,000 treated patients × 0.0080 annual probability of event avoidance=40 patients.

[d] "Primary prevention" refers to treatment in a group of patients with an abnormal biomarker (i.e., high cholesterol) but no disease. "Secondary prevention" refers to treatment of patients who have developed the disease of interest (i.e., cardiovascular disease).

[e] For the first three rows of the table (the meta-analysis and the LIPID trial), the final outcome reflects the estimated number of patients in whom at least 1 event is avoided. For the last row of the table (JUPITER), the final outcome reflects the estimated number of avoided events (i.e., 0.77 and 1.36 events per 100 person-years for rosuvastatin and placebo, respectively).[40]

JUPITER=Justification for the Use of Statins in Prevention: an Intervention Trial Evaluating Rosuvastatin; LIPID=Long-Term Intervention with Pravastatin in Ischaemic Disease; MI=myocardial infarction; NA=not applicable.

Limitations that were candidly acknowledged by the authors in their study report provide clues to the problem. **First**, the authors assessed *all-cause* medical service use without examining whether the medical conditions for which the patients were treated could reasonably have been caused by medication nonadherence. **Second** and related, the authors acknowledged that they did not assess the timing of the hospitalizations relative to the nonadherence that "caused" them.

These decisions were problematic because physicians may terminate drug therapy *after* the development of a new medical problem that is completely unrelated to the indication for the drug. For example, the physician of a patient who is hospitalized for kidney failure may, *after* the hospital stay, discontinue the patient's statin because of evidence that kidney disease affects the safety of treatment with hepatically cleared drugs.[42] (The analysis by Roebuck et al. adjusted for Charlson Comorbidity Index; however, moderate or severe renal disease increases the Charlson score by only 2 points on a scale of 0 to 37.[37]) This circumstance would cause a spurious association between "nonadherence" (actually, compliance with the physician order to terminate statin use *after* the hospital stay) and high medical cost (i.e., cost of hospitalization for kidney failure *prior to* termination of the statin). Similarly, a patient who is hospitalized for a problem unrelated to drug treatment will have no pharmacy claims for any medication during the hospital stay because facilities bill drugs using codes that do not identify the specific medication (Chapter 7). Thus, a patient could experience a high-cost medical event unrelated to drug treatment *followed by* an absence of pharmacy claims data for the drug.

In other words, the high-quality multivariate model used by the authors *assumed* fixed effects; however, it is possible that "healthy adherer" (or unhealthy nonadherer) behaviors may in fact vary over time because of life events or the development of new medical conditions. Validation of the multivariate results, including assessment of the timing and reasons for the medical care provided to the study patients, would have addressed those questions but was not performed.

In decision analytic modeling, validation of input assumptions is a standard of practice. Guidelines for high-quality modeling indicate that "model assumptions regarding causal structure and parameter estimates should be continually assessed against data, and models revised accordingly."[43] In other words, at the time that a model is developed, evidence may be uncertain; however, as the evidence base develops and assumptions are either confirmed or refuted, models should be updated.

Several model validation studies have found that replacement of model assumptions with empirical evidence resulted in dramatic changes in findings.[44] For example, when Cox et al. (2003) replaced assumptions about the use of gastroprotective agents (e.g., proton pump inhibitors, histamine-2 receptor antagonists) with actual utilization data in a decision analytic model of the economic effects of cyclooxygenase-2 (COX-2) use, the cost per year of life saved changed from $18,614 as calculated in the original model to $106,192 in the revised model.[44] Similarly, van Staa et al. (2009) found that the estimated cost of preventing an adverse upper gastrointestinal event by using a COX-2 instead of a traditional nonsteroidal anti-inflammatory drug was approximately $16,000 to $20,000 when using model inputs based on clinical trial adherence but increased to $104,000 after accounting for "real world" adherence based on data from the United Kingdom General Practice Research Database (UKGPRD).[44]

**Key Points:
Model Validation**

❖ Check diagnoses on all-cause health care claims.

❖ Check timing of events for reasonable attribution of causality.

❖ Update decision analytic models as new evidence becomes available.

❖ Compare results with those of previous work.

Rule of Thumb #6: Obtain and report a meaningful measure of overall model quality.

At *JMCP*, we sometimes receive papers in which the authors have statistically controlled for a woefully inadequate list of covariates—for example, age and sex alone in an analysis predicting total medical expenditures—but nonetheless confidently assert that a "controlled" analysis supported their hypotheses. Often, when we request a summary measure of model quality, a *JMCP* requirement and recommended metric for reporting multivariate results,[5,14] we find that the quality is poor—for example, an R^2 of 3%, indicating that only 3% of the variance in the dependent variable was explained by the predictors.

Although assessing model quality may seem to be an uninteresting and perhaps overly obsessive detail, it is quite important to the internal validity of study results. As Pedhazur has pointed out in discussing the importance of the R^2 statistic, a low percentage of variance explained is usually the sign of a specification error. That is, when a large percentage of the variance in the dependent variable is unaccounted for, it is likely that important variables have been omitted from the model, resulting in potentially biased findings.[14]

It is important to note that a low R^2 may represent the best that could be done using the predictors available to the researchers; thus, a low R^2 is not necessarily a sign of poor-quality work by the researchers. Additionally, a finding of poor model quality does not mean that the study results have no value. However, it does mean that in the study report, cautious interpretation and a candid discussion of the limitations of the multivariate analysis are warranted (Chapter 10).

Typically, multiple summary statistics for model quality are available, and the investigator must choose from among them. Ideal summary statistics have substantive meaning for both the investigator and the information users. For example, the c-statistic, formally known as the area under the receiver operating characteristics (ROC) curve, is often used to gauge the predictive accuracy of logistic regression analysis. This technique assesses every possible pairing of cases in the dataset (e.g., in a logistic regression model to predict hospitalization, every possible pairing of hospitalized with nonhospitalized cases) and measures the proportion of pairs for which the model prediction is consistent with the outcome (e.g., a higher score for a hospitalized than a nonhospitalized case).[45] A c-statistic of 0.50 indicates that the model performs no better than chance assignment (e.g., a coin toss) in prediction, whereas 1.0 indicates that the model correctly predicted every case outcome.[45] Statistics that measure only whether the model coefficients significantly differ from zero, such as the F value in linear regression analysis or the –2 log likelihood (–2LL) in logistic regression analysis, are less meaningful.[14,30]

The statistics literature contains many examples of proposed or commonly used "pseudo-R^2" measures,[46] but the easiest way to identify good model quality statistics is to review the options available in your statistical package and select those that are most commonly used and, more importantly, most substantively meaningful. The requirements of the journal to which a manuscript is being submitted should also be checked, as discussed in Chapter 10. Finally, when in doubt in making these decisions, consult a knowledgeable colleague or statistician.

Summing Up: What Have We Learned?

Sophisticated analytic techniques are best understood as tools that one might or might not choose to use in a given way for a given project, depending on the circumstances and the task. In this regard, they are no different than any other tools. For example, in putting a roof on a home, a builder does not throw a bucket of tools at the shingles hoping that they land in the right location to secure the roof in its proper place. Instead, the builder considers what each tool was designed to do safely and effectively and uses it for the specific purposes for which it was intended. The builder also checks his or her results periodically, ensuring that the work performed using the tools has achieved its intended objectives. This approach is a good general guideline for use of multivariate analysis—*plan* **for appropriate use of the tool,** *act* **in accordance with that plan, and** *validate* **the results.**

Additionally, the complexity and limitations of multivariate analyses intended to adjust for measured or unmeasured confounding factors should make the enormous benefits of randomized design apparent. Assuming that randomization has been performed properly, there is usually no need for complex statistical controls because the study groups should be equivalent at baseline.[5]

In Chapter 7, we "drill down" further into the source of research data, considering how the secondary-source databases used by so many of us were constructed and how, in turn, those construction methods may affect the validity of the research results that we produce. We begin with a surprising combination of events that have more in common than you might think: a petty theft from the back seat of a car parked in Phoenix and a dispute over the severity of hospitalizations reported to the United Kingdom's National Health Service.

Helpful Resources

- Dunteman and Ho. *An Introduction to Generalized Linear Models.*[12]
- Glynn and Schneeweiss. Indications for propensity scores and review of their use in pharmacoepidemiology.[13]
- Miller. *The Chicago Guide to Writing about Multivariate Analysis,*[5] especially Chapter 9 ("Quantitative Comparisons for Multivariate Models") and Chapter 14 ("Writing About Multivariate Models").
- Weinstein et al. (International Society for Pharmacoeconomics and Outcomes Research). Principles of good practice for decision analytic modeling in health-care evaluation[43]
- Greenland. An introduction to instrumental variables for epidemiologists.[47]

References

1. Freedman D. From association to causation: some remarks on the history of statistics. *Statist Sci.* 1999;14(3):243-58.

2. García-Ferrer A. Professor Zellner: An Interview for the International Journal of Forecasting. *International Journal of Forecasting.* 1998;14:303-12. Available at: http://personal.strath.ac.uk/gary.koop/ferrerinterview.pdf.

3. Rita Mae Brown quotes. Available at: http://www.brainyquote.com/quotes/quotes/r/ritamaebro107591.html.

4. Fairman KA. Differentiating effective data mining from fishing, trapping, and cruelty to numbers. *J Manag Care Pharm.* 2007;13(6):517-27. Available at: http://www.amcp.org/data/jmcp/pages%20517-27.pdf.

5. Miller J. *The Chicago Guide to Writing about Multivariate Analysis.* Chicago, IL: University of Chicago Press; 2005: quotation p. 317.

6. Dormuth CR, Patrick AR, Shrank WH, et al. Statin adherence and risk of accidents: a cautionary tale. *Circulation.* 2009;119(15):2051-57. Available at: http://circ.ahajournals.org/cgi/reprint/119/15/2051.

7. Vandenbroucke JP, von Elm E, Altman DG, et al. Strengthening the reporting of observational studies in epidemiology (STROBE): Explanation and elaboration. *Ann Intern Med.* 2007;147:W-163-W-194. Available at: http://www.annals.org/content/147/8/W-163.full.pdf.

8. Halpern R, Becker L, Iqbal SU, Kazis LE, Macarios D, Badamgarav E. The association of adherence to osteoporosis therapies with fracture, all-cause medical costs, and all-cause hospitalizations: a retrospective claims analysis of female health plan enrollees with osteoporosis. *J Manag Care Pharm.* 2011;17(1):25-39. Available at: http://www.amcp.org/data/jmcp/25-39.pdf.

9. Ballinger GA. Using generalized estimating equations for longitudinal data analysis. *Organizational Research Methods.* 2004;7(2):127-50. Available at: http://orm.sagepub.com/content/7/2/127.full.pdf+html.

10. Bosco JL, Silliman RA, Thwin SS, et al. A most stubborn bias: no adjustment method fully resolves confounding by indication in observational studies. *J Clin Epidemiol.* 2010;63(1):64-74.

11. Campbell MK, Torgerson DJ. Bootstrapping: estimating confidence intervals for cost-effectiveness ratios. *QJM.* 1999;92(3):177-82.

12. Dunteman GH, Ho MR. *An Introduction to Generalized Linear Models.* Thousand Oaks,

CA: Sage Publications; 2006.

13. Glynn RJ, Schneeweiss S, Stürmer T. Indications for propensity scores and review of their use in pharmacoepidemiology. *Basic Clin Pharmacol Toxicol.* 2006;98(3):253-59.

14. Pedhazur EJ. *Multiple Regression in Behavioral Research: Explanation and Prediction. Second Edition.* New York: CBS College Publishing; 1982.

15. Wooldridge JM. *Introductory Econometrics: A Modern Approach.* Mason, OH: Thomson South-Western; 2003.

16. Drake C. Effects of misspecification of the propensity score on estimators of treatment effect. *Biometrics.* 1993;49:1231-36.

17. Choudhry NK, Avorn J, Antman EM, Schneeweiss S, Shrank WH. Should patients receive secondary prevention medications for free after a myocardial infarction? An economic analysis. *Health Aff (Millwood).* 2007;26(1):186-94.

18. Goldman DP, Joyce GF, Escarce JJ, et al. Pharmacy benefits and the use of drugs by the chronically ill. *JAMA.* 2004;291(19):2344-50.

19. Fairman KA. The future of prescription drug cost-sharing: real progress or dropped opportunity? *J Manag Care Pharm.* 2008;14(1):70-82. Available at: http://www.amcp. org/data/jmcp/JMCPMaga_JanFeb%2008_070-082.pdf.

20. Based on a standard measure known as "price elasticity," the percentage change in quantity demanded ÷ the percentage change in price. See:

    • Moffat M. Price elasticity of demand. Available at: http://economics.about.com/cs/ micfrohelp/a/priceelasticity.htm.

    • Hodgkin D, Parks Thomas C, Simoni-Wastila L, Ritter GA, Lee S. The effect of a three-tier formulary on antidepressant utilization and expenditures. *J Ment Health Policy Econ.* 2008;11(2):67-77.

    • Landon BE, Rosenthal MB, Normand ST, et al. Incentive formularies and changes in prescription drug spending. *Am J Manag Care.* 2007;13(part 2):360-69.

    • Landsman PB, Yu W, Liu X, Teutsch SM, Berger ML. Impact of 3-tier pharmacy benefit design and increased consumer cost-sharing on drug utilization. *Am J Manag Care.* 2005;11(10):621-28.

    • Sedjo RL, Cox ER. Lowering copayments: impact of simvastatin patent expiration on patient adherence. *Am J Manag Care.* 2008;14(12):813-18.

21. Stukel TA, Fisher ES, Wennberg DE, Alter DA, Gottlieb DJ, Vermeulen MJ. Analysis of observational studies in the presence of treatment selection bias: effects of invasive cardiac management on AMI survival using propensity score and instrumental

variable methods. *JAMA*. 2007;297(3):278-85. Available at: http://www.ncbi.nlm.nih.gov/pmc/articles/PMC2170524/?tool=pubmed.

22. Leslie RS, Ghomrawi H. The use of propensity scores and instrumental variable methods to adjust for treatment selection bias. *SAS Global Forum 2008*. Available at: http://www2.sas.com/proceedings/forum2008/366-2008.pdf.

23. Hess G, Hill J, Lau H, Dastani H, Chaudhari P. Medical utilization patterns and hypertension-related expenditures among patients who were switched from fixed-dose to free-combination antihypertensive therapy. *P&T*. 2008;33(11):652-66.

24. McCall N, Cromwell J, Bernard S. Evaluation of Phase I of Medicare Health Support (formerly Voluntary Chronic Care Improvement) pilot program under traditional fee-for-service Medicare: report to Congress. June 2007. Available at: http://www.cms.gov/reports/downloads/McCall.pdf.

25. Summers AA, Wolfe BL. Which school resources help learning? Efficiency and equity in Philadelphia public schools. *Federal Reserve Bank of Philadelphia Business Review*. 1975. Available at: http://www.philadelphiafed.org/research-and-data/publications/business-review/1975/br75fas.pdf.

26. Summers AA, Wolfe BL. Do schools make a difference? *American Economic Review*. 1977;67:639-52.

27. Nobelprize.org. The Nobel Prize in Literature 1954: Ernest Hemingway. Available at: http://nobelprize.org/nobel_prizes/literature/laureates/1954/hemingway-bio.html.

28. Juddery M. 10 works of literature that were really hard to write. *Mental Floss*. January 16, 2011. Available at: http://www.cnn.com/2011/LIVING/01/16/mf.literature.hard.to.write/index.html.

29. Norušis M. *SPSS for Windows Base System User's Guide: Release 6.0*. Chicago, IL: SPSS Inc.;1993: quotation p. 337.

30. Norušis M. *SPSS Advanced Statistics 6.1*. Chicago, IL: SPSS Inc.; 1994: quotation p. 294.

31. Winship C, Radbill L. Sampling weights and regression analysis. *Sociological Methods and Research*. 1994; 23(2):230-57.

32. Hendrick B. Quitting smoking carries diabetes risk. WebMD. January 4, 2010. Available at: http://www.webmd.com/smoking-cessation/news/20100104/quitting-smoking-carries-diabetes-risk.

33. Yeh HC, Duncan BB, Schmidt MI, Wang NY, Brancati FL. Smoking, smoking cessation, and risk for type 2 diabetes mellitus: a cohort study. *Ann Int Med*. 2010;152(1):10-17.

34. National Security Agency/Central Security Service. The Battle of Midway: How cryptology enabled the United States to turn the tide in the Pacific war. Available at:

http://www.nsa.gov/about/cryptologic_heritage/center_crypt_history/publications/battle_midway.shtml.

35. Roebuck MC, Liberman JN, Gemmill-Toyama M, Brennan TA. Medication adherence leads to lower health care use and costs despite increased drug spending. *Health Aff (Millwood)*. 2011;30(1):91-98.

36. Charlson ME, Pompei P, Ales KL, MacKenzie CR. A new method of classifying prognostic comorbidity in longitudinal studies: development and validation. *J Chronic Dis*. 1987;40(5):373-83.

37. Christensen S, Johansen MB, Christiansen CF, Jensen R, Lemeshow S. Comparison of Charlson comorbidity index with SAPS and APACHE scores for prediction of mortality following intensive care. *Clin Epidemiol*. 2011;3:203-11.

38. Andrews RM. The national hospital bill: the most expensive conditions by payer, 2006. HCUP statistical brief #59. September 2008. Available at: http://www.hcup-us.ahrq.gov/reports/statbriefs/sb59.pdf.

39. Fairman KA, Curtiss FR. What do we really know about VBID? Quality of the evidence and ethical considerations for plan sponsors. *J Manag Care Pharm*. 2011;17(2):156-74. Available at: http://www.amcp.org/data/jmcp/156-174.pdf.

40. Sources include:
    - Ridker PM, Danielson E, Fonseca FAH, et al.; JUPITER Study Group. Rosuvastatin to prevent vascular events in men and women with elevated C-reactive protein. *N Engl J Med*. 2008;359(21):2195-207. Published online ahead of print on Nov 9, 2008. Available at: http://www.nejm.org/doi/pdf/10.1056/NEJMoa0807646.
    - No authors listed. Prevention of cardiovascular events and death with pravastatin in patients with coronary heart disease and a broad range of initial cholesterol levels. The Long-Term Intervention with Pravastatin in Ischaemic Disease (LIPID) Study Group. *N Engl J Med*. 1998;339(19):1349-57. Available at: http://www.nejm.org/doi/pdf/10.1056/NEJM199811053391902.
    - Baigent C, Keech A, Kearney PM, et al. Efficacy and safety of cholesterol-lowering treatment: prospective meta-analysis of data from 90,056 participants in 14 randomised trials of statins. *Lancet*. 2005;366(9493):1267-78

41. Kaul S, Diamond GA. Trial and error. How to avoid commonly encountered limitations of published clinical trials. *J Am Coll Cardiol*. 2010;55(5):415-27.

42. Dreisbach AW, Lertora JJ. The effect of chronic renal failure on drug metabolism and transport. *Expert Opin Drug Metab Toxicol*. 2008;4(8):1065-74.

43. Weinstein MC, O'Brien B, Hornberger J, et al.; ISPOR Task Force on Good Research

Practices—Modeling Studies. Principles of good practice for decision analytic modeling in health-care evaluation: Report of the ISPOR Task Force on Good Research Practices—Modeling Studies. *Value Health.* 2003;6(1):9-17. Available at: http://www.ispor.org/workpaper/research_practices/PrinciplesofGoodPracticeforDec isionAnalyticModeling-ModelingStudies.pdf.

44. See:
   - Cox ER, Motheral B, Mager D. Verification of a decision analytic model assumption using real-world practice data: implications for the cost effectiveness of cyclo-oxygenase 2 inhibitors (COX-2s). *Am J Manag Care.* 2003;9(12):785-94.
   - Fairman KA, Curtiss FR. It's only a pharmacoeconomic model—believe it or not. *J Manag Care Pharm.* 2008;14(1):83-85. Available at: http://www.amcp.org/data/jmcp/JMCPMaga_JanFeb%2008_083-085.pdf.
   - Fairman KA, Motheral BR. Do decision-analytic models identify cost-effective treatments? A retrospective look at *Helicobacter pylori* eradication. *J Manag Care Pharm.* 2003;9(5):430-40. Available at: http://www.amcp.org/data/jmcp/Formulary%20Management-430-440.pdf.
   - van Staa TP, Leufkens HG, Zhang B, Smeeth L. A comparison of cost-effectiveness using data from randomized trials or actual clinical practice: selective cox-2 inhibitors as an example. *PLoS Med.* 2009;6(12):e1000194. Available at: http://www.ncbi.nlm.nih.gov/pmc/articles/PMC2779340/pdf/pmed.1000194.pdf.

45. Peng CJ, Lee KL, Ingersoll GM. An introduction to logistic regression analysis and reporting. *Journal of Educational Research.* 2002;96(1):3-14. Available at: http://bit.csc.lsu.edu/~jianhua/emrah.pdf.

46. For example, see:
   - Schemper M. Further results on the explained variation in proportional hazards regression. *Biometrika.* 1992;79(1):202-04.
   - Shtatland ES, Moore S, Barton MB. Why we need an R^2 measure of fit (and not only one) in PROC LOGISTIC and PROC GENMOD. *Statistics and Data Analysis.* Available at: http://www2.sas.com/proceedings/sugi25/25/st/25p256.pdf.
   - Rouam S, Moreau T, Broët P. A pseudo-R^2 measure for selecting genomic markers with crossing hazards functions. *BMC Med Res Methodol.* 2011;11;28. Available at: http://www.ncbi.nlm.nih.gov/pmc/articles/PMC3068986/?tool=pubmed.

47. Greenland S. An introduction to instrumental variables for epidemiologists. *Int J Epidemiol.* 2000;29(4):722-29.

CHAPTER 7

Less Pain, Some Gain,
But Ask Questions When You Obtain:
Using Secondary Data Sources Appropriately

"For every problem, there is one solution which is simple, neat, and wrong."—American journalist Henry Louis Mencken[1]

"Isn't it time for a revenue boost? Improving your coding accuracy can do just that. ... More than 60,000 physicians rely on [our] coding software to maximize revenues."—Advertisement for software package used to generate medical claims (bills), which are commonly used in studies of numerous diseases and treatments[2]

"Under the most rigorously controlled conditions of pressure, temperature, humidity, and other variables, the organism will do as it damn well pleases."—Anonymous[3]

What You Will Learn in Chapter 7

✓ Important *advantages and pitfalls* in using secondary-source datasets
✓ Which *fields* in secondary-source datasets are most likely to be accurate and which require more cautious use
✓ 15 questions you should be able to answer about your dataset *before* you finalize plans for your study
✓ Why "no fishing" doesn't mean diving in blind: exploratory data analyses that you should *never* skip

---

On a sunny summer morning, I parked my car in front of a friend's house for a two-hour visit. Upon leaving her home, I discovered to my dismay that someone had smashed the car's back window and stolen my laptop computer from the rear seat. I immediately ran to my friend's house, intending to phone the police. Then I reconsidered. First, I knew from past experience that the police are too busy with serious crimes to solve small property thefts. If I called them, I would wait hours for their arrival and inconvenience my busy friend, with no hope of actually recovering the laptop. Second, because the replacement value of the laptop was far less than the deductible on our homeowner's policy, I did not need documentation of the theft for insurance purposes. Filing a police report would, I concluded, take time and effort but yield no benefit. So, I drove away, ordered a new laptop, and thought no more about the incident.

A few months later, I opened my morning paper to the local news page. "Phoenix police tout big drop in crime rates," read the headline. Police leaders, the article reported, had "heralded" the "20-year lows" for several types of crime, including thefts, which they had attributed to several factors that included "more emphasis on crime statistics to identify problem areas."[4] I realized in retrospect that I had done something that I try very hard not to do: I had contributed to the promulgation of inaccurate information. The crime database analysts knew nothing about the theft of my laptop because I had failed to report it.

At about the same time, the *British Medical Journal* spotlighted a scandal that had erupted in the United Kingdom's National Health Service (NHS) in 2009, when it was revealed that a large hospital, the Mid Staffordshire Foundation NHS Trust, had *both* been rated by government regulators as being in "urgent need" of quality-of-care improvement *and* ranked by a prominent health care guide, "Dr. Foster," as among the nation's safest and most improved facilities.[5] Investigation revealed that the primary cause of the incident, which caused "bruised egos"[5] throughout the NHS and prompted one commentary to pronounce the hospital ranking system "a bad idea that just won't go away,"[6] was surprisingly mundane. "Dr. Foster," the health analytics firm that reports standardized mortality rates for NHS facilities, relies on data provided by the hospitals themselves—and unbeknownst to the health analysts, workers in NHS hospitals, including Mid Staffordshire, had been making changes to the methods used to code the diagnoses of their patients. When asked by a reporter about the dramatic "improvement" in one quality-of-care metric, mortality following hip fracture, the administration of Mid Staffordshire provided a telling response: "We have not always had such a low [standardized mortality ratio] for fractured neck of femur. Our Clinical Coding department [advises us] that the change is due to substantially improved coding procedures."[5]

How can patient outcomes *seem* to improve based on coding alone? The answer in this instance was adjustment for case severity. For example, coding an increased number of diagnoses for each patient boosts the severity rating for the hospital's caseload, which in turn drives down the severity-adjusted mortality rate—even if no actual change in mortality has occurred. Similarly, applying codes for "palliative care" to patient records improves a hospital's mortality rating because it is assumed that an end-stage terminally ill patient would have died regardless of the inpatient care received; thus, these deaths do not "count against" the facility. In 2007-2008, 5% of hospital deaths in English facilities were coded as palliative care-related, but by 2009, that figure had risen to 11.3%. During that same time period, crude in-hospital death rates remained approximately unchanged.[5]

The moral of these two unrelated stories is that things are not always what they seem to be in a database. A crime statistics trend might reflect a true societal phenomenon—or it might mean nothing more than a change in reporting behavior. A decline in the adjusted death rate might mean that a patient really is medically safer in a hospital than he or she was five years ago—or it might represent a new method used to code clinical circumstances that haven't actually changed at all.

And, in a nutshell, these stories illustrate the challenge that researchers face when using secondary data sources. We have a handy package of information at our fingertips, usually on a personal computer, with the power to address our research questions at the touch of a button. Even better, we didn't have to collect the data ourselves—all we had to do was download the information and it was ready to go. It seems like a dream come true—or, as one of my graduate school professors more colorfully described it, like the proverbial pig rolling in ... well, what pigs roll in. But sometimes, in the rush to take advantage of convenient and readily available secondary-source data, it is easy to forget that we did not control—or even observe—the data collection process first-hand. Those beautifully packaged data were, ultimately, collected by human beings who might or might not have behaved in ways that we expect or want.

Fortunately, this limitation does not usually represent a fatal flaw in the work of a researcher; it simply means that it is important to be savvy about what the data—and therefore our results—do and do not mean. That is, we must attempt to determine what *unobserved* behaviors may have contributed to the data and how they might affect the validity of our research findings. This chapter reviews those behaviors and explains how to identify some of the most common problems in the use of secondary-source datasets.

In presenting this information, I assume that you are familiar with design features and terminology that were discussed in Chapter 3. If you have not yet read that chapter, you may wish to do so, or consult definitions of terms in the Glossary. I also assume that you are planning or have already started your project with a good basic research design that logically follows from what is already known about the subject (Chapter 4); thus, you know the hypotheses or research questions that you intend to address, and you have at least a basic data analysis plan. Finally, I assume that you completed initial verification upon receipt of your data (Chapter 2, Table 2A).

Why Use Secondary-Source Data?

A secondary-source database usually provides a number of important advantages for a busy researcher. **First**, its reputation as a reliable data source is often established, making it relatively easy to explain in ways that will be credible to formal or informal peer reviewers. For example, most policy researchers are familiar with data available from the National Opinion Research Center (NORC), which has been conducting the General Social Survey since 1972,[7] and with the Health and Retirement Study, a survey of Americans aged 51 years or older that has been conducted by the University of Michigan for nearly 20 years.[8] Most health care researchers are familiar with the Premier Perspective database, which contains complete billing data and associated codes for more than 45 million inpatient stays and more than 210 million outpatient hospital episodes nationwide,[9] and with numerous different commercially available databases of medical and pharmacy claims that represent the care provided to tens of millions of patients.[10,11]

Second, a database of this type usually provides an extremely large sample size, making it easy to identify and study sample subgroups—even those that represent a very small proportion of the population—and to conduct powerful statistical tests.[12] A **third** and related advantage is flexibility.[12] As discussed in more detail later in this chapter, when unexpected data patterns are identified in the data exploration phase of a project (e.g., a researcher plans to study an injectable drug using medical claims from physician offices but learns that the health plan requires most patients to obtain the medication from a pharmacy), corrections to the planned study methods can be made prior to beginning analyses of the study research questions. And, compared with primary data collection, using a secondary-source database is a low-cost or sometimes even no-cost option. For example, few of us could afford to pay survey researchers to interview more than 26,000 older adults every two years, but researchers can obtain the Health and Retirement Study survey data free of charge.[8]

Fourth, in addition to offering power, flexibility, and low cost, secondary-source data may enhance the usefulness of research project results. Because they represent "real-world" conditions, they may provide better **external validity** (applicability) in routine practice than data from a randomized trial, in which the sample and test conditions typically have been tightly controlled to enhance **internal validity** (accuracy of inference).[12] For example, a clinical trial of antipsychotic medication may exclude elderly patients, who metabolize drugs differently than do younger persons, and may also exclude patients who have comorbid mental health disorders (e.g., depression, anxiety disorder) because these conditions may make it more difficult to determine the true effects of the study drugs.[13] These are sound reasons for exclusion of patients from a drug study, but in real-world clinical practice, patients who are elderly or have comorbid conditions sometimes need antipsychotic medication. In fact, groups excluded from clinical trials prior to a drug's approval by the U.S. Food and Drug Administration (FDA) may represent a large proportion of those who will eventually use the medication after it is FDA-approved.[12] Secondary-source databases can help to fill these information gaps. (Of course, it is important to remember the research design principles that were described in Chapter 3; a study that is compromised by selection bias is likely to produce misleading results, even if it uses data that represent the "real world!")

Finally, secondary-source databases can provide information about phenomena that cannot be studied in more rigorous ways. For example, although a randomized trial might be the ideal test of the effects of different curricula on student achievement, randomization of children may be impossible because of school districting or parental preference. A database of standardized test scores for students whose schools use different curricula is a "second-best" option, *if* interpreted with appropriate caution. And, because the data are used retrospectively (after data generation), typically without the knowledge of the research subjects themselves,* there are no "Hawthorne effects," in which subjects adjust their behavior (e.g., medication adherence) during data collection because they know that they are being studied.[12]

Potential Pitfalls in Using Secondary-Source Data

Secondary-source data can be inappropriate for a researcher's intended purpose for many reasons. These reasons are illustrated below with examples, then described in more general terms and condensed into a list of questions that should be addressed **prior to**

---

* Generally, obtaining permission from research subjects is not required for use of a secondary-source database in health care; however, most database owners maintain the privacy of research subjects by using anonymized identifiers and prohibiting researchers from attempting to identify the people whom they are studying.

beginning analysis of your research questions. Although most of the examples are derived from databases of medical or pharmacy claims (bills), the problems illustrated by the examples apply to other types of data as well.

All these issues reflect the same general principle. *Accurate use of secondary-source data requires an understanding of how, by whom, and—most importantly—why they were collected.* *Always* obtain this type of information, even for databases that are widely used or have a great reputation. A data source may be ideally suited for its originally intended purpose (e.g., billing health plans for a particular medical service) but inappropriate for research purposes. As we'll see later in this chapter, a data source may even be appropriate for some research questions but inappropriate for others.

The Importance of Purpose

What do the results of standardized educational tests tell us about student ability? The answer may depend on the year in which the tests were taken. From the point of view of the school administrators and teachers who prepare students to take standardized tests, an important purpose of testing—albeit not the only purpose—is to obtain a favorable average score that can be shared with parents and the larger community. This incentive may result in a phenomenon known as "teaching to the test," in which schools adjust the content and method of instruction to facilitate better test performance by students, often after receiving a suboptimal ranking on a state educational performance measure. Changes in methods of "teaching to the test" may result in score increases that do not necessarily represent true improvements in academic achievement. In their commentary on regression to the mean, Smith and Smith (2005) described the phenomenon of the "Lake Woebegone Effect," humorously named after Garrison Keillor's fictional Minnesota town "where all the children are above average" because of the mathematical "flaw in claims made by states that all of their schools perform above average on state tests."[14] Thus, in interpreting test scores, it is important to remember the purposes of the test from the perspective of the state and school officials who may influence the data in unobserved ways.

Similarly, in health care research using administrative claims (billing) data, remembering the *original* purpose of data generation is critically important. *From the perspective of those who generate medical and pharmaceutical claims data* (i.e., health care providers who bill for services and health insurance companies that pay for them), *the purpose of a claim is to produce accurate payment for services rendered.* If a claim is good enough to generate the right payment to the right provider, it is good enough—*even if* a detail of the claim that may not affect payment, such as a secondary diagnosis code, is erroneous or missing. As we'll see in more detail throughout this chapter, the perspective of those who *generate* claims data may differ greatly from that of the researcher, whose ideal scenario is 100% accuracy for all fields on the claim. Thus, for the researcher using the data second-hand, it is important to know which fields are required to generate an accurate payment and how those fields are typically understood by their users.

Examples of Accuracy and Inaccuracy in Health Care Billing Data

Generally, the most reliable data in medical and pharmacy claims include:

1. The patient identifier;

2. The date of service;

3. The services provided, including procedure codes for medical claims and the national drug code (NDC) number indicating the specific drug dispensed for pharmacy claims;

4. The fields used in calculating payment, including allowed charge (which reflects the provider charge for the service after applying discounts), payments received from other sources (e.g., patient, other insurance), and final payment amount; and

5. The provider, sometimes an organization (e.g., medical group or hospital), to which payment was made.

Notably, many fields that are commonly used by researchers, such as secondary diagnosis (medical claims) and days supply (pharmacy claims), are often not essential to payment and are subject to a greater degree of inaccuracy. However, even essential fields are subject to error, unexpected discrepancies, or "gaming" (systematic coding practices intended to maximize reimbursement) for a variety of reasons (Table 7A).

Your Database Ain't Misbehavin'— Just Doing What It Was Designed to Do

Most problems that occur in the use of secondary-source databases in health care arise from root causes that are common in multiple database types. Each of these is discussed below.

Table 7A
Sources of Inaccuracy in Medical and Pharmacy Claims (Billing) Data

Name, Description, and Common Sources of Inaccuracy

Patient identifier: numeric or alpha-numeric brief identifier
- Changes in identification systems over time (e.g., change from SSNs to anonymized identifiers).
- Claims for newborn submitted using mother's identifier.
- "Test identifier" records that do not represent actual patients but are used by computer programmers to monitor system performance (e.g., enrollee name = "Mickey Mouse").

Date of service: date on which service was rendered[a]
- For laboratory and x-ray claims, DOS may represent the date on which a test was *read*, not the date on which the test was *performed*.
- For prescription drug claims, DOS represents the date on which the drug was *filled or picked up*, not the date on which the prescription was *written*.
- For therapy claims (e.g., PT, OT, speech, rehabilitation), DOS may represent a date span (e.g., 3 PT visits over a 1-week time frame).
- For inpatient hospital claims, end DOS may represent end-of-month billing or change from one unit to another (e.g., ICU to general medical ward); multiple claims may represent a single inpatient stay, depending on hospital's billing practices.

Provider identifier: numeric or alpha-numeric brief identifier for provider; identifier type varies depending on type of claim
- On pharmacy claims, the NCPDP number does accurately and uniquely identify the pharmacy.
- The prescriber's DEA number often contains errors because it is not needed to make an accurate payment to the pharmacy.
- Often, database vendors will "clean" DEA numbers and match them to internal files to provide provider information, such as specialty and years since medical school graduation; however, specific cleaning and matching procedures vary.
- On medical claims, although provider identifier is accurate for payment purposes (e.g., payment is made to the right person or group), it might not identify an individual provider; multiple physicians can bill under a single identifier (e.g., a clinic director or corporate office).
- NPI numbers were required by CMS on health care claims for small health plans by May 23, 2008, and for larger health plans by May 23, 2007; however, using an *individual* NPI for a provider who is in a medical *group* (e.g., clinic) is optional.[15]

Procedure code (medical bills only): CPT or ICD codes for professional services (e.g., physician visits, surgeries); revenue codes for facility services (e.g., ER); HCPCS codes for supplies, transportation, and some procedures and drugs
- Subject to "bundling" (the billing of multiple services under a single code) and "unbundling" (the use of multiple codes when a single code would more commonly be used).
- An important type of bundling is the "panel test," which encompasses multiple individual laboratory tests; for example, a CBC can be billed either separately or as part of a "general health panel" that also includes tests for liver and thyroid function.
- Coding changes are common over time in CPT; the same code may be accurate in one year and inaccurate in the next.
- Some types of injectable medications can be billed under either the medical benefit (using HCPCS codes) or the pharmacy benefit (using NDC numbers), depending on the health plan's benefit design and arrangements with providers.
- Injectable medications, especially newly approved medications, are sometimes billed using nonspecific HCPCS codes J3490 ("unclassified drugs") and J3590 ("unclassified biologics").

Table 7A *(continued)*
Sources of Inaccuracy in Medical and Pharmacy Claims (Billing) Data

Name, Description, and Common Sources of Inaccuracy
Diagnosis (ICD) code (medical bills only): primary, secondary, tertiary, and sometimes additional diagnoses • Can be subject to inaccuracy due to provider concerns about reimbursement or stigma. • Can be subject to "upcoding" (i.e., reported severity higher than actual severity) for enhancement of reimbursement and/or quality-of-care rating. • Sometimes represent symptoms (e.g., abdominal pain) rather than the underlying cause (e.g., appendicitis), especially early in the history of an illness. • Health plans may require only a single diagnosis code for payment of the claim, even if more than one code (e.g., a secondary diagnosis) would be clinically appropriate. • Diagnostic coding is generally more accurate in organizations that use professionally trained coders (e.g., hospitals). • Specific code billed by a provider may depend on the preprinted "superbill" fields typically used in the provider's field of specialty; the same medical condition could be coded in different ways depending on the "superbill" content.
Place of service: type of location in which service was rendered • Not a reliable field for determining the type of service provided (e.g., cannot reliably identify hospitalizations from place of service = inpatient hospital)—specific codes should be used instead (Appendix 7A).
Days supply (pharmacy claims only): the estimated number of days until the medication is expected to be depleted, based on the quantity dispensed and daily dose • Generally unrelated to payment, except that health plans sometimes have limits on number of days dispensed. • Manually entered by pharmacist and sometimes inaccurate. • Particularly problematic for "as needed" medications and products that may be difficult for the patient to self-administer (e.g., drugs administered using an inhaler, insulin); in these situations, the pharmacist's estimate is a guess. • Typographical errors can occur (e.g., dispensed days = 900 instead of 90).
NDC number (pharmacy claims only): 11-digit numeric code that uniquely identifies the drug dispensed to a patient • Not available on claims billed by a facility (e.g., a hospital) because facility revenue codes are general (e.g., "pharmacy, general" or "pharmacy, generic drugs"), not specific to drug. • Highly accurate at point of data generation, but can be cumbersome to use for research purposes because drugs, especially older drugs, can have many NDC numbers; many database vendors match NDC numbers to more user-friendly systems, such as GPI or GCN.

[a] Generally represents completion of the service from the provider's viewpoint.
CBC = complete blood count; CMS = Centers for Medicare & Medicaid Services; CPT = Current Procedural Terminology; DEA = Drug Enforcement Administration; DOS = date of service; ER = emergency room; GCN = generic code number (First DataBank); GPI = generic product identifier (Medi-Span); HCPCS = Healthcare Common Procedure Coding System; ICD = International Classification of Diseases, ICU = intensive care unit; NCPDP = National Council for Prescription Drug Programs; NDC = national drug code; NPI = national provider identifier; OT = occupational therapy; PT = physical therapy; SSN = social security number.

Root cause #1—Systematic omissions. *General principle: The most important record may be the one that you didn't receive.*

Parents of Bay County, Michigan, public school students may have been unhappy to learn in August 2010 that the average ACT score for Bay County high school juniors had been "below national average" for three consecutive years beginning in 2008.[16] And Bay County was not alone; from 2007 to 2008, the average ACT scores of high school juniors in the state of Michigan had dropped by a seemingly shocking 18% from 22.0 to 18.1 and had improved very little since then.[16] What was the problem underlying the decline? Was it bad instruction, deficient testing preparation, tougher questions, or a reduction in school funding? No, it was none of these. In fact, the problem wasn't really a "problem" at all—just a major change in the pool of students taking the test. In 2007, the ACT was optional and taken by 642 college-bound Bay County juniors. In 2008, when Michigan began requiring *all* high school juniors to take the ACT as part of its school merit system, the number of test-taking Bay County kids nearly doubled to 1,251. Naturally, as the pool of test-taking students expanded to include those not planning to attend college, average scores declined. And, just as naturally, the change caused consternation that was not merited after more careful consideration of the data generation process.

Situations of this type occur routinely in health care research. In a particularly remarkable example, the oft-cited (and often inaccurately described) 1991 New Hampshire Medicaid study that was discussed in Chapter 4 was the subject of a careful follow-up analysis by Martin et al. (1996).[17] The original study had found that imposition of a monthly "cap" (limit) on the number of prescriptions that could be obtained by Medicaid beneficiaries in New Hampshire had resulted in a precipitous drop in medication use, measured using paid pharmacy claims, for a group of elderly patients using multiple drugs for chronic health conditions.[17] The policy implications were clear in the view of the researchers: the cap was damaging to the health of Medicaid beneficiaries.

But Martin et al. took the original analytic concept a creative step further in an analysis of the Medicaid program in Georgia, which in November 1991 had reduced the maximum monthly number of prescriptions for which Medicaid would pay from six to five. In a sample of Medicaid beneficiaries who consumed at least six prescriptions per month, Martin et al. analyzed the data using a method similar to that of the New Hampshire study—with one important difference. Instead of looking only at prescriptions for which Medicaid paid, the investigators matched the Medicaid data set to computerized sales data gathered directly from the pharmacies and compared results based on claims data with those based on retail sales. They found that many drugs that would have been defined as "discontinued" based on claims data actually *had* been obtained by the Medicaid beneficiaries. However, instead of using their Medicaid benefit, thereby generating a claim, the patients had paid for the medication out-of-pocket in a transaction that was not visible to users of the Medicaid claims database. Thus, the analysis based solely on claims data underestimated actual medication use and overestimated the effect of the Georgia policy change greatly— by approximately two-fold. More importantly, for certain therapy classes, such as central nervous system agents and antidiabetic drugs, the statistically significant policy change effects observed when analyzing the Medicaid claims database became nonsignificant when the complete database of dispensed medications was analyzed.[17]

More recently in the fall of 2006, a large retail chain discount store announced that it would begin selling many generic medications for just $4 per month. Its competitors quickly followed suit, and within a few years numerous commonly used drugs were available for as little as $10-$12 for a three-month supply. Although a great bargain for consumers, the change caused problems for researchers who were accustomed to identifying medication discontinuation using pharmacy claims data alone.[18] That is, a patient who fills prescriptions using his or her pharmacy benefit and then seems to stop using the drug, as measured by the absence of a pharmacy claim, might actually be obtaining the medication (or a therapeutically appropriate generic substitute) elsewhere at a lower cost without using his or her drug benefit. The missing data pose a potential threat to quality assurance activities routinely conducted by health plans, such as monitoring adherence to drug therapy.[18]

Perhaps in part to encourage use of the drug benefit and submission of pharmacy claims, one large health insurance company announced in December 2010 that it would begin offering generic medications at $2 for a 30-day supply to its Medicare enrollees through several large retailers.[19] It is possible that additional solutions to the missing data problem, as well as more systematic measurement of the degree to which the problem affects quality assurance and research activities, will be available in the future. Suggested approaches include providing financial incentives to pharmacists for claims submission and developing new data information and transmission systems that are based on pharmacy transactions (i.e., a comprehensive dataset of medication use) instead of pharmacy claims (i.e., the data subset of medication use that is paid by insurance).[18] Meanwhile, though, a researcher who studies diseases that could be treated with generic medications must be mindful of the possibility of an incomplete dataset.

Services that are "missing" from the researcher's viewpoint (albeit not the patient's) can also be caused by "carveout" arrangements, in which certain types of care are provided by a subcontractor (e.g., a specialized psychiatric counseling organization) that does not report detailed billing data to the health plan. Mental health services, dental care, and vision care often fall into this category. It is not uncommon for a researcher who is attempting to evaluate the total cost of a particular psychiatric diagnosis, such as a psychosis, to find that it costs much less than national estimates would suggest. However, this finding almost certainly represents an incomplete dataset rather than a true pattern of care.

Root cause #2: Users of secondary-source databases almost never have the opportunity to observe common practices that affect them. *General principle: Data generators use the methods necessary to do their jobs and usually do not know about the methods that the researcher wants them to use. (And, even if they did know, they probably would not care.)*

When the State of Arizona launched its Medicaid program in 1982, state officials wanted to avoid what they saw as the cost overruns and inefficiencies that had occurred in other states. Arizona applied to the Centers for Medicare & Medicaid Services (now CMS, then called the Health Care Financing Administration) for a "waiver" from its usual program requirements so that most of the state's Medicaid beneficiaries could be enrolled in managed care health plans.[20] To obtain the waiver, the state had to agree to intensive examination of its patterns of care by federal evaluators, a term that it accepted.

The only problem was that the program, called the Arizona Health Care Cost Containment System (AHCCCS), was "capitated"—meaning that all health plans and many providers were paid "per member per month" (e.g., payment of $200 each month for each enrolled member), not "fee-for-service" (i.e., payment for each service rendered and billed by doctors, hospitals, and other providers).[21] The capitated arrangement meant that providers had no reason to submit bills for each service. However, federal evaluators needed utilization data for *individual* services to produce an accurate assessment of how managed care affected beneficiaries' medical service use patterns. If Arizona had permitted providers to forego utilization data submission, the threat to the federal government's evaluation of AHCCCS and, ultimately, to the future of Medicaid managed care, would have been enormous.

Thus, providers were required by AHCCCS to submit "encounter" data, pseudo-billing data that represented what they would have submitted if they were actually billing for the service. However, federal officials expressed lingering concerns about the possibility of inaccurate or incomplete encounter data. These concerns prompted federal evaluators to study a sample of AHCCCS beneficiaries, comparing the contents of their medical records with the encounter database files. Both federal and state officials were disappointed to learn that the database files seemed to contain numerous inaccuracies, with many services provided to beneficiaries and recorded in the medical records but not documented in the encounters. It seemed that the entire evaluation effort might fail because of missing data.

But then Arizona officials asked the evaluators to perform another analysis. This time, they suggested that the evaluators compare Arizona's encounter database with the *fee-for-service* Medicaid claims database in neighboring New Mexico, where providers were paid based on the service and had a financial incentive to submit each and every bill. To the surprise of the evaluators, this analysis revealed a very different picture of the accuracy of Arizona's data—they were actually slightly more complete than the data in New Mexico.

What happened? Investigation showed that many of the "missing" services, both in Arizona and in New Mexico, had been "bundled" by providers according to *routine billing practices*. In other words, they were services for which providers typically did not bill or, in some instances, were not permitted to bill. Examples included removal of sutures (stitches) by the provider who originally performed the suturing, post-operative examinations conducted by a surgeon, and prenatal care visits provided by the obstetrician who delivered a baby. In all of these examples, the services were part of a "package." For example, the Current Procedural Terminology (CPT) code 59400 represents a "global" package of obstetrical services that includes prenatal visits, the delivery, and postpartum care.[22]

With this information, AHCCCS officials were able to convince the federal regulators that it was neither feasible nor fair to expect providers to record services that nobody in their offices had ever recorded before, especially when doing so would ordinarily constitute billing fraud.[23] The "bundling" practices also imposed some unwelcome limitations on the research questions that federal evaluators could answer with the data available to them. For example, it would not be feasible to count the number of prenatal care visits using either encounter or claims data because providers almost never billed for them; thus, determining how many prenatal care visits had taken place would require a time-consuming medical records review.

Routine coding changes are another source of problems for researchers who use medical claims databases. Each year the American Medical Association, which promulgates CPT codes, adds new codes, some of which alter the way in which procedures are recorded by provider offices.[24] For example, in January 2007, 21 new integumentary (skin) system codes were added, many of which modified the way in which "the destruction of premalignant and benign lesions" was billed.[25] Prior to the change, destructions of premalignant *or* benign lesions were billed using CPT codes 17000-17004.[26] After the change, destructions of premalignant lesions continued to be coded using 17000-17004, but destructions of benign lesions were coded as 17110 and 17111—which previously had been used to code destruction of warts, viral skin infections, and small cysts. Thus, a researcher conducting a study of any of these skin disorders using a medical claims database that spanned the change date (e.g., from 2006 through 2007) would have to be aware of the coding changes to avoid making errors. These errors might include trying to identify destructions of benign lesions using 17110 and 17111 in both periods *or* concluding that a rapid decline in claims coded with 17000-17004 meant a change in the prevalence of premalignant lesions in the study sample (when actually it meant that benign lesions were coded as 17000-17004 in one year and 17110-17111 in the next).

Delivery of services and products in more than one venue represents another common source of confusion in research using health care databases. The most common example is injectable drugs. Many of these can be injected in the physician's office and billed under the medical benefit *or* dispensed by a pharmacy, billed under the pharmacy benefit, and administered by the patient (self-administration) or a caregiver. Examples are palivizumab (Synagis) for prevention of respiratory syncytial virus (RSV, which is dangerous to infants who are premature or have certain health conditions); interferon beta-1a (Rebif and Avonex), which is used to treat multiple sclerosis; and colony-stimulating factors, such as filgrastim (Neupogen), used to prevent infection in cancer patients undergoing certain types of chemotherapy.

The choice of where to receive an injectable medication may depend on multiple factors. For example, a patient might have mental or physical problems that prevent self-injection. Patients might also wish to "shop around" for the best available deal when, for example, the copayment is lower for an office visit than for a prescription drug dispensed by a pharmacy. Or patients might make the decision based on convenience. For example, if they have a physician's office visit scheduled one month, they might get the drug there, but choose to pick it up at the pharmacy the next month. In Medicare, following the implementation of the prescription drug benefit in 2006, some drugs that had been billed through Medicare Part B (outpatient medical benefit) were transitioned over time to Medicare Part D (drug benefit) in schedules that were not consistent nationwide but instead depended on the Medicare "intermediary" (subcontractor) operating in a given geographic area.[27,28]

In all these situations, a researcher with access to pharmacy claims but not medical claims, or vice versa, may be getting a markedly incomplete picture of the actual use of the injectable medication, posing a major threat to study validity. The key for a researcher who wants to study injectable medications is to ask questions and adjust study plans accordingly. If a researcher has access to only one of the two data sources, it is critically important to *determine the billing rules* of the health plan(s) included in the study. For example, sometimes health plans impose "blocks" that prohibit billing in one venue or another (e.g., they require use of the pharmacy benefit and prohibit injection of the medication in the physician's office). Some health plans allow patients to get a certain number of injections from the physician but require that any subsequent medication be dispensed through a pharmacy. Others have no rules.

Unfortunately, sometimes the data are simply not appropriate for the originally planned research question. For example, a researcher who wants to study the use of interferon beta-1a by Medicare beneficiaries nationwide using only pharmacy claims data might face an exceptionally difficult task because use of the pharmacy versus medical benefit may vary by geographic region depending on the time period.

Root cause #3—Secondary-source data generators may not view codes in the way that you do. *General principle: The mere fact that a code for your topic of interest exists does not mean that it was understood or used in the way that you, as a researcher, want it to be.*

Looking through an *International Classification of Diseases* (ICD) coding manual, a health care researcher could get positively giddy at the wealth of available information—hundreds of pages of codes representing every imaginable disease state or injury, defined at a level of detail that seemingly enables the exploration of any conceivable research question. Codes distinguish, for example, conjunctivitis caused by allergies from that caused by viruses, illegal from legal induced abortion, and major depressive disorder from the depressive phase of bipolar disorder. But only a naïve researcher assumes that all coded data are usable for every research question. The key to accuracy is to *understand the codes as the original users understood them* when the data were generated. In health care, several factors play a role in determining whether the code that appears on a provider bill precisely represents the condition(s) for which the patient was treated.

One is *financial incentives*. Providers understand that certain services may be reimbursed for some diagnoses and not for others; hence, the assertion in the advertisement quoted at the start of this chapter that many physicians rely on sophisticated coding systems to "maximize revenues."[2] A letter to the editor of *JMCP*, written in 2004 by a neurologist in private practice, summarized the problem of "GIGO" (garbage in, garbage out) in medical billing data and provided a cogent example:

> "In the early years of the use of [diagnosis] codes, physicians learned not to code patient visits for 'tension headache' because the diagnosis for migraine was in the 'organic disease' section while the diagnosis for tension headaches was in the 'psychiatric' section. Any use of a tension headache diagnosis would invite an insurance company to reduce its payments for the patient services (psychiatric illness was paid at a lower rate than structural disease). So, the outcome of coding 'accurately' for tension headache often resulted in an angry patient and lower payment rates for the physician. Miraculously, everyone seemed to have migraine."[29]

Another important factor in coding accuracy is concern about *stigma*, sometimes coupled with *diagnostic uncertainty*. When I was a 19-year-old college sophomore working as a hospital diagnostic coder on the night shift (perhaps that alone is a cautionary tale), I was told of a local general hospital that coded all of its psychiatric ward discharges as 300.4 (today, dysthymic disorder; then, neurotic depression) out of concern for the privacy of patients who might have a more stigmatized condition, such as a psychosis. This example is not isolated. In a survey reported in 1994, Rost et al. asked a sample of primary care physicians drawn from the membership of two professional organizations if they had on at least one occasion during the previous two weeks used "an alternative diagnosis when they recognized that a patient met [*Diagnostic and Statistical Manual of Mental Disorders*] criteria for major depression."[30] One-half of respondents acknowledged the substitution of alternate codes, typically fatigue/malaise, insomnia, and headache. When asked why they had made the substitution, 46% reported being uncertain about the diagnosis, 44% expressed concerns about receiving reimbursement for services if they coded the depression diagnosis, 29% said that accurately coding major depression might affect the patient's ability to get health insurance in the future, and 21% said that stigma associated with a depression diagnosis might delay the patient's recovery.[30]

Another factor in coding accuracy is *avoidable or unavoidable human error* caused by a variety of problems that are not observable by the researcher. Often, these situations are caused by the natural progression of the disease or typical diagnostic sequence for a particular illness. For example, bipolar disorder is commonly initially misdiagnosed as depression because the patient comes to the provider office complaining of depressive symptoms; and it is not until later (sometimes a long time later), when the patient has a manic episode, that a correct diagnosis is made.[31] Similarly, a patient with a myocardial infarction may initially come to an emergency room or physician office complaining of chest pain, or a patient with appendicitis may complain of another symptom, such as abdominal pain or nausea. Thus, a researcher who wants to track the sequence of events—including the total cost of care for the disorder—should remember to examine *both* codes for symptoms of the disorder and codes for the disorder itself.

Sometimes it is hard to determine the reason why a coding error occurs; all that a researcher can do is explore the data, adjust, and hope for the best. For example, in a study of patients with type 2 diabetes, Shetty et al. (2005) had to exclude 35% of patients from the initially selected sample because they had diagnoses for both type 1 and type 2 diabetes in the study period, and it was impossible for the researchers to determine which type of diabetes the patient actually had.[32] Similarly, in an analysis of data from 78 U.S. health plans, Ollendorf and Lidsky (2006) had to remove 2% of medical claims records for infliximab (Remicade), an infused therapy for rheumatoid arthritis and other conditions, because the number of vials billed during the visit was inconsistent with dosing standards.[33] In a study of the integrity of Medicaid claims databases for six states, Hennessy et al. (2003) found that pharmacy claims were "missing intermittently in some states;" that a "valid marker of inpatient hospitalizations" could be found in only three states; and that hospitalization data were "missing to varying degrees" for patients aged 65 years or older (presumably because some of their claims had been submitted to Medicare instead of Medicaid).[34] Hennessy et al. provided the good advice that researchers intending to use claims databases should perform "macro-level descriptive analyses," such as examining counts of hospitalizations and pharmacy claims over time to identify gaps in the data, or comparing diagnostic information with known prevalence data by age group, before using the database for research purposes.

Problems also arise when the data generators have *no incentive to produce accurate data*. For example, because it is common for some health plans to require only a single diagnosis code for payment of a claim, provider offices—especially those that are small and do not have professionally trained coding staff—may bill just one code when including a second or third code might be clinically appropriate (e.g., a secondary diagnosis of anemia that is a consequence of a primary diagnosis of bleeding ulcer). Researchers who want to study medical conditions that are often secondary to other disease states may be missing important claims of interest, depending on the health plan billing and payment rules. Fortunately, many studies of the accuracy of codes for various disease states have been published,[35] and a prudent researcher consults these during project planning (Chapter 4).

Complexity in the coding system itself is often a source of trouble. Even the most sophisticated and brilliantly detailed coding system will provide invalid information if its users do not make entries properly. Currently, the coding industry is undergoing a major shift

> **Key Points: Sources of Inaccuracy or Omission in Diagnosis and Procedure Codes**
>
> ❖ Routine billing practices and "bundling."
> ❖ Coding changes over time.
> ❖ Delivery of services or products in more than one venue.
> ❖ Financial incentives or disincentives to submit a claim or use a particular code.
> ❖ Concerns about stigma.
> ❖ Disease progression from symptoms to final, accurate diagnosis.
> ❖ Complexity in the coding system.

in anticipation of the October 2013 implementation of the ICD-10-CM coding system, which will have an enormous impact on provider offices because of its added complexity.[36] The current American Academy of Family Practice (AAFP) **superbill**, a preprinted form containing the most commonly used codes, will expand from two to nine pages as a result of the new scheme, which will increase the number of available ICD diagnosis and procedure codes, respectively, from 14,025 and 3,824 to a whopping 68,069 and 72,589.[37] Professional organizations objecting to the change note that for many diagnoses, the mapping of the old to the new coding method is far from straightforward and may introduce imprecision; for example, codes 919.0 (abrasion, unspecified) and 919.4 (insect bite) will map to one of two more general codes, T07 (unspecified multiple injuries) or T14.90 (unspecified injury of unspecified body region).[38]

And it is not as if coding is simple now. To get a sense of the complexity that office billing staff—the source of the data used in hundreds of health care studies every year—face on a daily basis, consider the following description from a coding news blog:

> *"Get ready for modifier GU (Waiver of liability statement issued as required by payer policy, routine notice). You might have times when it's appropriate to report modifier GU instead of the revised standby modifier GA (Waiver of*

liability statement on file, individual). Medicare hasn't yet provided instructions for correctly reporting modifier G, but watch for updates in future issues ... Three modifiers now include non-physician providers in the descriptors: 76 (Repeat procedure or service by same physician or non-physician provider), 77 (Repeat procedure or service by another physician or non-physician provider), and 78 (Unplanned return to the operating/procedure room by the same physician or non-physician provider following initial procedure for a related procedure during the postoperative period)."[39]

For database researchers, there are **two important likely outcomes** of the change from ICD-9 to ICD-10 if it is implemented according to the schedule that is planned as of this writing. **First**, for dates of service during the final quarter of 2013 and probably much of 2014, diagnoses and ICD procedure codes in administrative claims data may not be reliable because billing staff and providers will likely be adjusting to the new system. **Second**, when analyzing databases that span the change date (e.g., a study period from 2012 through 2014), researchers will have to familiarize themselves with coding "crosswalks"[37] and perform exploratory analyses to ensure that they have not misinterpreted the providers' coding intentions. These are major concerns.

Root cause #4—Form may (or may not) follow function. *General principle: The data that were requested of the data source by the data collector are the data that you as a researcher receive—whether they are what you wanted or not.*

Before using secondary-source data, a wise researcher obtains as much information as possible about the data collection process—that is, the requirements and procedures that dictated the data collection method and, therefore, the content of the data. Fortunately, most large-scale survey research operations, such as the NORC, maintain readily accessible copies of their survey text, along with all important documentation (e.g., instructions given to respondents, changes in methods over time) online. Owners of proprietary databases of medical and pharmacy claims are less likely to post their technical documentation publicly but should respond readily to questions from customers about the methods used to collect and process the data.

Among the most common and important sources of documentation in physician office billing data are preprinted ***superbills*** with "checkboxes" for each specialty's most commonly used codes. These forms have a profound impact on the data available to researchers because when completing the paperwork necessary for patient checkout, physicians are more likely to use a preprinted code than to research an alternative code, as long as the preprinted code is not incorrect. A comparison of the superbill forms for the American Academy of Family Physicians with a sample gastroenterology superbill (Appendix 7B) provides several good illustrations.

First, the AAFP superbill template contains a single ICD-9 code and description for diarrhea, 787.91 (diarrhea, not otherwise specified), whereas the gastroenterology template contains three codes and descriptions: 009.2 (diarrhea, infectious), 564.4 (diarrhea, postoperative), and 564.5 (diarrhea, functional). Notably, the code specified on the gastroenterology form for postoperative diarrhea, 564.4, is technically "other postoperative functional disorders" according to the ICD-9 manual.[40] Second, the AAFP template contains a single ICD-9 code for abdominal pain, 789.00 (abdominal pain, unspecified site), whereas the codes shown on the gastroenterology template are specific as to site of the pain (e.g., 789.01 for right upper quadrant abdominal pain, 789.04 for left lower quadrant abdominal pain, etc.). Do these superbill form differences mean that family practitioners rarely see patients with infectious diarrhea or commonly fail to ask patients about the site of their abdominal pain? No—these differences mean that use of the more specific codes is seldom necessary in family practice *billing*; therefore, the codes do not appear on the preprinted form. In other words, the family physician will be paid for the visit for abdominal pain regardless of whether the diagnosis codes for pain *site* are specified on the bill.

Note that the *medical record* will almost certainly indicate the site of the pain. *The issue is not whether the patient was properly diagnosed or treated; it is whether the most specific diagnosis was required for payment and therefore included on the bill that ultimately becomes the source of the data used by the researcher.*

Root cause #5—The form is only as reliable as its users. *General principle: Better training usually (but not always) equals better-quality data.*

When data are collected primarily or solely for research purposes, as in the NORC and Health and Retirement surveys, the data collectors are trained to meet the specific needs of researchers—that is, to gather the data in a way that maximizes reliability (i.e., consistency) and internal validity (i.e., avoiding bias or systematic discrepancies in data collection). Secondary-source data that were generated for nonresearch purposes are rarely as "clean." Typically, the training and skill level of the data collectors are more closely related to incentives important to the data generators—such as the desire to enhance quality ratings or maximize reimbursement—than to optimizing data quality, although *sometimes* the incentives of the data generators and the researchers are compatible.

For example, coding is generally more accurate for administrative claims from hospitals than from physician offices because most hospitals use professionally trained and certified coders. Additionally, hospitals do not use preprinted paper superbills; instead, they research and code each diagnosis to the maximum level of specificity available, using an electronic system. However, as we saw with the NHS example earlier in this chapter, the use of professionally trained coders can be associated with disadvantages if "gaming the system" or "upcoding" (the coding of a higher level of severity than is warranted) occurs, especially if these coding practices changed over time and the research is longitudinal.

Root cause #6: Better late than never. *General principle: Data generators are usually prompt only when there is an incentive to submit their information quickly.*

Most health care researchers are familiar with the "shoebox effect," named after the patient who stores his or her medical bills in a shoebox throughout the year and submits them for reimbursement, often in an enormous packet, to the insurer at year's end. Although most secondary-source databases provide more timely data than the proverbial shoebox, submission delays do sometimes occur. A wise researcher obtains as much information as possible about the incentives that might encourage or discourage prompt data submission (e.g., financial penalties for late claims submissions, capitation arrangements that provide no incentive for prompt submission) and checks counts of claims over time (e.g., crosstabulation of claims counts by month of service) in the project's data exploration phase.

Root cause #7—Stuff changes. *General principle: Fields of study march on, and sometimes these new developments are inconvenient for researchers (but we have to adjust).*

One of the most exciting aspects of the medical field is the development of new technologies that have the potential to extend life or enhance its quality. Yet, these developments can pose challenges to researchers because they may cause the *meaning* of data to change over time, even when codes have *not* changed.

One such development is recent enhancements to the **sensitivity** (case-finding ability) of laboratory tests and screening procedures used to detect cancer, such as digitally enhanced mammography and liquid-based cytology screening for cervical cancer.[41] These newer techniques are more likely to identify abnormal cells in their earliest stages. However, because they may improve *only* **sensitivity**, not **specificity**, their increasing use has changed the pool of patients identified for additional screening (e.g., additional imaging and/or biopsy) and changed treatment from later stage to earlier stage at diagnosis. A researcher using a secondary-source database of tests and treatments for these patients should be aware of changes in technology over time, especially when conducting longitudinal research or making comparisons with previously published work.

Another change that commonly affects secondary-source database researchers is the development of new drugs. For injectable medications that can be billed through the medical benefit, health plans do not always have a Healthcare Common Procedure Coding System (HCPCS) code available for the specific medication and may instruct their providers to bill the new drug using a nonspecific code, such as J3490 (unclassified drugs) or J3590 (unclassified biologics) on a temporary basis until a formal code becomes available from CMS.

15 Questions About Your Dataset That You Should Be Able to Answer

Although the number of different sources of error in a database can seem overwhelming, error-prone features can generally be identified by asking a series of revealing questions. It may not be necessary or appropriate to ask all of these questions directly, but they do represent items that you should research on your own using available published information (including material in this chapter). If necessary, you should ask your database vendor and/ or other researchers who have used the data previously for more information.

1. *What was the original purpose for collecting the data?* How do those who generated the data understand its purpose?
2. *What are the circumstances under which a data record is generated?* For example, a pharmacy claim may be generated when the patient picks up the prescription; a laboratory claim may be generated on the date that the test is read; a claim line on a hospital bill may be generated when a patient is transferred from an intensive care unit to a general ward.
3. *How, by whom, and using what type of coding system were the data generated/ collected?* How are the data generators trained? Do data generators in different settings have different levels of training (e.g., a professionally trained and certified coder in a hospital versus a receptionist in a small physician office)? Are the codes used to generate the data easy or difficult for the data generators to understand?
4. *Are there any incentives to generate inaccurate data?* For example, are there reasons to suppress use of certain diagnoses because they might stigmatize the

patient or to use a particular diagnosis code because the alternative code is not covered by the health plan?

5. *Have there been changes in coding methods during the time period covered by my study?* (Examples: changes in CPT or ICD codes, identifiers, or scoring methods).

6. *Have there been changes in the pool of people for whom data are available during the time period covered by my study?* (Examples: changes in pool of students taking the ACT from college-bound seniors to all graduating seniors, changes in pools of patients who screen positive for abnormal cells in laboratory tests because of changes in test sensitivity).

7. *Have the codes that I intend to use been validated?* For example, have administrative claims data ever been compared with medical records in a patient sample that is similar to mine? If so, what problems have been identified, and is it feasible to avoid these problems by changing the study methods?

8. *Are the data generally reported on a timely basis, or are there lags?* Are there incentives for those who provide records or who collect the data to record information completely and timely?

9. *What rules govern the recording of data in this data source?* What level of accuracy is required to achieve the purpose of the data as understood by users (e.g., does the health plan require the recording of all diagnoses, or just a single diagnosis, for payment to be made to the provider)?

10. *Under what circumstances are the data recorded in this source, and could they be recorded in more than one source?* Are there "blocks" or other rules in place that govern the use of one source versus another (e.g., the plan requires use of the medical benefit to obtain the study drug)? If the data could be in more than one source, do I have access to all of them (e.g., injectable medication claims that could be paid under either the medical or pharmacy benefit)?

11. *Is there any "farming out" of the data (e.g., service carveout arrangements) that could mean missing data for a proportion of my sample?*

12. *Were preprinted forms used to generate or collect these data?* If so, do the forms vary by setting (e.g., different superbills for family practitioners vs. specialists)? Are the forms clear, or do they contain ambiguities or complexities? Do the codes that I am planning to use in my research appear on the forms? Do alternate codes that might apply to my research topic appear on the forms?

13. **Does the natural history of my research topic produce changes in codes used over time (e.g., first abdominal pain, then appendicitis)?** Have I captured all those codes in my analysis plan?

14. **Does a vendor "clean" these data and, if so, how?** (Examples: checks for codes that do not exist, checks of allowed charge against service type, such as a $10,000 allowed charge for an office visit).

15. **Who can help answer questions about the data set?**

Does "No Fishing" Mean Diving in Blind?
A Common Conundrum in Secondary-Source Database Research

In Chapter 5, we saw that because of cumulative type 1 error, "long fishing expeditions" into a dataset are highly likely to generate at least one erroneous result and should be avoided. However, in working with secondary-source databases, simply barreling ahead with an analysis plan without first examining the data is fraught with hazards. As we have seen in this chapter, data generators sometimes behave in unexpected ways that threaten study validity; thus, making some kind of unavoidable adjustment to an *a priori* study plan is common in database research. For this reason, a wise secondary-source database researcher follows procedures to prevent diving sight unseen into the hazardous waters of unobserved data generation behaviors, while at the same time preventing the necessary data exploration from becoming an excuse to "go fish." The key is to know the planned approach in advance and follow it consistently.

First, begin with a preliminary *a priori* analysis plan (Chapter 4). Use previously published research, especially secondary-source database research in your topic area, along with examination of online sources, such as health plan billing instructions, treatment guidelines, or testing protocols, to develop a preliminary measurement plan—that is, how you will define and measure each of your study variables.

Second, *without performing the analyses for any of the study research questions*, explore the data for basic accuracy and make an assessment of whether the data appear to be reasonable. Suggestions and examples are in Table 7B.

Exploration may reveal the need for adjustments, either to the method for measuring study variables (e.g., adding a code of which you were previously unaware or modifying the analysis to account for an unexpected coding change) or, more seriously, to the analysis plan itself (e.g., changing your topic because your planned phenomenon of interest is not recorded in the database at all). After making those adjustments, proceed

Table 7B
Suggested Data Exploration Analyses[a]

Do This	To Catch These Common Problems
• Run basic descriptive statistics for the sample and compare with national statistics or results observed in previous research, for example: —Disease prevalence —Use prevalence for treatments (e.g., drugs, hospitalizations, office visits) —Scores (e.g., test scores by percentile, or measures of central tendency such as mean or median) • If you have obtained data from more than one source (e.g., health plan, state), run separately for each source if possible	• Systematic exclusions, such as "carveouts" • Requirements that you did not know about, such as a requirement that a patient use his/her pharmacy benefit instead of medical benefit to obtain an injectable medication • Unexpected patterns in the "pools" of cases (e.g., giving a test to all students in one state but to college-bound students in another) • Procedure codes that you did not know about and therefore failed to include in your analysis plan
• Run frequencies on all study variables or, for variables with too many levels to run frequencies, examine descriptive statistics[b]	• Typographical errors (e.g., prescription days supply of 900 instead of 90) • "Garbage" values (e.g., patient identifier = "0\$5##00*0") • Cases used by database staff for testing purposes (e.g., enrollee name = "Mickey Mouse")
• Run frequencies on key fields by periods of time (e.g., weekly or monthly).	• Change in data generation methods over time (e.g., coding practices, methods used by study subjects to carry out the activity of interest) • Change in coding requirements over time (e.g., ICD-9 vs. ICD-10) • Change in pool of subjects over time • Gaps in the data • Lags in data submission (i.e., data records dwindle over time)
• When examining a phenomenon of interest that you believe will be coded in a certain way, run frequencies on the actual codes used and research the meaning of the most commonly used codes.	• Unexpected coding procedures by data generators —You expected ICD codes for major depression for patients using antidepressant medications, but doctors coded these as fatigue or dysthymia. —You did not know that the health plan requires patients to have Diagnosis X in order to receive Drug Y. —Office administrators were unsure of how to code a particular diagnosis or treatment and used a nonspecific code instead of the expected (correct) code.
• When studying the cost of a phenomenon, run descriptive statistics, not only for the sample overall but also for each type of item (e.g., office visit, hospital stay, or whatever the key categories are).	• Identifies especially costly services that may require additional examination for better understanding of the phenomenon of interest. • Identifies outliers that may be appropriate for correction or exclusion.

[a] One client with whom I have worked combined items of this type with incoming data verification items (Chapter 2, Table 2A) into a single checklist. This approach has the advantage of simplicity because the analyst uses only a single tool; however, data verification should be performed immediately upon receipt of the data, whereas data exploration can take place at a later period of time (but prior to beginning analyses of the study research questions).
[b] For data exploration purposes, these usually include mean, median, interquartile range, minimum, and maximum. When looking for outliers, it is also common to run the fifth and 95th percentiles.
ICD = International Classification of Diseases.

with study analyses, following the *a priori* analysis plan to address the study research questions.

If after following these steps, you encounter a problem not detected at the data exploration phase, *do not* immediately adjust the *a priori* analysis plan, because doing so can take you on a "fishing expedition." Instead, discuss the situation with a knowledgeable and dispassionate observer who has no stake in the study outcome. Seek his or her opinion about whether it is necessary or prudent to change the analysis plan in response to the new information. If you and your observer agree that a change is necessary, report it transparently (see Chapter 10).

Summing Up: What Have We Learned?

As we saw in Chapter 3, there is no such thing as a perfect study or a perfect dataset. The keys to using secondary-source data—or any data—are to understand the purposes for which they were generated and the circumstances under which they were gathered, and interpret them accordingly. Exploratory analyses are critically important, and it may be necessary to adjust *a priori* research plans in response to an unexpected data pattern. However, these adjustments should be made at the earliest possible point in the project and, if at all possible, *before* analysis of study research questions has begun.

In Chapter 8, we will explore how to gather data from one of the most important sources available—the research subjects themselves. We begin with a predicament that is familiar to nearly anyone who follows politics—the missed election-day call.

Helpful Resources

- Motheral and Fairman. The use of claims databases for outcomes research[12]
- International Society for Pharmacoeconomics and Outcomes Research guidance on retrospective database studies[42]

References

1. Famous quotations network. Available at: http://www.famous-quotations.com/asp/ acquotes.asp?author=Henry+Louis+Mencken+%281880%2D1956%29&category=Mathematics+%2F+Statistics.

2. Ingenix advertisement. Available at: http://go.ingenix.com/webinars/ landing/10-25288/10-25288_landing.html.

3. Anonymous. Available at: http://www.todayinsci.com/QuotationsCategories/R_Cat/ Rigour-Quotations.htm.

4. Ferraresi M. Phoenix police tout big drop in crime rates. *The Arizona Republic.* September 16, 2010. B1.

5. Hawkes N. Patient coding and the ratings game. *BMJ.* 2010;340:950-52.

6. Lilford R, Pronovost P. Using hospital mortality rates to judge hospital performance: a bad idea that just won't go away. *BMJ.* 2010;340:955-57.

7. General Social Survey. Available at: http://www.norc.org/Research/Projects/Pages/ general-social-survey.aspx.

8. University of Michigan. Health and Retirement Study. Available at: http://hrsonline.isr. umich.edu/.

9. Premier Research Services. Available at: http://www.premierinc.com/quality/tools-services/prs/index.jsp.

10. IMSHealth. Pharmetrics database. Available at: http://www.imshealth.com/portal/site/ imshealth/menuitem.a46c6d4df3db4b3d88f6110194l8c22a/?vgnextoid=6d7660b6f5aa 0210VgnVCM100000ed152ca2RCRD&vgnextfmt=default.

11. ThomsonReuters Healthcare. Available at: http://thomsonreuters.com/products_ services/healthcare/.

12. Motheral BR, Fairman KA. The use of claims databases for outcomes research: rationale, challenges, and strategies. *Clin Ther.* 1997;19(2):346-66.

13. Canuso CM, Dirks B, Carothers J, et al. Randomized, double-blind, placebo-controlled study of paliperidone extended-release and quetiapine in inpatients with recently exacerbated schizophrenia. *Am J Psychiatry.* 2009;166(6):691-701.

14. Smith G, Smith J. Regression to the mean in average test scores. *Educational Assessment.* 10(4):377-99. Available at: http://economics-files.pomona.edu/GarySmith/ aveTestScores.pdf.

15. U.S. Department of Health and Human Services, Centers for Medicare & Medicaid Services. What is the purpose of the National Provider Identifier (NPI)? Who must

use it, and when? Available at: https://questions.cms.hhs.gov/app/answers/detail/a_ id/2623/kw/npi and https://questions.cms.hhs.gov/app/answers/detail/a_id/9419/kw/ npi .

16. Dodson A. Bay County ACT scores below national average, school officials say improvements on the horizon. August 1, 2010. Mlive.com.

17. See:

   • Martin BC, McMillan JA, Kotzan JA. Bias associated with missing out-of-plan prescription data for Medicaid recipients. *Journal of Research in Pharmaceutical Economics.* 1996;7(3):65-77.

   • Soumerai SB, Ross-Degnan D, Avorn J, McLaughlin T, Choodnovskiy I. Effects of Medicaid drug-payment limits on admissions to hospitals and nursing homes. *N Engl J Med.* 1991;325(15):1072-77.

18. Choudhry NK, Shrank WH. Four dollar generics—increased accessibility, impaired quality assurance. *N Engl J Med.* 2010;363(20):1885-87. Available at: http://www.nejm. org/doi/pdf/10.1056/NEJMp1006189?ssource=hcrc.

19. UnitedHealthcare. UnitedHealthcare expands Pharmacy Saver, bringing cost-savings opportunities to more Medicare plan members. December 13, 2010. Available at: http://www.uhc.com/news_room/2010_news_release_archive/unitedhealthcare_ expands_pharmacy_saver.htm.

20. Gleick E, Cohen A, Willwerth J. A tale of two states. *Time.* December 18, 1995.

21. This discussion is based on personal experience; I was hired as a researcher at AHCCCS in 1986 and was involved in the studies described here.

22. Blue Cross Blue Shield of Illinois. Obstetrical billing reference guide. Available at: http://www.bcbsil.com/PDF/ob_reference_guide.pdf.

23. Schwalm E. Unbundling: when to use modifier -59 and understanding CCI. August 6, 2006. Available at: http://www.ericacodes.com/Unbundling.htm.

24. Codingahead. 2011 CPT code changes. Available at: http://codingahead.blogspot. com/2010/11/2011-cpt-code-changes.html.

25. Bosler B. Coding changes for the integumentary system. *For The Record.* January 22, 2007;19(2):11. Available at: http://www.fortherecordmag.com/archives/ ftr_01222007p11.shtml.

26. For example, code 17000 was: "Destruction (e.g., laser surgery, electrosurgery, cryosurgery, chemosurgery, surgical curettement), all benign or premalignant lesions (e.g., actinic keratoses) other than skin tags or cutaneous vascular proliferative

lesions, first lesion." Anderson CA, Beebe M, Dalton JA, et al. *Current Procedural Terminology: CPT 2002.* Chicago, IL: American Medical Association; 2002.

27. Trailblazer. Self-administered drug exclusions – J4. Revised September 2011. Available at: http://www.trailblazerhealth.com/Specialty%20Services/Drugs%20and%20 Biologicals/SADExclusionJ4.aspx?DomainID=1.

28. Ward MM. Medicare reimbursement and the use of biologic agents: incentives, access, the public good, and optimal care. *Arthritis Care Res (Hoboken).* 2010;62(3):293-95.

29. Barbuto JP. Categorizing patients from medical claims data—the influence of GIGO. *J Manag Care Pharm.* 2004;10(6):559-60. Available at: http://www.amcp.org/data/jmcp/ Letters_559-566.pdf.

30. Rost K, Smith R, Matthews DB, Guise B. The deliberate misdiagnosis of major depression in primary care. *Arch Fam Med.* 1994;3(4):333-37. Available at: http:// archfami.ama-assn.org/cgi/reprint/3/4/333.

31. Manning JS. Tools to improve differential diagnosis of bipolar disorder in primary care. *Prim Care Companion J Clin Psychiatry.* 2010;12(Suppl 1):17-22.

32. Shetty S, Secnik K, Oglesby AK. Relationship of glycemic control to total diabetes-related costs for managed care health plan members with type 2 diabetes. *J Manag Care Pharm.* 2005;11(7):559-64. Available at: http://www.amcp.org/data/jmcp/ Original%20Research_559_564.pdf.

33. Ollendorf DA, Lidsky L. Infliximab drug and infusion costs among patients with Crohn's disease in a commercially-insured setting. *Am J Ther.* 2006;13(6):502-06.

34. Hennessy S, Bilker WB, Weber A, Strom BL. Descriptive analyses of the integrity of a US Medicaid claims database. *Pharmacoepidemiol Drug Saf.* 2003;12(2):103-11.

35. For example, see:
    - Curtis JR, Mudano AS, Solomon DH, Xi J, Melton ME, Saag KG. Identification and validation of vertebral compression fractures using administrative claims data. *Med Care.* 2009;47(1):69-72.
    - Damush TM, Jia H, Ried LD, et al. Case-finding algorithm for post-stroke depression in the veterans health administration. *Int J Geriatr Psychiatry.* 2008;23(5):517-22.
    - Dodds L, Spencer A, Shea S, et al. Validity of autism diagnoses using administrative health data. *Chronic Dis Can.* 2009;29(3):102-07.
    - Eichler AF, Lamont EB. Utility of administrative claims data for the study of brain metastases: a validation study. *J Neurooncol.* 2009;95(3):427-31.

- Ginde AA, Blanc PG, Lieberman RM, Camargo CA Jr. Validation of ICD-9-CM coding algorithm for improved identification of hypoglycemia visits. *BMC Endocr Disord.* 2008;8:4.
- Iezzoni LI. Using administrative data to study persons with disabilities. *Milbank Q.* 2002;80(2):347-79.
- Iezzoni LI, Greenberg MS. Capturing and classifying functional status information in administrative databases. *Health Care Financ Rev.* 2003;24(3):61-76.
- Iezzoni LI, Daley J, Heereen T, et al. Identifying complications of care using administrative data. *Med Care.* 1994;32(7):700-15.
- Quinn RR, Laupacis A, Austin PC, et al. Using administrative datasets to study outcomes in dialysis patients: a validation study. *Med Care.* 2010;48(8):745-50.
- Steele LS, Glazier RH, Lin E, Evans M. Using administrative data to measure ambulatory mental health service provision in primary care. *Med Care.* 2004;42(10):960-65.

36. Draak K. Don't procrastinate, ICD-10 will be here sooner than you expect. *AAPC News.* January 14, 2011. Available at: http://news.aapc.com/index.php/2011/01/dont-procrastinate-icd-10-will-be-here-sooner-than-you-expect/.

37. Centers for Medicare & Medicaid Services. General equivalence mappings: ICD-9-CM to and from ICD-10-CM and ICD-10-PCS. April 2010. Available at: http://www.cms.gov/ICD10/Downloads/GEMs-CrosswalksBasicFAQ.pdf. See also http://www.entnet.org/Practice/upload/Superbill-Template-ICD9.pdf and http://www.entnet.org/Practice/upload/Superbill-Template-ICD10.pdf.

38. American Academy of Otolaryngology—Head and Neck Surgery. Conversion of an ICD-9 superbill to ICD-10 superbill. Available at: http://www.entnet.org/Practice/Conversion-of-an-ICD-9-Superbill-to-ICD-10-Superbill.cfm.

39. CPT 2011: New modifier GU and revision to 76, 77, and 78 change your reporting. *Coding News: Medical Coding Advice & News for everyday use.* January 19, 2011. Available at: http://codingnews.inhealthcare.com/hot-coding-topics/cpt-2011-new-cpt-2011-modifier-gu-and-revisions-to-76-77-and-78-change-your-reporting/.

40. 2011 ICD-9-CM diagnosis code 564.4. ICD9Data.com. Available at: http://www.icd9data.com/2011/Volume1/520-579/560-569/564/564.4.htm.

41. See, for example:
- Bluekens AM, Karssemeijer N, Beijerinck D, et al. Consequences of digital mammography in population-based breast cancer screening: initial changes and

long-term impact on referral rates. *Eur Radiol.* 2010;20(9):2067-73.

- Ronco G, Cuzick J, Pierotti P, et al. Accuracy of liquid based versus conventional cytology: overall results of new technologies for cervical cancer screening: randomised controlled trial. *BMJ.* 2007;335(7609):28.

- Pisano ED, Hendrick RE, Yaffe MJ, et al.; DMIST Investigators Group. Diagnostic accuracy of digital versus film mammography: exploratory analysis of selected population subgroups in DMIST. *Radiology;* 2008;246(2):376-83.

42. See:

- Motheral B, Brooks J, Clark MA, et al. A checklist for retrospective database studies—report of the ISPOR Task Force on Retrospective Databases. *Value Health.* 2003;6(2):90-97. Available at: http://www.ispor.org/workpaper/research_practices/A_Checklist_for_Retroactive_Database_Studies-Retrospective_Database_Studies.pdf.

- Berger ML, Mamdani M, Atkins D, Johnson ML. Good research practices for comparative effectiveness research: defining, reporting and interpreting nonrandomized studies of treatment effects using secondary data sources: the ISPOR Good Research Practices for Retrospective Database Analysis Task Force Report—Part I. *Value Health.* 2009;12(8):1044-52. Available at: http://www.ispor.org/taskforces/documents/RDPartI.pdf.

- Cox E, Martin BC, Van Staa T, Garbe E, Siebert U, Johnson ML. Good research practices for comparative effectiveness research: approaches to mitigate bias and confounding in the design of nonrandomized studies of treatment effects using secondary data sources: The International Society for Pharmacoeconomics and Outcomes Research Good Research Practices for Retrospective Database Analysis Task Force Report—Part II. *Value Health.* 2009;12(8):1053-61. Available at: http://www.ispor.org/taskforces/documents/RDPartII.pdf.

- Johnson ML, Crown W, Martin BC, Dormuth CR, Siebert U. Good research practices for comparative effectiveness research: analytic methods to improve causal inference from nonrandomized studies of treatment effects using secondary data sources: the ISPOR Good Research Practices for Retrospective Database Analysis Task Force Report—Part III. 2009;12(8):1062-73. Available at: http://www.ispor.org/TaskForces/documents/RDPartIII.pdf.

Appendix 7A
How to Identify Common Services in a Medical Claims Dataset

Service and Summary of Identification Method

Office visits
- Use CPT EM codes indicating physician examination and assessment of the patient—"office or other outpatient services, new patient" (99201-99205) and "established patient" (99211-99215); "preventive medicine services, new patient" (99381-99387). Check EM codes for all years studied.
- Do not use EM codes specific to inpatient stays (e.g., hospital observation discharge services, 99218; initial hospital care, 99221-99223).
- Examine place of service codes (usually 11 for office and 20 for urgent care center) to look for discrepancies between EM codes and place of service; however, sometimes clinic visits on the campus of a hospital facility are coded with place of service 22 (hospital outpatient), and visits can take place in ambulatory surgical centers (place of service 24). There are also place-of-service codes for various types of clinics, mobile units, and other settings.
- To get the total charge for an office visit, sum the EM charge plus any charges for procedures or tests performed during the same visit (e.g., stitches, urinalysis); identify these by looking for same date of service and provider number as the EM claim.

Hospitalizations
- Use "room and board" codes (revenue codes 100-169 for various room and board types; 200-219 for ICU/CCU; and, for newborns, 170-179 for nursery). These indicate the dates of inpatient care.
- Note that multiple "room and board" claim lines for a single hospital stay are common—for example, a patient might spend the first five days on the ICU and the last three in a general surgical ward.
- Identify the start and end date of the hospital stay by looking for the earliest and latest dates of room and board services for each person, then check for gaps between the stays. For example, a person with room and board codes covering January 1 through January 10, then March 1 through March 10, has two hospital stays.
- For each stay, identify all of the services provided from the beginning through the ending date (e.g., surgeries, tests, EM, revenue codes indicating use of procedure rooms and laboratories—anything occurring during that span of days) and count these services as part of the hospital stay. Exceptions: Physician office visits and pharmacy claims on either the date of admission or the date of discharge should not be attributed to the hospital stay.
- Place of service code of 21 (inpatient) should *not* be used to identify hospital stays; this method is not reliable.

Emergency room
- Use revenue codes for ER use (revenue codes 450-459).
- Some ER services will span multiple days of service even though the patient was not admitted and was not an inpatient; this situation usually arises when a patient is admitted to the ER at nighttime and not discharged until after midnight (technically, the next day).
- Generally, all services provided during the date(s) of ER care are attributable to the ER visit, except for physician office visits and pharmacy claims.
- Some researchers use EM service codes for emergency care (99281-99288) to identify ER use, but this method is suboptimal because services may be missed (e.g., if EM code is not used during ER visit) or overcounted (e.g., if EM code for emergency care is erroneously used in an urgent care setting).
- Do *not* use place of service code of 23 (ER) to identify ER use because services with revenue codes 450-459 are sometimes billed with either place of service 21 (inpatient hospital) or place of service 22 (outpatient hospital).
- For patients admitted to the hospital from the ER, you will usually see both ER revenue codes (450-459) and room and board codes on the same day or one day apart. In this situation, most researchers count the ER visit as part of the inpatient stay.

CCU=coronary care unit; CPT=Current Procedural Terminology; EM=evaluation and management (a code classification in the CPT); ER=emergency room; ICU=intensive care unit.

Appendix 7B
Codes for Abdominal Pain and Diarrhea on
AAFP and Gastroenterology Superbills

AAFP:	789.00	Abdominal pain, unspec.
	787.91	Diarrhea, NOS
Gastroenterology:	789.01	Abd pain (RUQ)
	789.02	Abd pain (LUQ)
	789.03	Abd pain (RLQ)
	789.04	Abd pain (LLQ)
	009.2	Diarrhea, infectious
	564.4	Diarrhea, post-op
	564.5	Diarrhea, functional

Sources: Family practice superbill is available at: http://www.aafp.org/fpm/icd9/fpmsuperbill.pdf. Gastroenterology superbills are available at a variety of websites; because addresses may change, this chapter does not cite one in particular.

AAFP=American Academy of Family Physicians; Abd=abdominal; L=left; LQ=lower quadrant; NOS=not otherwise specified; R=right; UQ=upper quadrant.

CHAPTER 8

When in Doubt, Ask:
Writing and Administering an Effective Survey

"We make no claim to infallibility. We did not coin the phrase 'uncanny accuracy' which has been so freely applied to our Polls.... It would be a miracle if every State of the forty-eight behaved on Election Day exactly as forecast ..."—Editors of the *Literary Digest*, cautioning readers about their prediction that Alf Landon would defeat Franklin Roosevelt by a landslide margin in the Presidential election of 1936[1]

"There's a lot of room for humility in polling. Every time you get cocky, you lose."—Warren Mitofsky, widely considered to be the "father" of the exit poll[2]

"I don't think the government is out to get me or help someone else get me but it wouldn't surprise me if they were out to sell me something or help someone else sell me something. I mean, why else would the Census Bureau want to know my telephone number?"—Humorist Andy Rooney[3]

What You Will Learn in Chapter 8

✓ Why the choice to conduct a survey has ethical implications

✓ Why the *response rate* is among the most important measures of survey quality, and how to maximize it

✓ How *seeing the world through the eyes of your respondent* affects the reliability and validity of your survey

✓ What *total survey design* means and why you should practice it faithfully

✓ How to choose the best method of *administration* and write *questions* that will yield accurate results

---

"What's up with Nevada?" asked a daily report by respected pollster Scott Rasmussen on November 7, 2010.[4] Considered by politicians on both sides of the political aisle to be among the most consistently accurate prognosticators in U.S. politics,[5] Rasmussen's organization reported less than one week after the November

2010 election that it had missed—badly—in its prediction about the likely outcome of the Senate race between incumbent Harry Reid and challenger Sharron Angle. Like other polling organizations around the country, Rasmussen had picked Angle to win by several percentage points. Instead, Reid won by a margin of 5.6 points—in other words, a discrepancy of more than eight percentage points for a polling organization that rarely misses by as much as one.

Investigation of the missed call suggested a surprising explanation: unexpected election-day enthusiasm among voters who had described themselves *prior* to the election as less than enthusiastic. Rasmussen's final pre-election poll showed that among those who had already voted or described themselves as "absolutely certain to vote," Angle was in the lead, whereas Reid was the favorite among those who "said something might come up to prevent them from voting."[4] The same pattern appeared when voters were asked prior to the election how closely they were following election-related news; "the lower the rated level of interest" pre-election, "the higher the advantage was for Reid."[4] Yet, according to Rasmussen's current "working hypothesis" about the incident, a larger-than-expected group of those self-described disinterested voters turned out in force on Election Day and gave Reid the victory. Rasmussen indicated that, as good polling organizations typically do when errors of this type occur, it would evaluate "what changes we could have made in our sampling approach or Likely Voter [prediction] model to capture a more accurate sample."[4]

It was not the first time that a polling organization had experienced a prediction failure—and certainly it was not the most dramatic. Students of history know well the picture of a triumphantly grinning President Harry Truman two days after his re-election in November 1948, holding over his head the *Chicago Tribune* with its blaring headline: *DEWEY DEFEATS TRUMAN*.[6] Faced with an impending printer's strike on election night, the *Tribune*, which had previously denounced Truman as "a nincompoop," relied on predictions from several highly respected polling organizations instead of waiting for early election results and went to press with the news that Truman had lost his re-election bid to Governor Thomas Dewey.[6] The result was the now infamous headline error, which prompted one radio comedian to quip that Truman was the "first president to lose in a Gallup and win in a walk."[6] The causes of the mistake included premature termination of the Gallup polling efforts because "we had been lulled into thinking that nothing much changes in the last few weeks of the campaign," according to George Gallup, Jr., as well as use of "quota" (by-group) sampling instead of the **random sampling** (also known as **probability sampling**) methods favored today.[2]

Twelve years earlier, the *Literary Digest* had erred in predicting a landslide victory of Alf Landon over Franklin Roosevelt 57% to 43% in the 1936 Presidential election; instead, Roosevelt won 61% of the vote and defeated Landon handily.[1] That mistake was the result of **two problems. First** was an error in creating the **sampling frame**, that is, the list of study subjects used by the researcher in an attempt to represent the **target population,** the group of interest (voters in this example). The *Digest* poll had, in the midst of the Great Depression, made the mistake of drawing its sample from lists of telephone subscribers and automobile owners, who were wealthier than the population at large and therefore more likely to favor the Republican Landon. **Second**, the poll's **response rate** (i.e., the proportion of those asked to complete the survey who actually did so) was only 22%, indicating that the *actual* sample was only a small proportion of the *intended* sample and therefore might not represent the population well. Indeed, analysis of the prediction debacle revealed that Republicans were more likely to respond to the *Digest* survey than were Democrats—an early historical instance of **nonresponse bias**, in which those responding to a survey systematically differ from those who do not, producing misleading results.[1]

These accounts illustrate questions that arise frequently about surveys—not just political polls, but also market research, investigations of consumer behavior, satisfaction surveys, and quality-of-life measurements. Can survey data be trusted? Do survey findings accurately reflect the target population? Why do some surveys succeed in accurate measurement and/or prediction, whereas others fail?

In this chapter, we'll examine the strengths of surveys and potential pitfalls in conducting them. We'll look at how to select the type of survey to be performed and how to construct and administer a questionnaire that yields reliable and valid information.* We'll see that a survey is a powerful tool that, like any good tool, must be designed and used appropriately to produce the desired results. As in previous chapters, I assume that you have performed a literature review, are aware of what is known about your topic and what your survey is intended to add, and have a preliminary analysis plan (Chapter 4).

Should You Perform a Survey?

Among the most important decisions to be made in a survey project is whether to do

---

* Much of the material in this chapter was previously presented in Fairman KA. Going to the source: a guide to using surveys in health care research. *J Manag Care Pharm.* 1999;5(2):150-61. Available at: http://www.amcp.org/data/jmcp/ce_v2_150-161.pdf. It is used here with permission.

the survey at all. Careful consideration of "whether a survey would actually be the best way to acquire the information needed" is among the "best practices" recommendations of the American Association for Public Opinion Research (AAPOR), a good source of information about guidelines and strategies for survey research.[7] The AAPOR makes that recommendation in part because carrying out a survey project that yields valuable information, although certainly feasible, is harder than it looks. If you think that conducting a survey is the type of work that can be done "on the fly," sandwiched between database analyses intended to obtain more reliable information—please think again. Planning, writing, conducting, and interpreting a survey are tasks that take thought and considerable effort. More importantly, the decision to conduct a survey has ethical implications. As sociologist and survey research textbook author Earl Babbie (1986) notes:

> "Social research often, though not always, represents an intrusion into people's lives. The interviewer's knock on the door or the arrival of a questionnaire in the mail signals the beginning of an activity that the respondent has not requested and one that may require a significant portion of his or her time and energy. ... Social research, moreover, often requires that people reveal personal information about themselves—information that may be unknown to their friends and associates."[1]

In other words, a respondent's time and trust are valuable resources. It is incumbent upon a researcher to use these resources carefully and well, conducting a survey *only* when there is reason to believe that it will yield useful information. This ethical principle is among the reasons that the AAPOR "best practices" guidelines include the recommendation that researchers "have specific goals for the survey."[7]

For similar ethical reasons, surveys should *never* be used for purposes other than gathering information, such as marketing, persuasion, or even education. When prospective survey respondents are told about a "survey," their natural expectation is that the project's purpose is to determine their opinions and experiences—not to sell them a product or convince them to act in a particular way. To avoid misleading respondents, the investigator must fulfill that expectation. (Unfortunately, legitimate survey researchers must now contend with a notorious and especially troubling type of poor ethical behavior—the "push poll," in which political campaigning is disguised using a question that contains information or gossip about a candidate, such as "If you knew that [candidate name] had an illegitimate child, would you still vote for him?". Practices of this type discredit the survey research industry as a whole and make it harder for researchers to obtain responses to legitimate questionnaires.)

When is a survey most likely to produce accurate information? The key, as we will explore in more detail later in the chapter, is to remember what respondents *probably* know, what they *might* know, and what they *cannot reasonably be expected* to know. If respondents do not have the information that they need to answer the questions that you ask, *you might get responses anyway*—but they are unlikely to be worth much. This point leads to one key to an effective survey research project that will be explained in more detail throughout this chapter—try to **see the world through the eyes of your respondent** at every project phase.

What Information Can a Survey Provide?

Surveys contribute unique information because they go directly to consumers, voters, or whatever group is of interest. In an era in which all kinds of explanations and prognostications about public opinion can be (and are) distributed worldwide over the Internet at the push of a button, actually *obtaining* information directly from those who are the source of important decisions and beliefs can provide an important "reality check." In health care, consumers make numerous decisions that are critical to the clinical and economic outcomes of medical and pharmaceutical services. For example, consumers choose health plans and physicians, patronize particular pharmacies, request specific products or treatments, and decide whether to comply with the recommendations of medical professionals. Surveys can examine the reasons underlying those decisions.

Surveys can also play an important role in the interpretation of outcomes research using automated data, such as retrospective analyses of administrative claims databases, because they provide "process information." That is, by showing researchers not just *what* happened but *why* it happened, survey information can help researchers avoid the errors of confusing association with causation (Chapter 3) or of assuming that a pattern observed in claims data means one thing when actually it means something else entirely (Chapter 7).

Surveys in health care: a practical example. When one managed care organization (MCO) observed using its pharmacy claims (paid billing) data that some health plan members seemed to be getting no medication after receiving a "step-therapy" instruction (i.e., a requirement to try a lower-cost medication before receiving a higher-cost medication for the same condition) for proton pump inhibitors and nonsteroidal anti-inflammatory drugs, Cox et al. (2004) investigated the situation using a mailed survey. The sample comprised 201 patients who had received a step-therapy instruction during approximately the previous six months.[8] In the survey, 59% of patients reported obtaining medication through the health plan—not a surprising finding because the step-therapy process offered several ways to do so. But many respondents said that they had obtained medication in a different way, without using their health plan benefit. Eleven percent said that they paid the total cost themselves; 8% switched to an over-the-counter (nonprescription) drug; and 9% used samples from a physician or filled the prescription using their spouse's insurance. Only 11% said that they obtained no medication to treat their condition.

Still concerned about the 11% who reported receiving no medication in the mailed survey, the MCO used a small-sample telephone survey to contact members who had a step-therapy instruction followed by no pharmacy claim and ask them what had happened. Of those who remembered and confirmed receiving no medication (n=25), about one-third reported that they *had* actually taken medication to treat their condition but had obtained it another way—including having the drug on hand already before trying to fill the prescription, a response not anticipated by the research team and therefore not included in the original mailed survey. Additionally, 16% told the survey interviewers that they "did not need the medication or the issue resolved itself."[8]

Despite low response rates (23% by mail, 33% by telephone) that made the value of the survey results primarily qualitative, this study illustrated the benefits of obtaining information directly from consumers in several respects. **First**, the mailed survey showed that of the large minority (41%) who did not obtain medication through the health plan and therefore had no medication purchasing activity (i.e., no claims paid by the health plan), a majority—about 68%—reported obtaining medication through other sources that were not reflected in the plan's database. The health plan had no way to learn about these sources without asking patients about them. **Second**, the health plan discovered that it had missed an important point in interpreting its original analysis; sometimes patients keep on hand medication that was purchased previously and use it as needed. **Third**, the plan learned that a small proportion of patients saw no need for the drug that had been prescribed for them, at least at the time of the survey.

Total Survey Design

Early in any survey project, the principal investigator(s) must make important decisions that will affect both accuracy and cost. For reasons explained in more detail throughout this chapter, these decisions are interrelated. They include the following:

- **Mode of administration**—whether the survey will be administered by telephone, mail, interactive voice response (IVR, i.e., automated telephone), or Internet.
- **Content and source of questionnaire**—topics to be covered on the survey and whether an existing **survey instrument** (questionnaire) can be used or writing a new questionnaire is necessary.
- **Whom to survey**—decision rules to be used in drawing the sample.
- **How many to survey**—both the starting sample size (the number of attempts to be made) and the anticipated final sample size.
- **Response rate protocols**—methods that will be used to encourage response to the survey, such as postcard reminders, follow-up telephone calls to initial nonrespondents, or small monetary incentives mailed with the survey.
- **Professional help**—whether professional assistance is needed to write, pretest, or administer the survey and, if so, which professionals to choose.

In making all these decisions, a key concept is **total survey design**,[9] a perspective that emphasizes the quality of the survey research project *overall*. That is, total survey design incorporates the literature review, the text and ordering of survey questions, the pretesting process, the professionalism of materials and personnel that are presented to potential respondents, and the appropriateness of data collection methods for the sample and for the study topic. For example, a beautifully written questionnaire won't yield accurate information if it is printed with type so tiny that respondents can't read it, or if it is sent with a cover letter containing so many grammatical errors that respondents throw the whole packet in a trash can. Even a huge initial sample of 10,000 potential respondents will yield questionable information if the investigator invests so little time and money on follow-up to nonrespondents that the survey response rate is a meager 10%. Although small monetary incentives provided to respondents increase response rates,[10,11] even a survey that uses substantial incentives won't produce valid and reliable information if respondents become offended or confused by unclear language in the survey questions. And—a point to remember well—even a well-written questionnaire that yields highly accurate data will produce worthless information if the investigator neglected to determine before launching the project what the intended audience actually needed to know. Good planning is critical (Chapter 4).

Thus, to summarize "total design" as survey researcher Floyd Fowler (2002) describes it, "the quality of data will be no better than the most error-prone feature of the survey design."[9] The basic idea is to focus on *excellence* throughout the entire process, from beginning to end.

Planning the Survey

Literature review. After the initial study planning phase, including determination of the necessary sample size (Chapter 4), the first step in any survey project is to search previously published peer-reviewed research articles and the Internet for existing questionnaires that have been used to investigate similar research topics, particularly questionnaires that are standard in the field. This search has **two purposes**. **First**, if an acceptable questionnaire has already been developed, it might be unnecessary to incur the expense and effort of "reinventing the wheel." Using an already existing questionnaire is particularly appropriate if it has been subjected to tests of *reliability* (the degree to which a tool measures a phenomenon consistently) and **construct validity** (the degree to which a tool measures the concepts that it is intended to measure).[1,12] **Second**, if it is necessary to write a questionnaire, a solid understanding of previous work will help the investigator to write appropriate questions.

Two points about **using an existing questionnaire** are noteworthy. **First**, selection of a particular questionnaire may "force" the decision about how the survey will be administered. For reasons explained in more detail later in this chapter, some question formats are appropriate for mailed or Internet surveys but inappropriate for telephone or IVR, and vice versa. Thus, for example, if the existing questionnaire was validated in a mailed survey process, an investigator who wishes to use that questionnaire should also conduct a mailed survey if feasible. **Second**, for copyrighted questionnaires, it is important to incorporate user fees, if any, into the project budget and to allow sufficient time to obtain permission from the instrument source.

The importance of response rate in survey planning. At this and every project phase, the investigator must carefully consider the methods that will be necessary to maximize the survey response rate, which is rightly considered to be one of the most important measures of the **external validity** (applicability) and **internal validity** (accuracy of inference) of a survey. Why? *Response rates are a key measure of the degree to which the* *sample accurately represents the target population*, for **two reasons**.

First, low response rates often signal that only those who felt strongly about the survey topic took the time to respond.[1] In surveys of customer satisfaction with services or products, satisfaction rates commonly increase when an investigator introduces a new method that greatly enhances response rate—for example, a change from a postcard mailed with a shipment, which requires the recipient to seek out an opportunity to comment, to a telephone survey, which makes commenting easier.[13] This phenomenon occurs because when response rates are low, especially if suboptimal response is attributable to problems in the survey process, the respondents tend to be those whose dissatisfaction prompted them to make the effort to respond—the "unhappy customers."

An example of this phenomenon appears to have occurred in a 2008 Kaiser Family Foundation (KFF) survey of the effects of the economic downturn on families. KFF reported that when respondents were asked if they or anyone in the household had "decided to get married mainly to have access to your spouse's health care benefits" or "mainly so your spouse could have access to your health care benefits" in the past year, 7% answered yes.[14] That result certainly sounds as if lack of health insurance produced troubling unintended consequences—except that the *total* number of marriages in the United States that year was about 2,204,000, far less than 1% of the adult population, making the 7% estimate of *insurance-related* marriages implausible.[15] KFF advanced several explanations for the discrepancy, focused primarily on how respondents understood the question,[14] but a more likely explanation is that families with unusual experiences and/or especially strong feelings about economic hardship were particularly likely to respond to the survey. (Unfortunately, KFF did not report the survey response rate, a standard that will be discussed in Chapter 10.)

Second, nonrespondents tend to differ systematically from respondents in a variety of ways that are not always apparent to the investigator but could affect study results. For example, those aged 65 years or older are easier to contact for a survey—but less likely to consent to it—than are younger prospective respondents.[16,17] The resulting age bias is particularly problematic in a health care survey because number of medical conditions and use of medical services increase with age.

The effects of nonresponse bias on the accuracy of survey results can be devastating. In his brief and helpful book, *Survey Research Methods*, Fowler provides a great illustration of the problem, modified and explained in more detail in Table 8A.[9]

Table 8A
Range of Possible True Percentages for an Answer of 50%[a]

	Method	RR=90%	RR=70%	RR=50%	RR=30%	RR=10%
Bottom of range[b]	(A X RR) + (0% X NRR)= (50% X RR) + (0% X NRR)	45%	35%	25%	15%	5%
Top of range[b]	(A X RR) + (100% X NRR)= (50% X RR) + (100% X NRR)	55%	65%	75%	85%	95%

[a] For example, assume that 50% of respondents answer "yes" when asked "Do you plan to purchase Product X in the coming 4 weeks?"

[b] "Bottom of range" is calculated on the assumption that all nonrespondents would have answered "no" (multiply rate of nonresponse by 0%). "Top of range" is calculated on the assumption that all nonrespondents would have answered "yes" (multiply rate of nonresponse by 100%).

A=answer obtained in the survey (50% in this example); NRR=nonresponse rate; RR=response rate.

In fact, this was part of the painful lesson learned by the *Literary Digest* in its erroneous prediction that 57% of voters would support Landon in 1936. With a 22% response rate (remember, that's 78% *nonresponse*!), Landon's actual support as predicted by the survey ranged from 12.5% if all nonrespondents voted for Roosevelt (57% X 22%) to 90.5% if all nonrespondents voted for Landon ([57% X 22%] + [100% X 78%]). Thus, good intentions and reputation aside, the *Digest* poll results were highly unreliable—and on Election Day, it showed.

Response rate calculation and planning. Calculating the response rate is simple but requires good project documentation (Chapter 2). The response rate is defined as the proportion of eligible respondents (those who meet study criteria) who actually complete the questionnaire.[18] Respondents who are inappropriate for study are excluded from the calculation.

For example, assume that Health-R-Us HMO is conducting a member satisfaction survey. Because the HMO has determined in advance that, for privacy reasons, members cannot be telephoned at work, an eligible respondent is defined as a Health-R-Us member with an accurate home telephone number. Of 1,000 members telephoned, 600 complete the interview, 100 are not reached, 100 advise the interviewer that they no longer belong to Health-R-Us, and 100 refuse to complete the survey. For an additional 100, the telephone number provided to the health plan is determined to be a business, so the call is terminated without attempting an interview. The response rate is 75%, derived as follows:

$$\textbf{numerator} = \underline{600 \text{ completed interviews}}$$
$$\textbf{denominator} = 1,000 \text{ attempts} -$$
$$(100 \text{ nonmembers} + 100 \text{ business telephone number}) = 800$$

Note that only those ineligible for study are removed from the denominator. *Both* refusals *and* members who were not reached are *included* in the denominator, because there is no information to suggest they are ineligible for study. Only completed interviews are included in the numerator.[17,18]

The *anticipated* response rate should also be used in determining the starting sample size (the number of initial survey attempts). Assume, for example, that an investigator has used a standard formula for sample size calculation (Chapter 4) to determine that the number of cases needed for analysis is 300. If the expected response rate is 80%, the number of attempted interviews should be 300 ÷ 0.80=375.

Choosing whom to survey. At this stage, the investigator must also choose the *sampling frame*. The general rule of thumb is that the sampling frame should, as closely as possible, represent the population to which the results of the project will be applied.[7] Yet despite the apparent simplicity of this decision rule, actually achieving this standard is not always easy, as described well by Graham Kalton in his book, *Introduction to Survey Sampling* (1983):[19]

> *"Consider, for instance, a survey to be carried out in a city to discover the degree of support for the introduction of a new bus system. Should the survey be confined to persons living within the city boundaries? What is the minimum age for the population to be surveyed? Should residents ineligible to vote in city elections be included? Should visitors living temporarily in the city be excluded, and if so, how are they to be defined? A variety of questions like these arise in defining most populations, making the definitional task less straightforward than it might at first appear."[19]*

Even after making decisions about the *intended* sampling frame, choices about how to **operationalize** the sampling frame—that is, translate the concept into specific decision rules—may be difficult. For example, suppose a researcher wants to perform a survey to ask people who are prescribed Drug A about their experiences, such as ease or difficulty in filling the initial prescription, side effects, how long they took Drug A, and why they stopped taking Drug A. First, the researcher must determine how to identify patients who are prescribed Drug A. Should the researcher target for sampling those patients who fill at least one prescription for Drug A during a certain period of time?* That is a relatively easy way to identify patients—but that sampling method will miss patients who obtained free samples of Drug A from their physicians, received Drug A as part of a "patient assistance program," or failed to fill their initial prescription for Drug A. Should the researcher use medical records review to identify patients whose physicians prescribed Drug A for them? That is a good way to measure all prescribed medication—but it requires obtaining permission from the physician offices and possibly the patients to audit medical records, not an easy task. Apart from the role that patient privacy standards may play in making these decisions,[20] patients and physicians who assent to such requests may differ systematically from those who refuse, posing threats to internal and external validity (Chapter 3).

Once those hurdles are overcome, the researcher must determine whether to study patients who receive Drug A for *any* diagnosis or for only certain diagnoses. If the latter, the researcher must determine how to identify the diagnoses and whether the diagnoses should be selected according to U.S. Food and Drug Administration-approved indications, published guidelines for treating particular diseases, or something else.

These decisions can become complex, making it particularly important to incorporate feedback from knowledgeable colleagues and professionals into the planning process (Chapter 4). Three rules of thumb, as described by Fowler, are **comprehensiveness**, **efficiency**, and **probability of selection**.[9]

Comprehensiveness refers to whether the planned procedures will yield a sample that is reasonably representative of the population of interest. For example, a sample that is drawn from telephone directories omits those with unlisted numbers, and a survey administered over the Internet omits those without computers (unless the researcher provides them to respondents, as some Internet survey firms do).

Efficiency refers to the amount of effort that must be expended by researchers and respondents to determine if a potential subject meets the sampling requirements for the survey. This process is known as **sample screening**, that is, asking questions to determine if the potential respondent is or is not a member of the sampling frame *before* beginning the

---

* Recall from Chapter 7 an advantage of using secondary-source databases—when the data are anonymized (i.e., contain no identifying information), obtaining specific permission from the patient to use the data for research purposes is generally not required. However, using anonymized data to identify patients for a survey is obviously impossible. At this writing, the legality of using medical or pharmacy claims data to contact patients is highly controversial. Generally, according to the Health Insurance Portability and Accountability Act (HIPAA) of 1996, health care organizations can legally use "protected health information" as part of their "treatment, payment, and health care operations" (i.e., normal course of business to maintain and improve health plan services).[20] However, use of protected health information to identify potential survey respondents requires review by an internal or external consultant who has expertise in HIPAA requirements.

survey. For example, a survey that is targeted to pharmacy customers might ask potential respondents if they have made at least one purchase at any pharmacy in the past month. Chances are that a majority will answer yes, making the screening process efficient. In contrast, a screening process that eliminates many potential respondents—such as requiring that a potential respondent has a rare disease, filled prescriptions for drugs to treat that disease in the past week, and filled no prescriptions to treat the disease in the previous six months— is highly inefficient. Surprisingly, efficiency sometimes has ethical implications. For example, requiring that a respondent answer 30 minutes of questions to determine if he or she is eligible for a project that will pay $25 for each completed survey is ethically questionable because it requires a great deal of the respondent's time for potentially no benefit.

Probability of selection refers to knowledge of the mathematical likelihood that a particular research subject was selected for a sample. For example, purchasing a database of individuals living within a 5-mile radius of a pharmacy, identifying a 5% sample using a random number generator, and then sending a mailed survey to those individuals yields a sample of potential pharmacy customers for whom the probability of selection is known, that is, a **probability sample**. A commonly used probability sampling

> ### Key Points: Survey Sampling
>
> ❖ Choice of sampling frame is not always straightforward—seek advice.
> ❖ Check for comprehensiveness (accurate representation) and screening efficiency.
> ❖ Probability samples yield more valid results than convenience samples.
> ❖ Samples with low response rates or unknown probability of selection may indicate a biased group of respondents.

method in telephone surveying is random digit dialing, in which a computer sets some digits to a fixed value (often the first six digits) and then chooses the remaining digits using a random number generator. The randomly generated number is dialed and, when someone in the household answers the telephone, an individual within the household is then chosen at random using one of a variety of algorithms (e.g., the family member with the most recent birthday).

In contrast, selecting pharmacy customers by standing in the pharmacy parking lot, looking friendly, and administering the survey to anyone who approaches is a **convenience sampling** method, in which administration of the survey is based on the convenience of the investigator and/or study subjects. Using this method, there is no record of who did or did not respond and no way to determine the probability of selection or, by extension, the degree of potential nonresponse bias.

Probability of selection is **important for three reasons. First**, as we saw in Chapter 5, for appropriate use of statistical testing and other mathematical operations, the probability of selection need not be *equal* for all research subjects, but it must be *known* so that appropriate weighting procedures can be performed if necessary (e.g., for stratified samples). More complex survey sampling designs, such as *cluster sampling* (e.g., sampling a group of physicians, then surveying all patients treated by those physicians) and *multistage sampling* (e.g., sampling a group of MCOs, then sampling physicians within each MCO, then sampling a proportion of patients treated by those physicians) require special analytic techniques.[19,21] These techniques adjust both for probability of selection and for homogeneity within clusters—for example, similar patterns of care for a group of patients treated by the same physician.[21]

Second, inferential statistical tests (i.e., tests of statistical significance) assume a probability sample of the population, making tests performed in convenience samples of questionable validity (although they are commonly performed, nonetheless). **Third**, partly because convenience sampling methods tend to attract respondents who are particularly interested in and/or knowledgeable about the survey topic, comparisons of convenience samples with probability samples have shown that the latter produce much more accurate results,[22,23] although these comparisons are controversial.[24]

Choosing how to survey: mode of administration. For a researcher who has not selected an existing instrument with a particular mode of administration, the choice of mail, telephone, IVR, or Internet can be extremely important. A good general rule of thumb in choosing the survey mode is articulated in the AAPOR best practices guidelines—the researcher should use an approach that will balance the cost of the project, including budgetary considerations and staff availability, against the need for accuracy.[7] The keys to a good decision are knowledge of the advantages and disadvantages of the chosen method *and* the willingness to invest the monetary and/or human resources that are necessary to use the method well. For example, a successful telephone interview project requires highly trained interviewers and multiple follow-up calls for initial nonrespondents. A successful mailed survey project requires high-quality printed materials, as well as mailed and/or telephone follow-up reminders to complete the survey. These elements require the expenditure of time and/or money. Nonetheless, if the study results are to be used to make important policy decisions (e.g., a decision by a health plan about preferred drugs for a formulary) or are intended for publication, resources should be made available to maximize response quantity and quality.

Table 8B provides a summary comparison of the four methods.

Table 8B
Key Features of Four Survey Modes

Mail	Telephone	IVR	Internet
Response rates in a well-done project[a]			
~70%-80%	~70%-80%	Information is limited, but one well-done project found a response rate of ~30% initially and ~50% after intensive telephone follow-up[10]	Usually at least 20 percentage points less than mail or telephone, and often less than 10%-15%
Staff/consultant time/cost assuming a well-done project			
Survey package assembly time, plus follow-up for initial nonresponse	Extensive interviewer training time plus interview time; follow-up calls for initial nonresponse	Extensive computer programming time plus telephone follow-up for initial nonresponse	Extensive computer programming time plus telephone follow-up for initial nonresponse
Physical overhead costs			
Office space for assembly of survey packets (usually a survey and cover letter)	Adequate number of telephones	Little or none	Little or none
Materials costs[b]			
Introductory postcards and postage, printed questionnaires, postage for mail-outs, postage-paid return envelopes	None, or introductory postcards and postage	None, or introductory postcards and postage	None, or introductory postcards and postage
Questions presented exactly as worded by investigator			
Always	Depends on training	Always	Always
Best question response scales (Appendix 8A)			
• Labeled scale points • Matrix formats • Graphic depictions • Simple response choices	• Polar-end scales • Open-ended • Simple response choices	• Polar-end scales • Simple response choices	• Labeled scale points • Matrix formats • Graphic depictions, especially complex or interactive • Simple response choices
Strengths			
• Can include monetary incentive with the mailing to boost response rate. • Respondent can answer at his or her own pace. • Familiar format for many respondents.	• Permits probing questions to make sense of topics that are not well understood. • If CATI is used, it is easy to skip respondents over questions that do not apply to them.	• No "interviewer effect." • Once initial programming is completed, costs are low. • Foreign-language speakers can be surveyed without hiring bilingual or multilingual interviewers.	• Permits the use of "panels" of respondents with rare conditions or situations (e.g., a disease with a low prevalence rate), increasing efficiency. • Easy to skip respondents over questions that do not apply to them.

Table 8B *(continued)*
Key Features of Four Survey Modes

Mail	Telephone	IVR	Internet
Strengths (continued)			
	• If CATI is used, data entry is unnecessary—the interviewer does it.	• Good for respondents with limited reading ability (including visual impairment). • Data entry is unnecessary—the respondent does it.	• If programming is done well, respondent can answer questions at his or her own pace. • Data entry is unnecessary—the respondent does it. • Especially good when a convenience sample is acceptable.
Weaknesses			
• Can frustrate respondents whose answers do not fit neatly into the choices shown on the survey—they may want to explain their answers. • Requires respondents to be able to read questions. • Open-ended questions may be difficult for respondents if the answer is lengthy. • Data entry can introduce error.	• Particularly vulnerable to "social desirability bias" (i.e., giving answers that the respondent thinks the interviewer wants to hear). • Subject to "interviewer effect"—answers may depend on which interviewer the respondent happens to get (mitigated or eliminated with good interviewer training). • *Might* be subject to "primacy effect" (respondent selects first choice that is read to him/her) or "recency effect" (respondent selects last choice read).	• Start-up programming costs can be high. • Premature survey termination is much more likely with IVR than with a live telephone interview. • Responses are constrained to particular words or response choices—can frustrate respondents who may want to explain their answers. • Respondents dislike long IVR surveys; better suited to short questionnaires. • *Might* be subject to "primacy effect" (respondent selects first choice that is read to him/her) or "recency effect" (respondent selects last choice read).	• Start-up programming costs can be high. • For efficiency, usually requires an existing email database or a panel. • Some Internet survey firms use convenience samples, making accuracy and statistical inference problematic. • Requires respondents to be able to read questions. • Requires respondents to be computer literate and to have computer access; however, some Internet survey firms provide computers to respondent panels.

[a] The definition of "well-done" refers to the "total design" approach, including advance notice of the survey (e.g., an introductory postcard), professionalism, well-written questionnaire, small monetary incentives when possible, follow-up to those who do not respond initially, and trained interviewers if applicable.
[b] Use of a copyrighted instrument may require paying use fees to the instrument's owner regardless of mode of administration.
Sources:
Best and Radcliff. *Polling America.*[25]
Chang and Krosnick. National surveys via RDD telephone interviewing versus the Internet.[22]
Dillman. *The Total Design Method.*[26]
Dillman et al. Response rate and measurement differences in mixed-mode surveys.[10]
Fowler. *Survey Research Methods.*[9]
Schonlau et al. *Conducting Research Surveys via E-Mail and the Web.*[27]
CATI=computer-assisted telephone interviewing; panel=a group of people identified in advance of survey administration who agree to participate in survey projects periodically; RDD=random digit dialing.

Several decision-making factors in the table are noteworthy. First, the choice of mode depends in part on the sampling frame and the type of information that the investigator wants to obtain. For example, for respondents whose reading ability is limited (including those who are visually impaired), either telephone or IVR will be necessary. In an exploratory survey, such as the step-therapy survey performed by the MCO described earlier in this chapter, telephone interviewing can be exceptionally helpful because a well-trained interviewer can ask follow-up questions, typically using neutrally worded probes (e.g., "Can you tell me more about that?" "And why was that?") to get more information about a relatively unknown topic. For sensitive topics (e.g., drug addictions, sexually transmitted disease, medication compliance), mail, IVR, or Internet administration may be more appropriate than telephone because of *social desirability*, the tendency of respondents to present themselves in the best possible light or to provide what they believe is the desired response in the presence of an interviewer.

The scales that are best suited to address the study topic should also be taken into account when selecting the administration mode (Appendix 8A). Any administration mode can be used for questions with two or three simple response choices (e.g., yes/no, agree/disagree/not sure). Topics that can be addressed well with "polar end" numeric scales (e.g., "On a scale of 0 to 10, where 0 is worst, and 10 is best …") are especially well-suited to auditory modes (i.e., telephone and IVR) but can be used well in visual modes (i.e., mail or Internet). Likert-type scales, in which ordered categories are used (e.g., Strongly Agree, Somewhat Agree, Somewhat Disagree, Strongly Disagree), can be used for either auditory or visual modes. However, if the Likert-type scale changes mid-questionnaire (e.g., from Strongly Agree, Somewhat Agree, etc., to Excellent, Good, Fair, or Poor), auditory administration is likely to become cumbersome and confusing. Mail or Internet administration is necessary for topics that require the use of graphics to illustrate one or more questions.

For multipart questions, in which there is a single "root" question (e.g., "Which of the following strategies did you use during the past year to save on prescription drug costs?") followed by multiple subparts (e.g., shopped at a discount pharmacy, obtained samples from the physician, skipped at least one dose), a matrix format is clearer and much more succinct than repeating the root question for every subpart (e.g., "Did you shop at a discount pharmacy to save on prescription drug costs during the past year? Did you obtain samples from a physician to save on prescription drug costs during the past year?"). When a matrix format is optimal, a mailed or Internet survey should be used.

Mixed mode: if at first you don't succeed. An approach that is becoming increasingly popular is the **mixed mode** survey, in which a researcher begins with one mode of administration and then, if that does not produce a response, offers the respondent the opportunity to take the survey using a different mode. The rationale underlying the mixed mode approach is that respondents who feel uncomfortable with one mode of administration (e.g., mail) might feel more comfortable with another (e.g., telephone).[10]

Intuitively, the mixed mode concept makes sense; we all know people who "don't like the telephone" or "lose mail" in a heaping pile on the dining room table. Experimental data suggest that this approach increases response rates. Dillman et al. and Gallup (2009) conducted a well-done study in which potential survey respondents were randomized to one of four administration modes, followed by switching initial nonrespondents to a different administration mode.[10] The questionnaire content was identical for all four groups. The groups and response rates are summarized in Table 8C.

Table 8C
Results of Gallup "Mixed-Mode" Experiment

Group	First Mode	Second Mode (For Those Not Responding to First)	RR After First Mode	RR After Second Mode
1	**Mail:** Mailed advance notice of survey, mailed questionnaire with personalized letter and $2 bill, follow-up reminder postcard	**Telephone:** Contact from Gallup by telephone with at least four callbacks at different days/times if necessary to complete interview	75.0%	82.8%
2	**Telephone:** Contact from Gallup by telephone with at least four callbacks at different days/times if necessary to complete interview[a]	**Mail:** Mailed questionnaire with personalized letter and $2 bill, follow-up reminder postcard	43.3%-43.4%[a]	80.4%
3	**IVR:** Contact from Gallup by telephone using live interviewer, with invitation to complete remainder of survey using IVR	**Telephone:** Contact from Gallup by telephone with at least four callbacks at different days/times if necessary to complete interview	28.5%	50.4%
4	**Internet:** Contact from Gallup by telephone using live interviewer, with invitation to complete remainder of survey using Internet. Those who agreed were sent a letter with survey completion instructions and a $2 bill. Follow-up email was sent to initial nonrespondents	**Telephone:** Contact from Gallup by telephone with at least four callbacks at different days/times if necessary to complete interview	12.7%	47.7%

[a] Two separate telephone conditions were employed to test the effects of the order in which response choices were heard; this distinction is not important for this table and is not shown.
Source: Dillman et al. Response rate and measurement differences in mixed-mode surveys.[10]
IVR=interactive voice response; RR=response rate.

Three points should be highlighted. **First**, even using the mixed mode approach, the use of the Internet or IVR as the initial mode ultimately yielded response rates much lower than those achieved with initial data collection by mail or telephone. However, the results should be interpreted in light of the years in which the data were collected (from late 1999 to early 2000), when automated methods were not as widely used as they are today. **Second**, as Dillman has observed, switches from one mode to another must be made cautiously because question formats may not always "translate" well.[28] For example, questions asked and answered easily using a matrix format on the Internet may become quite cumbersome when asked over the telephone (Appendix 8A). **Third**, the effectiveness of the mixed-mode approach in the Dillman/Gallup study is consistent with the results of previously published work. Shettle and Mooney (1999) found that after two mailed survey attempts with a small monetary incentive, their response rate was 73%; offering a telephone interview increased the response rate to 81%; and in-person interviewing yielded a final cumulative 88% rate of response.[11]

Hiring a professional. Another important decision to be made at the planning stage is whether to use a professional or conduct the survey using only "in-house" staff. A review of any survey project by a well-trained professional survey researcher will likely enhance the quality of results obtained. However, such a review may be unnecessary or too costly, especially for small-scale or low-budget projects. How does an investigator know whether the expenditure and effort to employ a professional are necessary?

Generally, the services of a survey researcher should be employed when results are to be used to make particularly important decisions (e.g., to identify physicians who will receive a "high-quality" designation in a provider network directory) or to fulfill statutory, contractual, or external quality review requirements, such as for accreditation. Obtaining professional services is prudent when results are intended for publication or when the questionnaire will discuss sensitive or potentially threatening topics. Services could range from full-scale project administration to brief review/consultant arrangements, depending on project budget, complexity, and scope.

Choosing a professional. If the choice is made to outsource all or part of a survey project, the principal investigator must choose the individuals and firms to be used. If you are responsible for hiring a questionnaire writer, ask to see a copy of one or more of the writer's surveys and cover letters. Compare these materials with the measures of quality that are described in the next section. Additionally, try to take the surveys yourself; and ask a few others, preferably of different educational levels and backgrounds, to do the same. If all the items and response choices are clear, that is a good sign of high-quality work. On the other hand, if you find yourself confused about how to respond, your respondents probably will be confused, too—and you might want to look elsewhere to find your survey writer.

To choose a telephone interviewing firm, ask about interviewer training procedures, and compare the firm's procedures with the best practices that are described later in this chapter. Additionally, ask about monitoring procedures. High-quality telephone survey firms monitor data collection on a regular basis to ensure that study protocols are strictly followed and that results are reliable, an AAPOR best practice recommendation.[7] If legally permissible (depending on the state), some firms even monitor interviews by telephone in "real-time," so that if they hear a problem with an interviewer's technique, they can correct it on the spot.

To choose an Internet survey firm, take one or more questionnaires online to assess clarity and check for "bugs" and problems in administration. Examples of common problems include being unable to return to the previous question after submitting the answer or becoming "stuck" because you are required to give a response to an item that you cannot answer before moving to the next page.

Additionally, one of the most important questions to ask an Internet survey firm is what sampling method it uses. Some Internet survey firms use random digit dialing to telephone potential respondents and offer the chance to participate in the survey. Although this method generally yields a lower response rate than traditional telephone interviewing (because some respondents do not complete the Internet survey), it does yield a probability sample.[22,27] In contrast, some Internet firms use online advertisements to recruit survey participants; anyone who volunteers is accepted into the survey panel.[22,27] This is a convenience sampling method that, like all convenience sampling, tends to attract those especially interested in the topic and may overrepresent certain groups, such as those with better educations and higher incomes.[22] Although a survey sample drawn in this way might yield useful information, a firm that uses this approach should be selected with caution and a clear understanding of the risks of mischaracterizing the population.[22-24] It is also important to ask about weighting methods that the firm recommends or uses to account for potential biases; however, Internet convenience sample results may be inaccurate even after "best practice" weighting.[24]

Writing a High-Quality Questionnaire

Five principles of questionnaire construction should guide the survey writer:

1. Enlist the respondent's interest and trust.
2. Maintain trust by keeping respondent burden (the degree of difficulty in completing the survey) to a minimum.
3. Provide an attractive product.
4. See the world through your respondent's eyes—this will increase the accuracy of data collection *and* reassure the respondent that you understand his or her perspective.
5. Use open-ended items strategically and in a way that is consistent with the level of effort necessary to answer them.

If the first four of these principles sound like marketing advice, it's because they are; conducting a survey is, in a sense, a sales task. The investigator wants something (information) and in return must provide something—the opportunity to be involved in an interesting project, the rewarding feeling of helping others, and/or the chance to express an opinion. For the respondent to feel confident that the promised "goods" will be delivered, the investigator, associates (e.g., telephone interviewers), and all written materials must be highly professional and must appeal to the respondent. Methods used to operationalize each of these principles are summarized in Table 8D and discussed in more detail below.

Enlist the Respondent's Interest and Trust: How to Write Introductory Material

The old saying that first impressions are important applies nowhere more than in an introduction to a survey. *The initial study description provided to prospective respondents tells them what the project and the investigator are all about. Their decision about whether to participate will be based on the beliefs generated by that description.* A number of techniques enhance the likelihood of enlisting the respondent's trust. It is usually not feasible to use all of these, but as many as possible should be employed.[1,9,26,29] These principles apply to all types of introductory material, such as a cover letter for a mailed survey or opening script for a telephone survey.

First, it is important to make the prospective respondent aware that the investigator is credible. If the survey is sponsored or commissioned by a respected organization,

Table 8D
Checklist of Key Principles and Practices in Questionnaire Writing

Respondent's interest and trust
➤ Investigator's credentials, organizational sponsorship
➤ Importance of project (use nonbiased language)
➤ Personalized communications
➤ Ethical principles of voluntarism and confidentiality
➤ Material incentives if possible (e.g., small reward, drawing for a prize available only to survey participants)

Minimizing respondent burden
➤ Survey as brief as possible, without repetition
➤ Minimal effort with no financial cost for respondents
➤ Contingency questions when appropriate
➤ Process as convenient as possible for respondents using whatever means are necessary (e.g., for a telephone interview survey, interviewers available at nights and on weekends)

Attractive, professional product
➤ "Advance notice" provided to respondents (e.g., a postcard prior to mailing a full questionnaire or initiating a telephone interview)
➤ Weight, color of mailed materials
➤ Spacious feeling—plenty of "white space" on each page of a mailed survey, only a few questions per screen on an Internet survey
➤ Carefully trained interviewers

Clarity and ease of completion
➤ Terms, questions that respondents are able to understand
➤ Refer to specific time frames, events when possible
➤ Response choices mutually exclusive and appropriate for population
➤ No "double-barrelled" items
➤ Questionnaire in logical order
➤ Introduction to every major section
➤ Items with similar topics, response choices grouped together
➤ Attention to "order effects"
➤ Simple, attractive graphics

Handling open-ended items
➤ Open-ended items "precoded" if necessary
➤ Consistency and accuracy of precoding verified
➤ Careful screening of quotations for presentation or publication to ensure that they do not identify individual respondents

Sources:
Babbie. *The Practice of Social Research.*[1]
Dillman. *The Total Design Method.*[26]
Fowler. *Survey Research Methods.*[9]
Schonlau et al. *Conducting Research Surveys via E-Mail and the Web.*[27]

particularly one to which prospective respondents belong, this should be mentioned (e.g., "The Pharmaceutical Treatment Association asked me to conduct this survey because..."). Researchers commonly put a cover letter or introductory postcard on the sponsoring organization's official stationary or use its official seal (with permission, of course). Mentioning the investigator's credentials is helpful as well (e.g., "As a Professor of Pharmacology with Halls-of-Learning University, I know the importance of...").

Second, the introductory material should explain the importance of the project. For example, the introduction to a survey of enrollee attitudes toward a proposed benefit change might mention that the change is being considered for implementation next year. The introduction to a survey measuring satisfaction with a particular subcontracting firm might mention that its contract is up for renewal. These descriptions must be completely honest. Additionally, they must not bias the respondent in any way. For example, it would be inappropriate to tell respondents, "We would like to know what problems people are having with the Healthy-U Center so that we can decide whether to terminate their contract" (even if that is one purpose of the survey). Instead, it would be better to say, "We would like to know about your experiences with the Healthy-U Center, so that we can make an informed decision when it is time to reissue our contracts on July 1, 2010."

Third, the introductory material should be personalized with the respondent's name if possible (i.e., "Dear Mr. Smith" instead of "Dear Health Plan Member") and should emphasize the respondent's value to the project (e.g., "I know that your time is valuable, but hearing your point of view would help us greatly."). This information signals to respondents that you respect them and would not allow them to incur unnecessary burdens. The respondent's individual contribution should be emphasized (e.g., "We need your answers to these important questions to help us make sound policy decisions."). If the respondent is part of a carefully selected sample of, for example, leaders in the physician community or successful health plan executives, emphasize this.

Fourth, the introductory material should never imply in any way that the respondent is obligated to complete the survey. Ethical principles dictate that all research participation is voluntary. In addition, attempting to coerce respondents may annoy them. It is better to inform the respondent fully, including a truthful assessment of how long it takes to complete the survey (e.g., "Do you have about five minutes to speak with me now?"). Let the respondent know of the right to refuse in a way that emphasizes the respondent's importance to the project (e.g., "You do not have to answer my questions, but your answers will help us to learn about the experiences of people who belong to the Health-

R-Us Healthplan.").

Fifth, ethical principles also require that assurances of confidentiality be provided, and investigators must maintain strict control over study data to ensure that these promises are kept.[1,7,9] The methods necessary to achieve confidentiality will vary depending on the mode of data collection. For example, in their helpful guide to Internet surveys, Schonlau et al. (2002) recommend that a password be required for entry into the survey to protect respondents.[27]

Finally, providing a *material incentive* to participate is a proven technique for enlisting respondents.[11,26,30] Some researchers include one or two dollars in every mailed survey. Others enter participants in a drawing for a prize. Additionally, respondents may be offered a copy of the report of study results, as long as the report will present no information that would violate the confidentiality of any other respondents.

Maintain Trust by Minimizing Respondent Burden[1]

Several techniques strengthen the trust and interest of respondents by minimizing their cost of participation. **First,** the survey should be as brief as possible, asking only necessary questions. However, the need for a longer survey in order to cover a topic adequately is not cause for alarm. Respondents will complete lengthy surveys if they are interesting and attractively presented. It is not uncommon for good survey research organizations to achieve response rates in excess of 80% for interviews of one-half hour or longer. However, questions should not appear repetitious, a flaw that makes respondents feel that they are wasting time.

Second, respondents should never incur any financial cost for participation, and time expenditures for administrative tasks should be kept to a minimum. Mailed surveys should include a pre-addressed, postage-paid envelope for easy return. If respondents need to return calls to participate in a telephone survey, a toll-free number should be provided. For Internet surveys, the program should permit respondents to stop, save their work, and re-enter the survey at a later time, especially if the survey is lengthy.[27]

Finally, respondents should never have to expend effort figuring out whether a question applies to them.[1] To avoid this problem, surveys use **contingency questions** that are ordered using **skip patterns.** For example, in a satisfaction survey of health plan members, there might be a series of items regarding pharmacy services. The investigator might want answers from those members who have used the pharmacy within the past month. Asking, "If you used a pharmacy within the past month, please rate the services provided by the pharmacist." "If you used a pharmacy within the past month, please rate the convenience of the location." is incorrect. This question format is repetitious, and requires respondents to make decisions about whether to answer the questions, which can be confusing and time-consuming, particularly in a multiquestion series. In contrast, the correct format tells the respondent exactly what to do by having the respondent "skip" over inapplicable questions. For example:

4. Have you used the Health-R-Us pharmacy within the past month?

[   ] Yes—*Continue with Question 5*
[   ] No—*Skip to Question 10*

5. I'd like you to think about your most recent visit to the Health-R-Us pharmacy. How would you rate the *overall quality of service* that you received? Would you say that it was Excellent, Good, Fair, or Poor?

Additionally, language used in the survey should be understandable to the target population, an AAPOR best practice.[7,32] Respondents who are baffled by terminology will quickly give up, denying you the opportunity to receive valuable information.

Provide an Attractive Product

To promote respondents' trust and willingness to participate, a professional appearance is essential.[1,26] Surveys mailed using first-class postage generate higher response rates than bulk-rate mailings. The weight and color of the paper should have a professional, not flimsy, feel. Booklet formats are easy to construct and make an attractive presentation. An attractive logo is often helpful. If graphics within the questionnaire itself are necessary, they should be visually appealing and clear. For the return envelope (in which the survey will be mailed back), sometimes researchers use a first-class stamp instead of business-reply postage. The advantage of this approach is that the stamp may prompt the prospective respondent to feel obligated to complete and return the questionnaire. The disadvantage is the higher cost of purchasing a first-class stamp for every prospective respondent (even those who will not return a questionnaire).

The spacing of the questionnaire makes a particularly important contribution to professional appearance. It is sometimes tempting to think that cramming as many questions as possible into a small number of pages will make the questionnaire appear shorter and thus enhance response rate. In fact, the opposite is true; respondents are likely to be irritated or overwhelmed by a messy or difficult form. Questionnaires should have plenty of blank space between each question, with easy-to-see brackets for making response choices. Respondents generally feel encouraged by progressing quickly through the pages, rather than spending a great deal of time on numerous questions on a single page. For Internet surveys, showing the respondent's progress using a bar placed in a prominent location on the screen is recommended.[27]

In telephone interviews, the primary way to enhance professional appearance is using an effective interviewer. The interviewer's demeanor affects the quality of information obtained in several ways. First, the interviewer's voice characteristics, including the speed and pitch of speech as well as accuracy of pronunciation, affect the likelihood that a prospective respondent will participate in the survey. Additionally, the interviewer's attitude about the project and expectations about the interview affect both the likelihood and quality of response to questions.[31]

The interviewer's technique for "probing" (asking follow-up questions when necessary) also affects results. For example, in response to the question, "How would you rate your health today—would you say it is excellent, good, fair, or poor?" a respondent might answer "Oh, it's all right." A correct interview technique would be to probe politely by repeating the response options: "And would you say that it is excellent, good, fair, or poor?" It would be incorrect technique to assume that the respondent meant to say "fair" or to ask, "So do you mean your health is fair?" These approaches could bias study results. Findings are particularly affected by interviewer technique when sensitive questions are being asked, as is common in health care surveys.[31] The term **interviewer effect** refers to the unhappy situation in which the findings of an interview are the result not only of the questions asked, but also of the demeanor of the particular interviewer who happens to be on duty that day.

To avoid interviewer effect, it is essential for a qualified instructor to provide formal structured training of every interviewer, an AAPOR best practice.[7] Training should include methods for reading questions and for asking follow-up questions in an unbiased and nonjudgmental way. Additional training should be provided on the purpose of the project and how its data will be used. Emphasizing the importance of confidentiality is a must. A detailed review of each survey question should be included, and *supervised* practice interviews are also critically important. Although training and

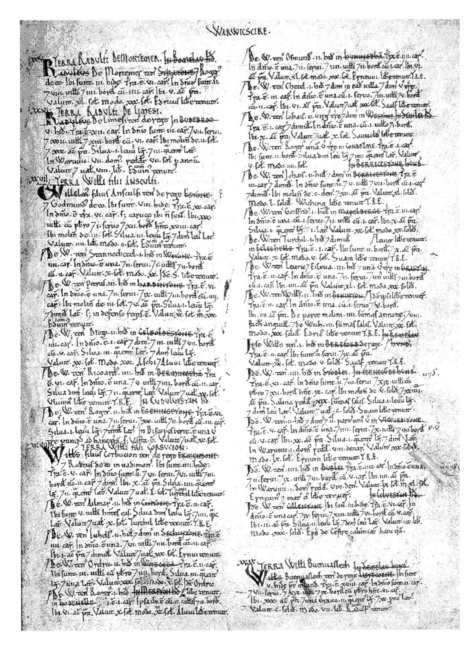

Page from Domesday Book for Warwickshire, anonymous artist. Resistance to survey data collection efforts is nothing new. In 1086, the Domesday Survey of recently conquered property throughout England, ordered by William of Normandy, reportedly generated resistance to what was perceived as "a bitterly resented onset of bureaucratic feudal rule."[17] Public domain image from Wikimedia Commons.

monitoring interviewers may appear to be time-consuming, it is better to spend the time in training than to struggle to interpret baffling results after data collection, only to find that those results are attributable to the effect of one or more interviewers with suboptimal skills.

Clarity and Ease of Completion

Competence. One of the most important principles to remember in writing questionnaire items is that respondents must be asked only those questions that they are **competent to answer**—meaning that they have enough information about the question to answer it accurately. To do this, try to see the world through your respondent's eyes. For example, in writing a survey that will be administered to consumers of a good or a service, consider what they *do* (i.e., their roles), which affects what they *know* (Table 8E).

A typical health care enrollee is capable of telling you whether the waiting time in an emergency room was satisfactory, but likely has no knowledge of whether the triage system was medically appropriate. Typical patients can answer questions about how they have been feeling, but most cannot answer questions about the medical reasons for their sensations. For example, the question "While taking Drug A, did you ever experience a situation in which you stood up and suddenly felt dizzy or lightheaded?" is more appropriately worded than "While taking Drug A, did you ever experience orthostatic hypotension?" When asking about diagnoses, it might be helpful to review language from validated surveys, such as the National Health Interview Survey.[33]

Specificity. Questions should be as specific as possible. For example, instead of asking about satisfaction with physician office visits in general, it is better to direct the respondent's attention to a particular visit: "I'd like you to think back to your most recent visit to your Health-R-Us primary care provider." If there is a concern that the most recent visit might be atypical, respondents can be asked if it was a typical visit. Because recall diminishes with time, it is better to ask about recent rather than distant events, particularly when eliciting detail.[34]

For clarity and accuracy, response choices must be mutually exclusive. For example, the following response choices for age are incorrect: 1 to 20 years; 20 to 30 years; 30 to 40 years; 40 years or older. Respondents who are 20, 30, or 40 years old fit into two categories. Correct response choices are: 1 to 20 years; 21 to 30 years; 31 to 40 years; 41 years or older.[1]

Table 8E
Roles Played by Consumers

What Consumers Do	Examples of What They Probably Can Report Accurately	Examples of What They Probably Cannot Report Accurately
• Interact with staff and personnel	• Their opinions about whether staff members were courteous, knowledgeable, and friendly	• Whether staff members are paid adequately • How long staff have been with the employer • How other customers feel about the staff • Details about staff knowledge in technical fields (e.g., the medical knowledge level of a physician)
• Make purchasing decisions • Request certain services or treatments	• Their reasons for purchasing or not purchasing a particular product recently • Their reasons for requesting a particular service recently • How they heard about the service • Why they chose a particular organization or location to obtain the services or goods that they purchased	• Their purchasing history for all products of that type during the past year • Whether their purchasing decision was wise (i.e., whether the product was available elsewhere at a lower price) • How someone else in their household made a similar purchasing decision
• Choose whether to read materials sent to them • Choose whether to speak with an organizational representative (e.g., a customer service representative) by telephone	• Whether they remember receiving the mailed materials or the call • If so, whether they read the materials or spoke with the representative • If so, what they remember about the mailing or the call	• The content of a mailing or call that they do not remember receiving • The content of a mailing or call that took place too long ago for them to remember it
• Receive services, such as medications and treatments	• What the service felt like to them (e.g., medication side effects, medication taste) • When they stopped using the service or treatment, if it was not too long ago • Why they stopped using the service or treatment, if it was not too long ago	• The side effects of the medication or treatment that are reported in the medical literature • Why they made a decision that was so long ago that they no longer recall it • How much the service or medication cost, if they did not pay for it (e.g., if a health plan paid for the service or medication)
• Experience various health conditions and events	• Whether the health condition is a problem for them and, if so, why and to what extent • How long they have had the health condition (within a margin of error for those who have had the condition for a long time) • Circumstances and approximate time frame for an event that was important to them (e.g., emergency room visit, hospital stay)	• Costs of treatments and medications for the health condition, if they did not pay for them • Their prognosis (and even if they know, you shouldn't ask them) • Events that weren't sufficiently important or unusual for them to remember (e.g., routine physician office visit that took place two years ago)

Additionally, the range of response choices should be appropriate for the sample. For example, the age breakdowns for a survey of retirees might be younger than 65 years, 65 to 74 years, 75 to 84 years, and 85 years or older. In contrast, the age breakdowns for an employed population probably will include only one or two categories for those aged 65 years or older, but multiple age categories for those younger than age 65. Although this example is relatively straightforward, it is sometimes more difficult to identify the appropriate range. For example, in measuring income in a Medicaid population, it would be helpful to know the financial requirements for eligibility so that the range of possible incomes is understood prior to writing response choices. Failure to identify the appropriate range can result in either confusing the respondents or missing potentially important information. For example, in a survey of Medicare beneficiaries, nearly all respondents would check a box marked "65 years or older."

Double-barrelling, threatening, and other foibles. It is important to avoid "double-barrelled" questions, which confuse and sometimes frustrate respondents by including more than one concept in the same item.[1] For example, the question, "Do you believe that Health-R-Us Healthplan's services are courteous and timely?" asks the respondent two questions at once. A respondent who believes that services are courteous but not timely, or timely but not courteous, does not know how to answer. Although separating this question into two items takes more time and space, it yields much more interpretable results.

In addition to being clear, terms used in questionnaires must be nonthreatening and nonbiased. The question, "What do you think of the outrageously excessive dispensing fees being charged by pharmacies today?" is both threatening in tone and unclear. What are the definitions of the terms "excessive" and "outrageous?" Does the respondent have any way to know what dispensing fees are charged by pharmacies (or even what a dispensing fee is)? The question, "What is your opinion of a policy that compels physicians to prescribe generic drugs even if their medical judgment tells them that the brand drug is better?" uses value-laden terms (compels and medical judgment) and biases the respondent toward a negative assessment of a generic substitution program. A better approach would be to describe the program briefly and neutrally, including a description of prior authorization options if they are available, and then ask, "What is your opinion of a program like this one?" Similarly, the question, "Has your financial situation deteriorated in the past year?" is both confusing because there is no point of comparison (deteriorated compared with what?) and biasing because it presents only one option to the respondent (how does a respondent whose financial situation has improved answer the question?). A better approach would be to say "Which of the following describes how your financial situation in 2011 compares with 2010—is it better, worse, or about the same?"[1,35]

Examples of problematic questionnaire items, along with explanations of better approaches, are in Table 8F.

Order as your respondent (not you) understands it. To further enhance respondents' willingness and ability to complete the survey, the organization of the questionnaire should be logical, interesting, and nonthreatening. To be logical, the questionnaire should present items in an order *that will make sense to the respondent*. For example, in asking about satisfaction with Health-R-Us primary care services, items might progress chronologically through questions about making appointments, spending time in the waiting room, having conversations with the nurse and doctor, and filling prescriptions at the in-house pharmacy following the visit. In a survey of opinions or experiences, questions about each major topic area (e.g., satisfaction, symptoms, subjective well-being) should be grouped together, if possible. Ideally, items with similar scales should be grouped together as well, because respondents become confused by repetitive changes from one scale format (Excellent, Good, Fair, Poor) to another (Very Satisfied, Somewhat Satisfied, Somewhat Dissatisfied, Very Dissatisfied).

Major sections should begin with a brief description of what the group of questions is about and how it fits into the overall theme of the questionnaire. For example, the opening section might begin with: "First, I would like to ask your opinions about the services provided by Health-R-Us." The next section might begin: "Now, I would like to know about some of our specific services. To begin, I have some questions about your opinions of our pharmacy." The next section might begin, "My next set of questions asks about your use of Health-R-Us services during the past year."

Generally, the questionnaire should progress from easier to more difficult, less threatening to more threatening, less specific to more specific, and more interesting to less interesting items. It is often helpful to open the questionnaire with an easy item that will apply to and interest every respondent, such as, "We would like to begin by asking your opinion about the pharmacy benefits provided by our company. Would you rate them as excellent, good, fair, or poor?" Questions such as this suggest to respondents that you are interested in hearing their points of view. They also encourage respondents to begin thinking about the survey topic. Typically, demographic items such as age and gender should be in the final major section of the questionnaire, because demographic items are

Table 8F
Examples of Common Questionnaire Problems and Solutions

Question	Biased and/or Unclear Because ...	Better Approach
"Five people in our company have complained frequently to us about the services provided by We-B-PBM. What problems have you had?"	• Question is biased because it begins by advising the respondents of other employees' complaints. • Question is unclear because it asks about *which* problems were experienced before asking *whether* any problems were experienced; a respondent without problems will not know how to answer.	Begin by asking a general question about satisfaction with We-B-PBM using balanced response choices—for example: "On a scale of 0 to 10, where 0 is the worst possible service and 10 is the best possible service, how would you rate the services provided by We-B-PBM?" Respondents who answer below 5 could be asked questions about reasons for dissatisfaction.
"Taking all antibiotic medication until it is gone is one of the most important determinants of successful bacterial eradication. People who prematurely terminate antimicrobial pharmacotherapy risk expensive and often painful recrudescence. Did you take all your medication?"	• Question signals to the respondent that people who fail to take antibiotic medication are irresponsible and/or not very bright. This approach puts considerable pressure on the respondent to answer that all medication has been consumed. • The terminology used in the question would baffle a typical respondent. • "Did you take all your medication?" requires a yes or no response, treating a respondent who missed one dose in the same way as a respondent who missed every dose.	Begin the item with a neutrally worded introduction, such as "Some patients taken medicine exactly as prescribed, while others do not. We would like to know about your experiences." Then ask respondent about the number of days on which he or she took medication and whether doses were taken on time or late.
"Do you favor or oppose illegal immigration laws?"	• The question is too vague to be understandable; many immigration laws have been proposed.	Briefly describe a specific legal proposal, *then* ask the respondent his or her opinion about it.
"Please provide the dates and a detailed description of every physician office visit you have had since 1982."	• The question asks for an impossible level of recall.	If this is the information that the researcher needs, he or she should not be using a survey to get it. A medical records review or database analysis is required.

boring and occasionally can be threatening, such as questions about income. A single, final open-ended item asking for comments leaves a pleasant impression with respondents.

Order effect. It is also important to consider the possibility of **order effect**, a circumstance in which the answer to a question is based not only on the wording of the question itself but also on where the question is placed in the survey. For example, consider a survey that asks women who have just had a baby 15 questions about their experiences in obtaining prenatal care, then asks their opinion about whether prenatal care is important. Respondents' answers to the last question will be biased because they will likely conclude, "Prenatal care must be important; otherwise, that interviewer wouldn't have just asked me all those questions about it."

Similarly, respondents' ratings of general satisfaction (e.g., with services provided to them) will sometimes differ depending on where in the questionnaire the general satisfaction item is placed. If specific satisfaction questions are asked first, before the general satisfaction question, respondents will tend to frame their assessment of general satisfaction based on the specific items.[36] For instance, if asked, "How satisfied or dissatisfied are you with the speed of our mail order delivery service?" before being asked about overall satisfaction, respondents will tend to consider mail order delivery speed in making their overall assessment. Whether this tendency is helpful or harmful depends on the circumstances. On the one hand, if respondents' memories on a particular topic might be weak, it is appropriate to mention specifics before trying to measure a general opinion. On the other hand, it may be important for the respondents' opinions to be completely fresh and unaffected by the investigator's preconceived notions of which specific items promote general satisfaction.

Handling Open-Ended Items
Although open-ended items (questions without response choices) appeal to many respondents who wish to explain or embellish their answers, they sometimes pose an analytical challenge. There are a number of possible uses for the information gleaned from an item such as, "We welcome any comments you have about our services." If the information is to be used only for quotations that will illustrate key points made in the quantitative data presentation, clerical workers are needed to type and organize the quotations. Even with this minimal use, a senior investigator should be responsible for reviewing all quotations intended for presentation or publication to ensure that none reveals the identity of any participant (e.g., "I was the only employee in my company to

have triplets last year, and I thought the OB service was terrific!").

A more sophisticated use of responses to open-ended questions requires more human resources. For example, if the investigator wishes to quantify the open-ended responses received, two qualified staff members should independently assign the responses to categories for data analysis, a process known as "precoding." To ensure that the precoding is reliable and valid, the codes assigned by the staff members should be compared for consistency and discrepancies resolved prior to analysis.

The intended use for open-ended items, and the workload necessary for that intended use, should be considered *during the questionnaire-writing phase* of the project. In other words, if the investigator does not intend to use an open-ended item on which a respondent may spend a great deal of time, the open-ended question probably should not be asked.

Pretesting the Survey

A ***pretest***, sometimes called a "pilot test," prior to full-scale implementation of the survey is an important tool to help the investigator see the world through the eyes of the respondent and is an AAPOR best practice.[7] The pretesting process helps the investigator to identify and correct problems, such as faulty questions, flawed response options, or interviewer training deficiencies. To conduct a pretest, the investigator (or a designated interviewer) administers the questionnaire to a small sample of perhaps 10 to 50 cases, depending on the size and complexity of the project. Different approaches are used to determine whether changes are needed. Sometimes, the clarity, intrusiveness, and meaning of the items are discussed directly with the pretest sample members (e.g., "Did any items on the survey confuse or upset you?"). Sometimes, in debriefings following completion of the pretest interviews, interviewers are asked about respondents' reactions.

A pretest is often a good way to resolve disputes that arise during questionnaire construction. For example, a disagreement over whether a particular item is confusing can be resolved easily by asking pretest respondents or interviewers their opinions about how the item was perceived. Alternatively, a "split-sample" pretest, in which one-half of respondents are asked the question using one approach and the other one-half are asked the question using a different approach, can be helpful.[7]

Another approach that is sometimes used in handling controversial or difficult topics is the ***slow start.*** In a "slow-start" arrangement, the survey goes into the field on a very limited initial basis (e.g., less than 5 interviews per interviewer during the first day). Issues that arise during that phase—for example, interviewer instructions that require additional clarification—are addressed prior to massive fielding. Generally, lack of clarity should be handled in the pretest phase, but the "slow start" provides a helpful double-check on procedures, especially in exploratory work.

Pretest surveys should never be used in calculating the final project results. These surveys were obtained under different circumstances, and in some cases using different questions, than the production interviews. However, "slow-start" surveys are typically usable, as long as the "slow start" did not result in major changes in the questionnaire or survey procedures.

Follow-Up with Initial Nonrespondents

Generally, repeated contacts with those who fail to respond to the initial survey attempt will yield much higher response rates and more accurate results than single attempts with little or no follow-up. For mailed surveys, it is sometimes helpful to send a reminder postcard to all respondents one or two days after the original mailing. The postcard can remind respondents that a survey was recently sent to them, briefly reiterate the importance of the project, and offer a telephone number to call with any questions, concerns, or requests for a replacement questionnaire. The first set of initial responses usually comes in a cluster sometime during the first week or two after mailing. A second mailing to initial nonrespondents, preferably including another copy of the questionnaire if the budget permits, can be sent when that first set of returns begins to taper off. To avoid annoying respondents who have already returned their questionnaires, it is important to include in these materials a statement such as, "If this letter and your completed questionnaire have crossed in the mail, please accept this as our sincere thank you for your participation!"

In telephone interview follow-ups, attempts to reach respondents should be made on different days of the week and times of day.[37] If a respondent is reached but is unable to conduct the survey at that time, the interviewer should attempt to make an appointment to complete the interview. Consistent with the principle of maintaining respondent trust, and as a matter of basic courtesy, the interviewer or a colleague must keep that appointment at (nearly) any cost.

No matter what mode of administration has been chosen, a follow-up telephone call is often an opportunity to answer questions that potential respondents might have or to provide reassurances about confidentiality, use of information, or other concerns.

Reliability Assessment

Several types of reliability (consistency) are potentially important in health care surveys, depending on study methods and questions.[12] Foremost among these is ***interviewer reliability***; the investigator should compare response rates and key findings, such as overall satisfaction levels or reported compliance rates, across interviewers, and enhance training or make other adjustments if discrepancies are found. Additionally, if interviewers are responsible for making assessments, such as a respondent's ability to perform certain tasks, two or more interviewers should independently assess a subsample of respondents, and a test of their ***inter-rater reliability*** should be performed. Consistency among conceptually related items, such as components of a scale, is ***internal reliability***. The consistency of measurement of the same subject at two different points in time, known as ***test-retest reliability***, is important in studies that measure trends. For example, if a respondent reports in January that his appendix was removed two years previously, but in June reports no previous surgeries, there is a problem.

Statistics to measure test-retest and inter-rater reliability include Pearson correlations, intraclass correlations, kappa, and weighted kappa. Internal reliability is commonly assessed using the Cronbach's alpha statistic. [38,39]

Validity Assessment

Even if the investigator has performed a careful pretest, assessment of the ***construct validity*** of survey questions is important. For example, a survey might ask patients who filled antibiotic prescriptions whether they took all medication as prescribed by the doctor. Some patients may erroneously believe that taking the antibiotic on a precise schedule—but only until their symptoms were gone—does not remove them from the "as prescribed" category; in this instance, the item lacks construct validity because its meaning to the patient is not as intended by the investigator. To assess and, if necessary, correct the construct validity of the item, patients who answer "yes" to the "as prescribed" question might be asked additional, more specific questions pertaining to use of the medication, such as whether all doses were taken, the timing of doses taken, and whether instructions to avoid certain foods were followed.

The terms ***criterion validity*** and ***predictive validity*** refer to the accuracy of a measure relative to an external criterion or benchmark that may include an event occurring after the survey (predictive validity).[1] In health care surveys, criterion validity is commonly assessed by comparing patient-reported data with information about actual behaviors and outcomes, perhaps for a subsample of patients depending on project budget. For example, investigators have compared patient-reported perceptions of health status with medical utilization, subsequent mortality, laboratory values, medical records, or other clinical criteria.[40] Limited validation of survey findings can be performed even for an anonymous survey (one in which respondents' identities are completely unknown to the investigator). For example, if survey findings suggest that a particular group increased utilization in response to a benefit design change, a claims analysis could confirm that, in the aggregate, utilization grew for that group.

Content validity refers to the degree to which a tool assesses all important dimensions of a concept. A good example used by Babbie is a survey tool to assess mathematics skills. The tool should not assess only addition; it must also assess subtraction, multiplication, and division because these are important components of basic mathematics.[1] In a health care research example, a survey intended to assess satisfaction with a hospital stay should not be limited to questions about the nurses; it should also include items pertaining to the physical environment (e.g., cleanliness, comfort), the food, the physicians, and any other element that affects overall satisfaction.

Good Reporting

A final AAPOR best practice recommendation is that the survey report should fully "disclose all methods of the survey to permit evaluation and replication."[7] This important admonition will be taken up in Chapter 10.

Summing Up: What Have We Learned?

Objectively measuring experiences and opinions can be a time-consuming and sometimes expensive task. However, making the effort to conduct a high-quality survey can yield enormous benefits *if* the investigator remembers the total design principle—excellence and attention to detail at every stage of the survey research process—to encourage accurate and candid expression of respondents' points of view. Like many complex tasks, this effort is greatly enhanced by collaboration and taking advantage of opportunities to obtain feedback, not only from respondents but also from colleagues.

In Chapter 9, we examine the use of constructive (and sometimes not so constructive) feedback to improve research quality. We begin with an auspicious group that includes internationally known economists, Nobel Prize-winners, and "Darwin's bulldog."

Helpful Resources

- American Association for Public Opinion Research. Best practices.[7]

- Babbie. *The Practice of Social Research*, especially Chapter 7 (the logic of sampling); Chapter 9 (survey research); and Chapter 19 (the ethics and politics of social research).[1]
- Fowler. *Survey Research.*[9]
- National Council on Public Polls: 20 questions a journalist should ask about poll results.[41] This is a user-friendly and informative summary of much of the material in this chapter, viewed from the perspective of those who use survey results.

References

1. Babbie E. *The Practice of Social Research. Fourth Edition.* Belmont, CA: Wadsworth Publishing Company; 1986: quotations pp. 138, 450-51.

2. Lester W. "Dewey Defeats Truman" disaster haunts pollsters. *Los Angeles Times.* November 1, 1998. Available at: http://articles.latimes.com/print/1998/nov/01/news/mn-38174.

3. Andy Rooney quotations. Available at: http://www.brainyquote.com/quotes/authors/a/andy_rooney.html.

4. Rasmussen Reports. What's up with Nevada? November 7, 2010. Available at: http://www.rasmussenreports.com/public_content/politics/general_politics/november_2010/what_s_up_with_nevada.

5. Rasmussen Reports. About us. Available at: http://www.rasmussenreports.com/public_content/about_us.

6. Jones T. Dewey defeats Truman: well, everyone makes mistakes. *Chicago Tribune.* Available at: http://www.chicagotribune.com/news/politics/chi-chicagodays-deweydefeats-story,0,6484067.story.

7. American Association for Public Opinion Research. Best practices. Available at: http://www.aapor.org/Best_Practices1.htm.

8. Cox ER, Henderson R, Motheral BR. Health plan member experience with point-of-service prescription step therapy. *J Manag Care Pharm.* 2004;10(4):291-98. Available at: http://www.amcp.org/data/jmcp/Research-291-298.pdf.

9. Fowler FJ. *Survey Research Methods. Third Edition.* Thousand Oaks, CA: Sage Publications, Inc.; 2002: quotation p. 8.

10. Dillman DA, Phelps G, Tortora R, et al. Response rate and measurement differences in mixed-mode surveys using mail, telephone, interactive voice response (IVR) and the Internet. *Social Science Research.* 2009;38:1-18. Available at: http://152.2.32.107/odum/content/pdf/Dillman%20Mixed%20Mode%20Soc%20Sci%20Research%202009.pdf.

11. Shettle C, Mooney G. Monetary incentives in U.S. government surveys. *Journal of Official Statistics.* 1999;15(2):231-50.

12. Motheral BR. Research methodology: hypotheses, measurement, reliability, and validity. *J Manag Care Pharm.* 1998;4(4):382-90. Available at: http://www.amcp.org/data/jmcp/ce_v4_382-390.pdf.

13. Author experience. For example, I once recommended that a company change from a postcard measure, which was yielding a 5% response rate and a 30% rate of

dissatisfaction, to a telephone survey method, which yielded a 90% response rate and an 80%-90% rate of satisfaction.

14. The Henry J. Kaiser Family Foundation. Data note: rush to the altar? April 2008. Available at: http://www.kff.org/kaiserpolls/upload/7773DataNote.pdf.

15. Tejada-Vera B, Sutton PD. Births, marriages, divorces, and deaths: provisional data for 2007. National vital statistics reports. 2008;56(21). Available at: http://www.cdc.gov/nchs/data/nvsr/nvsr56/nvsr56_21.htm#T2.

16. O'Neil M. Estimating the nonresponse bias due to refusals in telephone surveys. *Public Opin Q.* 1979;43(2):218-32.

17. Goyder J. *The Silent Minority: Nonrespondents on Sample Surveys.* Oxford, UK: Polity Press; 1987.

18. Kviz FJ. Toward a standard definition of response rate. *Public Opin Q.* 1977;41(2):265-67.

19. Kalton G. *Introduction to Survey Sampling.* Newbury Park, CA: Sage Publications, Inc.; 1983: quotation p. 6.

20. Department of Health and Human Services. 45 CFR Parts 160 and 164. Standards for privacy of individually identifiable health information. August 14, 2002. Available at: http://www.hhs.gov/ocr/privacy/hipaa/administrative/privacyrule/privrulepd.pdf.

21. Lee ES, Forthover RN. *Analyzing Complex Survey Data. Second Edition.* Thousand Oaks, CA: Sage Publications, Inc.; 2006.

22. Chang L, Krosnick JA. National surveys via RDD telephone interviewing versus the Internet: comparing sample representativeness and response quality. *Public Opin Q.* 2009;73(4):641-78.

23. Yeager DS, Krosnick JA, Chang L, et al. Comparing the accuracy of RDD telephone surveys and Internet surveys conducted with probability and non-probability samples. August 2009. Available at: http://comm.stanford.edu/faculty/krosnick/Mode%2004.pdf.

24. Langer G. More on the problems with opt-in Internet surveys. September 28, 2009. Available at: http://blogs.abcnews.com/thenumbers/2009/09/guest-blog-more-on-the-problems-with-optin-internet-surveys.html.

25. Best SJ, Radcliff B. *Polling America: An Encyclopedia of Public Opinion.* Westport CT: Greenwood Press; 2005.

26. Dillman DA. *Mail and Telephone Surveys: The Total Design Method.* New York: Wiley Interscience; 1978.

27. Schonlau M, Fricker RD, Elliott MN. *Conducting Research Surveys via E-Mail and the*

Web. Santa Monica, CA: RAND; 2002.

28. Dillman DA. Why choice of survey mode makes a difference. *Public Health Reports.* 2006;121(1):11-13.

29. Dillman DA, Sinclair MD, Clark JR. Effects of questionnaire length, respondent-friendly design, and a difficult question on response rates for occupant-addressed census mail surveys. *Public Opin Q.* 1993;57(3):289-304.

30. Church AH. Estimating the effect of incentives on mail survey response rates: a meta-analysis. *Public Opin Q.* 1993;57(1):62-79.

31. See for example:
    - Billiet J, Loosveldt G. Improvement of the quality of responses to factual survey questions by interviewer training. *Public Opin Q.* 1988;52(2):190-211.
    - Oksenberg L, Coleman L, Cannell CF. Interviewers' voices and refusal rates in telephone surveys. *Public Opin Q.* 1986;50(1):97-111.
    - Singer E, Frankel MR, Glassman MB. The effect of interviewer characteristics and expectations on response. *Public Opin Q.* 1983;47:68-83.
    - Singer E, Kohnke-Aguirre L. Interviewer expectation effects: a replication and extension. *Public Opin Q.* 1979;43:245-60.
    - Tucker C. Interviewer effects in telephone surveys. *Public Opin Q.* 1983;47(1):84-95.

32. Fowler FJ. How unclear terms affect survey data. *Public Opin Q.* 1992;56(2):218-31.

33. Centers for Disease Control and Prevention. About the National Health Interview Survey. Available at: http://www.cdc.gov/nchs/nhis/about_nhis.htm.

34. Bachman JG, O'Malley PM. When four months equal a year: inconsistencies in student reports of drug use. *Public Opin Q.* 1981;45(4):536-48.

35. See, for example:
    - Bishop GJ, Oldendick RW, Tuchfarber AJ. Effects of presenting one versus two sides of an issue in survey questions. *Public Opin Q.* 1982;46:69-85.
    - Bradburn NM, Sudman S, Blair E, Stocking C. Question threat and response bias. *Public Opin Q.* 1978;42(2):221-34.
    - Rasmussen S. What you can learn about Wisconsin dispute from differences in poll questions. March 7, 2011. Available at: http://www.rasmussenreports.com/public_content/political_commentary/commentary_by_scott_rasmussen/what_you_can_learn_about_wisconsin_dispute_from_differences_in_poll_questions
    - Smith TW. That which we call welfare by any other name would smell sweeter: an analysis of the impact of question wording on response patterns. *Public Opin Q.* 1987;51(1):75-83.

36. See, for example:
- Benton JE, Daly JL. A question order effect in a local government survey. *Public Opin Q.* 1991;55(4):640-42.
- McClendon MJ, O'Brien DJ. Question-order effects on the determinants of subjective well-being. *Public Opin Q.* 1988;52:351-64.
- McFarland SG. Effects of question order on survey responses. *Public Opin Q.* 1981;45(2):208-15.

37. Weeks MF, Kulka RA, Pierson SA. Optimal call scheduling for a telephone survey. *Public Opin Q.* 1987;51(4):540-49.

38. Feinstein AR. Clinimetric perspectives. *J Chronic Dis.* 1987;40(6):635-40.

39. Main DS, Pace WD. Measuring health: guidelines for reliability assessment. *Fam Med.* 1991; 23(3):227-30.

40. See, for example:
- Ford DE, Anthony JC, Nestadt GR, Romanoski AJ. The General Health Questionnaire by interview. Performance in relation to recent use of health services. *Med Care.* 1989;27(4):367-75.
- Idler EL, Kasl SV, Lemke JH. Self-evaluated health and mortality among the elderly in New Haven, Connecticut, and Iowa and Washington Counties, Iowa, 1982-1986. *Am J Epidemiol.* 1990;131(1):91-103.
- Kaplan SH. Patient reports of health status as predictors of physiologic health measures in chronic disease. *J Chronic Dis.* 1987;40(Suppl 1):27S-35S.
- Burns RB, Moskowitz MA, Ash A, Kane RL, Finch MD, Bak SM. Self-report versus medical record functional status. *Med Care.* 1992;30(5 Suppl):MS85-MS95.
- McHorney CA, Ware JE, Raczek AE. The MOS 36-Item Short-Form Health Survey (SF-36): II. Psychometric and clinical tests of validity in measuring physical and mental health constructs. *Med Care.* 1993;31(3):247-63.

41. Gawiser SR, Witt GE. 20 questions a journalist should ask about poll results: 3rd edition. National Council on Public Polls. Available at: htt8p://www.ncpp.org/files/20%20Questions%203rd%20edition_Web%20ver_2006.pdf.

Appendix 8A
Sample Questionnaire Scale Formats

Two or Three Simple Response Choices (telephone survey example)
2. How old were you when your asthma first began?

[　] Respondent remembers age: *Record age in years here _____ and skip to Item 4.*
[　] Respondent does not remember exact age: *Continue with Item 3.*

3. Would you say you were younger than 6 years old, 6 to 18 years old, or 19 years or older when your asthma first began?

[　] Younger than 6 years old
[　] 6 to 18 years old
[　] 19 years or older
[　] Respondent does not know

Two or Three Simple Response Choices (mailed survey example)
2. Last week, [employer name] mailed a packet to your home address. The packet described your Open Enrollment choices for 2012. Do you remember receiving the packet?

[　] Yes – *Continue with Item 3*
[　] No – *Skip to Item 4*
[　] Not sure – *Skip to Item 4*

3. Which of the following best describes what you have done with the packet so far?

[　] You read the packet.
[　] You still have the packet, but you have not read it yet.
[　] You threw the packet away.
[　] Something else (what?)_____

Labeled Scale Points (Likert-Type Scale)

You said that you filled a prescription at the Pills-R-Us Pharmacy during the past week. Please rate the service provided to you by the Pills-R-Us Pharmacy staff during your most recent visit—would you say that it was Excellent, Good, Fair, or Poor?

[   ] Excellent
[   ] Good
[   ] Fair
[   ] Poor

Matrix

We are interested in methods that you might or might not use to save money on prescription drugs. For each method listed below, please tell us whether and how often you used the method during the past year. If you did not use the method during the past year, please answer "Never."

Method	How Often Did You Do This to Save Money on Prescription Drugs in the Past Year?			
	Never (Did Not Do This)	Rarely	Sometimes	Often
a. Called different pharmacies to find the best price for your medication	[ ]	[ ]	[ ]	[ ]
b. Switched from a more expensive prescription drug to a less expensive prescription drug	[ ]	[ ]	[ ]	[ ]
c. Switched from a prescription drug to an over-the-counter (nonprescription) drug	[ ]	[ ]	[ ]	[ ]
d. Stopped taking a drug without asking your doctor first	[ ]	[ ]	[ ]	[ ]
e. Took less medication than your doctor recommended you take	[ ]	[ ]	[ ]	[ ]
f. Used a mail order pharmacy	[ ]	[ ]	[ ]	[ ]
g. Used a pharmacy that fills a generic drug prescription at a low cost (e.g., $4 for one month or $10-$12 for three months)	[ ]	[ ]	[ ]	[ ]

Polar End Numeric Scales

You have indicated that you filled a prescription at the Pills-R-Us Pharmacy during the past week. **On a scale of 0 to 10**, where **0 is the worst possible service** and **10 is the best possible service**, how would you rate the service provided to you by the staff of Pills-R-Us Pharmacy during your most recent visit?

Worst   **Best**

  0   1   2   3   4   5   6   7   8   9   10

Probing

We are interested in methods that are used by some people and not others to save on prescription drug costs. During the past year, have you used any methods to save on prescription drug costs?

[   ] No

[   ] Yes – *Interviewer: please probe for more detail. Ask: "What methods have you used?" For each method listed, ask the respondent, "Can you tell me more about why you used NAME OF METHOD?" and record the answer in Box Q10A. Then ask "Were there any other methods that you used?" and repeat the process for each of these.*

Appendix 8B
Sample Questionnaire Cover Letter

Dear Mr. [lastname]:

You're the expert, and we need your opinions!

All of us at the Healthy-U Plan are committed to providing you with high-quality service. To do that, we need to learn about our strengths and weaknesses—and nobody can tell us about that better than you.

Please take a few minutes to complete the enclosed opinion survey and return it in the postage-paid envelope that we've provided. We ask that you take the survey *whether or not you currently use your health plan benefit.* To get an accurate picture of all members' opinions, we need to hear from everyone in our scientifically selected sample.

The survey is completely confidential. Reports will be in summary form only, and will not identify you in any way.

If you have any questions or comments about the survey, please feel free to call Sally Survey at 1-800-555-5555, extension 555.

You are not required to complete this survey, and participation will not affect your benefits at all. Still, we hope you share your point of view with us. We value and respect your opinion!

Sincerely,

John Q. Executive
Really Impressive Title
Healthy-U Plan

CHAPTER 9

An Attitude of Gratitude:
Making the Most of Difficult Feedback

"You have no idea of the intrigues that go on in this blessed world of science ... I know that the paper I have just sent in (to the Royal Society) is very original and of some importance, and I am equally sure that if it is referred to the judgement of my 'particular friend' ... that it will not be published. ... Why? Because for the last twenty years ... [he] has been regarded as the great authority on these matters, and has had no one to tread on his heels, until at last, I think, he has come to look upon the Natural World as his special preserve, and 'no poachers allowed.' So I must manoeuvre a little to get my poor memoir kept out of his hands." —English biologist and "Darwin's bulldog" Thomas Henry Huxley in 1852, describing the prospect of review by a peer[1,2]

"Sometimes one has to tell an author where and why he is being illogical, inaccurate, sloppy or trivial: and there is no doubt that adverse criticisms rouse personal animus at the time. Having been at the receiving end of referees' comments, I've usually found on reflection that they were worth heeding; and I am grateful now to these anonymous colleagues for their candour. ... [As] the old saying goes, your best friends won't tell you."—Scientist J.W. Conforth, commenting on peer review one year before winning the Nobel Prize for Chemistry[1]

What You Will Learn in Chapter 9

✓ Why you should seek out—and *never* avoid—criticism of your work

✓ Why every comment—even an erroneous comment—is an opportunity to get information that you really need

✓ Why *diverse opinions* about your work are not only expected but also particularly valuable

✓ What *questions you should ask* during informal peer review opportunities, such as poster sessions and meetings

✓ How to respond when given feedback that seems to be erroneous or unethical

"Your manuscript gave us heartburn. Have you ever thought of needlepoint?"—Text of rejection letter sent by Thunder's Mouth Press, as reported by author Peter Benjaminson[3]

You work for months on a research project that you firmly believe is first-rate and potentially influential, perhaps even groundbreaking. Wanting to share what you have learned with others, you search for weeks for an appropriate target journal, carefully craft a persuasive cover letter explaining the import of your work to the editors, and await the results of peer review. But when the reviews come in, you are disappointed to realize that at least one reviewer completely misunderstood the point of your paper. "Did they *read* this manuscript?" you wonder. "They just don't understand much about *my* specialty. What was that editor thinking?"

Has that ever happened to you? If so, you are in prestigious company. In 1994, Gans and Shepherd, then doctoral students in economics, queried Nobel Prize and Clark Medal winners about past rejections of their papers by leading economic journals and "hit a nerve. More than 60 percent responded, many with several blistering pages."[4] Articles deemed unworthy by the economic journals to which they were initially submitted included a groundbreaking paper by James Tobin on the extension of probit regression analysis to multiple regressors, a technique that eventually became well-known as "Tobit," and William Sharpe's "Capital Asset Prices: A Theory of Equilibrium Under Conditions of Risk," which, after being described by an editor as "preposterous" and "uninteresting," was subsequently accepted for publication by a different editor for the same journal and cited more than 2,000 times.[4]

You may also have received reviews that are internally inconsistent. One reviewer raved about your work, whereas the other panned it and recommended immediate rejection. This experience is common. Journal editor and widely published author J. Scott Armstrong recalled in 1997 that the first reviewer on one of his papers opined that the paper "is not deemed scientific enough to merit publication," whereas the second determined that the paper "follows in the best tradition of science... ."[5] It is widely acknowledged by editors of top journals that inconsistency in peer reviewer opinion is the rule rather than the exception and that on average, "agreement among reviewers for biological journals is no greater than would be expected by chance alone."[1,6] At *JMCP*, our most common pattern of recommendations provided by three peer reviewers is one "publish with minor revisions," one "publish with major revisions," and one "do not publish."

Have you ever felt angry after receiving comments on your work with which you disagreed? You are not alone in this, either. In responding to the Gans and Shepherd survey, economist Richard Freeman described "the relief one normally gets from a rejection: the certain knowledge that the editor and referees are blind baseball umpires, members of The Three Stooges, or incompetents in even more drastic ways."[4] Such high emotions about the outcomes of peer review are as old as science itself. In a particularly amusing example recounted by scientific historians, Albert Einstein received in 1936 a ten-page report written by a peer reviewer for the journal *Physical Review*, who carefully explained why the conclusions of Einstein's paper on gravitational waves were incorrect.[7,8] The plainly irritated Einstein wrote to the editor:

> "[My coauthor and I] had sent you our manuscript for publication and had not authorized you to show it to specialists before it is printed. I see no reason to address the—in any case erroneous—comments of your anonymous expert. On the basis of this incident I prefer to publish the paper elsewhere."[7]

Notably, however, the revised paper, which was eventually published in the *Journal of the Franklin Institute*, contained "dramatically" different findings. And, much to Einstein's credit, it also contained a thankful acknowledgement for the "friendly assistance" of the man who is believed to have been the original peer reviewer.[7]

You are also not alone if you have found yourself wondering at times whether the entire peer review system should be scrapped as a "straitjacket" that "[hinders] the progress of knowledge generation."[9] Organizers of the Third International Symposium on Peer Review, which in 2009 brought together participants from multiple engineering and scientific disciplines, argued that "[far] from filtering out junk science, peer review may be blocking the flow of innovation… ."[10] Noting that "research should be evaluated by people bound by mutual trust and respect who are socially recognized as expert in a given field of knowledge," the conference announcement contended that peer review in practice had failed to achieve this mandate and that "more effective methodologies and support systems" were needed.[10]

Even peer review's strongest supporters acknowledge the need for continuous quality improvement in the art and science of reviewing the work of others. Since 1990, the International Congress on Peer Review and Biomedical Publication has held six meetings, most recently in 2009, to "improve the quality and credibility of biomedical peer review and publication and to help advance the efficiency, effectiveness, and equitability of the dissemination of biomedical information throughout the world."[11] Topics prominent in the 2009 conference included detection of "ghost writing" (the inappropriate practice of writing an article without being named as an author); the effects of financial conflicts of interest on research results; methods of "mentoring" new peer reviewers to improve the quality of their assessments; and monitoring of time from submission to publication.

Peer review is of such interest to the general public that the United Kingdom House of Commons commissioned an investigation, conducted by its Science and Technology Committee (2011), to assess the performance of peer review in improving the quality of published scientific work.[12] Its summary report noted that errors and biases in the peer review process were inevitable and that innovative approaches to peer review and publishing, such as "open" peer review (in which the authors and peer reviewers know one another's identity), should be carefully considered by journals, depending on their purpose and audience. However, the committee's summary conclusion was that the peer review system is essential to the quality of scientific information:

> "Peer review in scholarly publishing, in one form or another, is crucial to the reputation and reliability of scientific research. ... The process, as used by most traditional journals prior to publication, is not perfect, and it is clear that considerable differences in quality exist. However, despite the many criticisms and the little solid evidence on its efficacy, editorial peer review is considered by many as important and not something that can be dispensed with."[12]

Why Bother? The Enormous Benefits of Formal or Informal Peer Review

Debates over the validity and necessity of peer review have occurred periodically in cycles dating back many years and seem to be on the resurgence now.[9,10,12] Although the dialogue is informative, at least in historical context, the real question for a typical author today is fundamentally pragmatic and immediate. If some measure of dissatisfaction with the peer review process is widespread, if at least occasional anger at the real or perceived errors of peer reviewers or editors is normal, if encountering seemingly inconsistent peer reviews is a nearly ubiquitous experience, then why bother with it at all? Why not self-publish online—easy enough nowadays—or, faced with difficult reviewer comments, simply pick up your marbles and go elsewhere, to a different journal? Let me suggest that despite—no, actually, *because of*—those seeming flaws in the peer review process, it is not only worthwhile but also essential.

First, peer review provides immensely valuable information about the *perspective of the reader*. To understand this point, recall from Chapter 1 the fundamental principle of Booth, Colomb, and Williams in *The Craft of Research* (2008) that research should be considered a profoundly social activity.[13] To make an effective argument, Booth et al. suggest, think of your research report as a conversation with your readers. In that conversation, a key question that will be asked (and answered) by readers is whether and how you acknowledge and address alternative points of view.[13] Why? Because, Booth et al. explain:

> *"Readers judge your arguments not just by the facts you offer, but by how well you anticipate their questions and concerns. In so doing, they also judge the quality of your mind, even your implied character, traditionally called your 'ethos.' Do you seem to be the sort of person who considers issues from all sides, who supports claims with evidence that readers accept, and who thoughtfully considers other points of view? Or do you seem to be someone who sees only what matters to her and dismisses or even ignores the views of others? ... In the long run, the ethos you project in individual arguments hardens into your reputation, something every researcher must care about, because your reputation is the tacit sixth element in every argument you write. It answers the unspoken question, 'Can I trust you?' That answer must be '**Yes**.'"* (emphasis in original)[13]

In contrast, Booth et al. argue, a researcher who plans an argument without considering the reader's viewpoint risks producing a feeling in readers that "your argument is not only thin but, worse, ignorant or dismissive of their views. You must respond to their predictable questions and objections."[13] Booth et al. suggest that a researcher should "read your argument as someone who has a stake in a different outcome—who *wants* you to be wrong"[13] and write or edit the paper accordingly: "Show readers that you put your argument through your own wringer, before they put it through theirs."[13] For example, if you believe that certain evidence is "irrelevant or unreliable" but you know that your readers may find it credible, your report should "acknowledge it but explain why you didn't use it."[13]

In treating anticipated objections to your work in this way, Booth et al. observe that you "'thicken' your argument, making it increasingly rich and complex, thereby enhancing your credibility as someone who does not oversimplify complex issues."[13] To facilitate this task, Booth et al. suggest that the researcher must "imagine" the questions and objections that will be raised by the target audience.[13]

And that, in a nutshell, is the beauty of peer review—*you don't have to "imagine" the objections of your readers. You know what they are, and if you use that knowledge well, the presentation of your work will be enhanced by this understanding.*

Second, internal inconsistency in reviewers' opinions is typically a strength—not a weakness—of the process. That is, diversity among peer reviewers probably reflects diversity in the pool of a journal's *readers*—your target audience. For example, in evaluating the report of an intervention to improve adherence to treatment with Drug A, it is entirely possible that a health plan executive (e.g., chief executive officer or medical director) will ask why a researcher failed to consider the cost of the intervention in evaluating the program, whereas a clinical pharmacist might ask why Drug A was chosen for the study when Drug B is more tolerable. Despite the difference in the reviewer perspectives, both of these questions are legitimate and merit consideration by the researcher—especially if the target audience consists both of executives and clinical pharmacists!

Additionally, divergence of reviewers' opinions often reflects the different areas of specialized expertise that must be tapped in evaluating a project that has multiple dimensions.[1] For example, it is possible that a methodologist will enthusiastically recommend acceptance of a research report on Disease X because of its sound, randomized design and technically appropriate statistical analysis, whereas a clinician with expertise in diagnosing and treating Disease X will identify the study design as inconsistent with evidence-based treatment guidelines and recommend rejection or major revisions.

There is nothing wrong with this pattern at all. *Bringing different perspectives to bear on a research project is healthy—it is what peer review is supposed to do.* If your paper is likely to be believed by some readers and not others, or if you can alleviate the concerns of various factions of the target audience—perhaps by providing more detailed explanations of your rationale or by changing a problematic data analysis—it is to your advantage to address those concerns prior to dissemination of the work. After putting in what was probably a substantial effort to produce your research results, you want them to be credible and understood. For this reason, *Journal of Clinical Investigation (JCI)* editor Jean Wilson asserted in a 1978 address to the American Society for Clinical Investigation that in the evaluation of a paper by reviewers from different disciplines or with varying areas of expertise, "concurrence of [reviewers'] opinion may be irrelevant."[1]

Third, peer review does screen out poorer-quality papers, and authors who heed the advice of peer reviewers improve the quality of their work.[4,5] Generally, studies that are accepted by high-quality journals are cited more often than studies that are rejected and subsequently published elsewhere.[1,14] Although, as we shall see in more detail in Chapter 11, publication in a high-quality journal is no guarantee of high-quality work,[12] it does *usually* indicate a better-quality research product.

More importantly, in an assessment of the consequences of ignoring the comments of peer reviewers, Armstrong et al. (2008) examined the subsequent publication history of manuscripts that had been declined by the *Journal of the American Academy of Dermatology (JAAD)* from March 2004 through June 2004. Of studies that were published in another journal following the *JAAD* rejection, 82% "incorporated at least one change suggested by the *JAAD* reviewers." Compared with manuscripts not incorporating the *JAAD* peer review feedback, manuscripts that incorporated the feedback were published in "higher impact" journals.[15] Additionally, suggesting an often overlooked role of peer review in protecting not only journals, but also *authors*, many of the respondents to the Gans and Shepherd survey expressed gratitude for those peer review rejections that had "[preserved] the reputations of famous economists by keeping their bad work unpublished."[4]

To those who would argue that the "gatekeeper" role of peer review is inappropriately adversarial because "reviewers seem to take the attitude that they are police, and if they find [a flaw in the paper] they can reject it from publication," surgeon David Gorski replied in a spicy August 2010 commentary that these claims are made "as though that were a *bad* thing. There is no inherent right to publish in the scientific literature, and papers with major flaws should be rejected."[16] Political scientist Gregory Weeks (2006) expressed a similar view, from a more philosophical perspective, in an interesting commentary on appropriate responses to failure in the journal peer review process.[17] Failure, Weeks suggested:

> "... *should be a tool used for the greater goal of intellectual and analytic advancement ... [Most] rejection letters can be used for gain. They are written by people with detailed knowledge of the field, and can yield critical insights that the author has failed to take into consideration. Failure to address those concerns may lead the author to resubmit to a different journal, but with essentially the same results.*"[17]

Even harsh critics of the journal peer review process openly acknowledge its positive effect on the quality of research articles. For example, management professor Arthur Bedeian has expressed concern that requiring authors to make changes in response to reviewer comments can result in loss of "a clear authorial voice."[18] Yet, in 2003, Bedeian reported mostly favorable assessments of the peer review process in his analysis of a survey that was administered to lead authors of articles published in the *Academy of Management Journal* and *Academy of Management Review* from 1999 to 2001 (response rate 61.1%).[19] Bedeian found that the vast majority of authors strongly agreed (57.2%) or agreed (31.8%) that "the net effect of the review process was to improve the quality of the manuscript," and only 4.1% disagreed. Similarly, the majority strongly agreed (33.3%) or agreed (40.9%) that "the required revisions to the manuscript improved it enough to justify the additional labor and delay in publication," with 14.0% disagreeing. Remarkably, more than 90% agreed that "the referees seemed to have carefully read the manuscript."[19] Bedeian's overall conclusion was that "by and large, the [peer review] system does work."[19] However, he expressed concern about the finding that more than one-third of respondents strongly disagreed (9.2%) or disagreed (24.9%) with the statement that "no pressure whatsoever was exerted by the editor or referees on me to make the revision conform to their personal preference," arguing that his findings pointed to "enormous coercive power in the hands of editors and referees."[19] (Note that the double-negative wording in this item/response combination was suboptimal—see Chapter 8.)

Let me add a thought about this latter point from the editor's perspective. An editor who exerts "no pressure whatsoever" on authors is highly likely to publish work that is, quite simply, wrong. For example, mathematical errors or deeply flawed assessments of products or services—which are sometimes a thinly disguised "sales pitch" to a journal's readers—are not edifying and do not belong in peer-reviewed literature. In health care research, this point is particularly important today, when patients and their families are able to access many research articles on the Internet, often without the educational background to evaluate the scientific validity of what they are reading. A small but vocal minority of authors may not like being required to correct mistakes prior to publication, but I know of no other way to protect a journal's readership from misleading or downright erroneous information. As *JCI* editor Wilson has said well, "Not all the unpleasant things that are said [by peer reviewers] from behind the cloak of anonymity are said from a desire to do mischief. Some need to be said."[1]

Opportunity Lost or Valuable Information Gained? It's Your Choice

To make the most of feedback from others, I offer the following **four key principles**:

First, view peer review (formal or informal) as the valuable tool that it is. Don't avoid it—seek it out. The single most important action that you can take to improve the quality of your research is to open your work to criticism early and often in the process, preferably before you begin data collection and analysis, and definitely before you write the first draft of your report. Options for obtaining this indispensable input include (1) regular workgroup meetings at which various members of a research team present their studies in progress and seek feedback; (2) periodic updates provided to supervisors and those who will eventually use the research findings; and (3) poster sessions and presentations made at scientific meetings, usually after completion of preliminary data analysis. Questions that you might ask of those from whom you are seeking input include the following:

1. *What do you see as the key take-away point of my work for your organization?* (Hint: Check to see if you and your listener have the same take-away point. If not, perhaps adjustments are in order, or perhaps your listener has come up with a good idea that you missed.)

2. *Do you have any concerns about what you see here?* (Hint: Your listener may be reluctant to raise the point with you. Ask directly, and you may receive helpful information in return.)

3. *Does my sample represent the group in which this type of study is most needed? Should I have included different group(s)?* (Hint: For example, if your listener tells you that your topic has been studied many times in your target group [Group A] but has not been studied in Group B, it may be wise to change the sampling plan to include at least a subsample of persons from Group B.)

4. *Does the study follow-up time adequately represent the time period during which my study outcomes are reasonably likely to occur?* (Hint: For example, if you plan to study change in the results of Laboratory Test X after a six-month period, but your listener tells you that your planned intervention cannot possibly affect Laboratory Test X in less than one year, it may be wise to change the study follow-up period.)

5. *Do you see any potential sources of bias in this work? If so, can they be addressed (how?) or do they represent an insurmountable limitation to the work? If a limitation, is this a major or minor problem for the validity of my conclusions?*

6. *Should I make any changes to the analysis before writing my final paper and, if so, what?*

7. *Is any part of this presentation (or paper) unclear? What specific aspects of the background, methods, or findings are not understandable? What questions did you have after initially reading this presentation/paper?*

Remember that in seeking this feedback, you are not required to adopt the suggestions made by your listener. However, even if you determine that the input of your listener is erroneous, you can use the feedback as an opportunity to learn about potential misunderstandings that your audience may have and adjust your write-up to increase its clarity and persuasiveness.

A practical example may be helpful. In 2000, my supervisor sent me to a scientific conference to present work that we knew would be controversial. Our research had examined the predictive accuracy of **decision analytic models**, hypothetical but often highly complex mathematical models that rely on assumptions to generate estimates of the likely results of various policies or treatments. We had replicated a widely cited decision analytic model of the likely economic and clinical outcomes of treatment for *Helicobacter pylori*, a cause of peptic ulcer disease. We had then replaced the model's assumptions about treatment patterns for *H pylori* infection with utilization data from a database of medical and drug claims. We found that replacing the *assumed* treatment patterns with *actual* treatment patterns resulted in the reversal of the findings of the originally published model.[20]

I presented our results in a hot and stuffy room to a group of professionals who were already annoyed because failure of the conference audiovisual equipment had resulted in a 20-minute delay in the session start time. After I finished speaking, I paused a few moments, wondering what would happen. I had anticipated some negative reaction, but nothing like the actual outcome—the room seemed to explode into polarization, with several audience members nearly shouting at one another over whether our findings were groundbreaking or worthless to a field accustomed routinely to making important decisions based on the models that we had criticized.

None of the controversy mattered to me, though, because I had what I'd come for. By the time I walked out of the room, I knew nearly every objection that would be raised about our paper before we wrote it. We incorporated these concerns into the manuscript, which was published a few years later, won the 2003 Academy of Managed Care Pharmacy's *Award for Excellence*, and, eventually, resulted in my employment at *JMCP* as an associate editor. Not a bad outcome for a rough 20 minutes—but it required an intentional decision.

That is, *nobody* wakes up in the morning and thinks "gee, it would be fun to be criticized today." *Instead, opening work to criticism is a decision that must be made intentionally, knowing that doing so will ultimately improve the quality of the final product.*

Second and related, every comment—positive or negative, right or wrong—should be viewed as an opportunity to learn, for which you are grateful. Most reviewers are probably *not* experts in every detail of your work. Neither are most readers. That's the point. If your article is unclear to a reasonably competent reader who is unfamiliar with the topic, your article is probably not publishable in its current form because it is not understandable to the journal audience.

So, if the person who is giving you feedback missed a key point in your report, chances are that others will, too. Correct these problems while you have the chance to make the work clearer. For example, an important detail of the methodology might be "lost to the reader" because of its placement in the paper. If a peer reviewer misses the detail, it is much more productive to say "how can I present this information so that it comes through more clearly?" instead of "it was on page 20; what's wrong with this guy?" As political scientist Weeks noted in his commentary on the effective use of failure: "In the heat of reading, it is easy to denounce the reviewers as 'idiots,' but even a poorly written review may contain good advice."[17]

There will also be times when you are asked to perform analyses that you know are unnecessary. For the most part, it is better simply to do these and report the results rather than arguing the point because, again, readers may share the reviewers' concerns. For example, I was once part of a team that performed a quasi-experimental study in which we compared two groups of health care enrollees, mostly employees of small businesses and their dependents, who were part of the same health plan.[21] For one group of enrollees, the sponsoring employers had made a benefit design change; the other group's employers had left the benefit design unchanged. We performed a ***difference-in-difference*** analysis in which we calculated utilization changes from pre-intervention to post-intervention for both groups and tested the statistical significance of the between-group differences in the change amounts. We used bivariate testing without statistical adjustments because, as we showed in the study report, at baseline the groups were virtually identical on all of the demographic and clinical factors that we measured.

Nonetheless, one reviewer asked us to perform multivariate analyses. We knew that statistically controlling for nonexistent differences would not change the findings and was therefore a pointless exercise. However, because we had a good documentation system (see Chapter 2), we also knew that performing the requested analyses would take only about one hour. We did so, added a sentence to the study report indicating that multivariate analyses had produced similar findings, and the paper was published.

Third, disagree without being disagreeable. There will, of course, be times when you must respectfully offer a response that takes exception with feedback received from others—but the key words are *respectfully* and *response*. A *respectful response* is factual and delivered in an objective tone, for example: "We appreciate the reviewer's remarks about Study A. However, Study B, which produced the opposite finding, was published more recently using a larger sample size and updated recommendations from Organization Q. Thus, we continue to believe that Study B is a more appropriate benchmark than Study A. Nonetheless, because readers may have the same concern as the reviewer, we included a sentence about the methods and findings of Study A versus Study B in our discussion section."

Fourth, recognize and plan for exceptions to the general rule that peer review is helpful. An important caveat to the "attitude of gratitude" is that there *are* times when journal peer reviewers behave badly. Some reviewers are simply unpleasant; I was once advised by an anonymous peer reviewer for a scientific journal that I should resubmit my paper to "a trade publication" once I had learned to "form coherent thoughts."

Sometimes the problem is financial interest. In one infamous instance, a prominent researcher who reviewed a paper for the prestigious *New England Journal of Medicine*, knowing that the paper was likely to disadvantage a particular pharmaceutical manufacturer for which he was a consultant, allegedly contacted the manufacturer in advance of publication to provide a highly unethical "heads up."[22] In other situations, the problem is professional competition—that is, a peer reviewer recommends rejection of a manuscript partly because it offers a point of view that competes with that of the peer reviewer or because the author is a professional rival.[1]

As suggested by the 160-year-old observations of Thomas Huxley, which are quoted at the start of this chapter and reflect an obviously intense professional rivalry, conflicts of this type are nothing new and are probably at least somewhat inevitable in any review process (or in any human interaction, for that matter). However, to protect yourself as much as possible from negative comments that are based primarily on competitive or financial concerns, I strongly recommend that in considering where to submit your work, you give preference to journals that offer "double-blind" review—that is, just as you do not know the identity of the peer reviewers, they do not know who you are. Is this a guarantee of fair treatment or a perfect process? No, but it is helpful. To find out whether a journal's process is "double-blind," you can read its "instructions for authors" page, or send the editor or peer review administrator a query; they should be happy to provide this information.

Speaking Truth to Power: How to Respond to Erroneous Feedback from Supervisors or Decision Makers

Ask any methodologist or statistician about the times when he or she has been asked by someone with authority over a research project (a "decision maker") to do something that was either incorrect or unethical. You will almost certainly hear at least one long story. Some will be funny; others will be painful. In their engaging book, *The Human Side of Statistical Consulting*, statisticians James Boen and Douglas Zahn (1982) describe a distressing incident involving what they call a "client crook"—a paying customer who knowingly misrepresents the data:

> *"He was in charge of a human services program in which he wholeheartedly believed. Someone was asked to arrange a panel discussion to discuss the merits of the human service. The panel consisted of four service recipients, two of whom testified that the service was vital to them; the other two said they could take it or leave it. Somehow the word got out that a study had been done, and it showed that 50 percent of the people need the service. I told the client, whom I know very well, that he should set the record straight and tell the world that a good needs assessment should be done. He disagreed. He said it's too easy to get bogged down in statistical details. He said there's a great need for the program and more good than harm is being done by the '50 percent result.' ... I saw in print a year later that the need rate was 80 percent. I did some checking and found the 80 percent was just a misquote of the 50 percent. I called the client and pushed him hard on the point, but he never yielded. He thought I was just hung up."*[23]

Methodologists may describe these experiences using entertaining terms: HARKing (Hypothesizing After Results are Known), Texas sharp-shooting (analogous to the "marksman" who draws a target around holes that he has already shot in the side of a barn),[24] torturing a data set until it confesses to anything,[25] and, last but not least, the "sample size samba," described by biostatistician Andrew Vickers in a commentary on power calculations.[26] The dance begins when the sample size calculation based on standard statistical factors, such as anticipated effect size and alpha, produces an infeasible case count:

> "[We] can't possibly do a trial with 774 patients, but hang on—who is to say that [the initial estimate of standard deviation] is right, and what if the standard deviation was 1.5? Oh, we'd need 380 patients, which is still too many. What if we change the between-group difference to 0.75? And now the sample size calculation spits out 170 patients, which is just about doable ... so we agree on that."[26]

In more serious evidence of the sometimes inappropriate influence that decision makers may exert on the results of biomedical studies, Rising et al. (2008) compared efficacy trials submitted to the U.S. Food and Drug Administration as part of new drug applications (NDAs) from 2001 to 2002 with published trial reports through 2007.[27] The investigators found strong evidence that study methods had been changed prior to final analyses and publication. Odds of publication were 4.8 times as high (95% CI=1.3-17.1) for trials with favorable results on the primary outcome measure than for trials with results that were nonsignificant or favored the comparator drug. Even more seriously, 41 primary outcomes were omitted from the 128 published papers; only 23 of 43 (53.5%) outcomes not favorable to the NDA drug were published; and among those 23, the statistical significance results for 4 outcomes had been changed to favor the NDA drug. Rising et al.'s findings are far from isolated; numerous studies have documented misconduct of this kind, including suppression of negative findings and unexplained modifications of the *a priori* analysis plan prior to publication of study results.[24]

So, what should *you* do when you have been asked by a supervisor or decision maker to do something that you believe to be wrong—for example, report the results of a multivariate analysis as conclusive even though summary statistics reveal it to be of poor quality (see Chapter 6) or report as definitive the results of a survey to which the response rate was so low that the results don't represent the target population (see Chapter 8)? Knowing that others have gone through the same experience is perhaps a little comforting but does not address the most pressing question: how do you respond, especially when you (like most of us) need to make a living? I suggest the following "do's and don'ts:"

1. *DO get more information before responding.* Begin by asking questions about the *specific* approach that the decision maker wants to take, as well as any concerns that he or she has about your proposed approach. Be willing to listen to the decision maker's viewpoint. You might have missed something in the analysis or interpretation. *DO NOT* simply assume that you know the decision maker's viewpoint before hearing it.

2. *DO explain clearly.* If the decision maker is unfamiliar with the technique that you used, explain it in factual and specific terms. *DO NOT* become offended when the decision maker does not just "take your word for it" because of your expertise. Yes, you might have more expertise than the decision maker, but it is still incumbent upon you to explain the issues in terms that the decision maker can understand. And *DO NOT* assume that your inability to explain a technical issue to a decision maker is indicative of his or her incompetence to render a judgment on the matter. If you understand it, you should be able to explain it. If you can't, rework your explanation, perhaps with the help of a knowledgeable colleague, and try again.

3. *DO have your facts straight and well-supported.* Have references on hand that describe the technical problem and appropriate solutions. For example, if asked to repeat analyses using multiple different scenarios, have in your hand (literally) articles or calculations that show the effects of multiple comparisons on type I error and advise the decision maker of the need to use adjustments to *P* values for multiple comparisons. *DO NOT* tell the decision maker only that "text books show this" or "studies show that" without being able to present at least one or two cogent examples.

4. *DO give the decision maker the benefit of the doubt.* Often these situations arise because the decision maker lacks one or more key pieces of information. *DO NOT* assume nefarious motives unless and until you have evidence about them.

5. *DO be polite, respectful, and responsive.* Always. No matter what.

6. *DO* incorporate the decision maker's specific concerns into any write-ups that you produce. Remember the advice of Booth et al. that open consideration of alternative points of view is one of the most important tools you can use to improve your own credibility.[13]

7. *DO NOT equate a single "slip-up" on a decision maker's part with a flawed character.* Everyone makes mistakes. Sometimes there is a need to "agree to disagree" and move on to an otherwise productive professional relationship, even when you

feel strongly. *However,* if inappropriate or unethical requests become a pattern of behavior, it may be time to think about looking for another job.

Summing Up: What Have We Learned?

In general, feedback that seems erroneous or offensive is often the best tool that researchers have to improve the quality of a research work product, because it can reveal points that are unclear or were missed in planning or write-up. Take it seriously, and adopt an "attitude of gratitude" for the input. Find opportunities—early and often in the research process—to seek out and use criticism from others. Your work will surely be improved as a result.

In Chapter 10, we examine good research-reporting practices that will help formal and informal peer reviewers do their job of evaluating the importance and validity of your work. We begin with a popular fictional tale about a murder—and a leg of lamb.

References

1. Wilson JD. Peer review and publication: Presidential address before the 70th Annual Meeting of the American Society for Clinical Investigation. *J Clin Invest.* 1978;61(6):1697-701.

2. Thomas Henry Huxley. Available at: http://www.ucmp.berkeley.edu/history/thuxley.html.

3. Benjaminson P. *Publish Without Perishing: A Practical Handbook for Academic Authors.* Washington, DC: National Education Association; 1992: quotation p. 50.

4. Gans JS, Shepherd GB. How are the mighty fallen: rejected classic articles by leading economists. *Journal of Economic Perspectives.* 1994;8(1):165-79.

5. Armstrong JS. Peer review for journals: evidence on quality control, fairness, and innovation. *Science and Engineering Ethics.* 1997;3(1):63-84. Available at: http://repository.upenn.edu/cgi/viewcontent.cgi?article=1110&context=marketing_papers.

6. Inglefinger FJ. Peer review in biomedical publication. *Am J Med.* 1974;56:686-92.

7. Goldman A. Smoking gun discovered in Einstein controversy. *University of Minnesota School of Physics and Astronomy Newsletter.* Spring 2005:3,8. Available at: http://www.physics.umn.edu/alumni/Newsletter5.pdf.

8. Blog posting. Einstein vs. Physical Review. *Discover* blog. September 16, 2005. Available at: http://blogs.discovermagazine.com/cosmicvariance/2005/09/16/einstein-vs-physical-review/.

9. Tsang EWK, Frey BS. The as-is-journal review process: let authors own their ideas. *Academy of Management Learning & Education.* 2007;6(1):128-36. Available at: http://www.iew.uzh.ch/wp/iewwp280.pdf.

10. International Symposium on Peer Reviewing: ISPR 2009. July 10th through 13th, 2009. Available at: http://www.ictconfer.org/ispr.

11. Sixth International Congress on Peer Review and Biomedical Publication. Available at: http://www.ama-assn.org/public/peer/previous.html.

12. House of Commons, Science and Technology Committee. Peer review in scientific publications: Eighth report of Session 2010-12. HC856. July 18, 2011. Available at: http://www.publications.parliament.uk/pa/cm201012/cmselect/cmsctech/856/856.pdf.

13. Booth WC, Colomb GG, Williams JM. *The Craft of Research. Third Edition.* Chicago, IL: University of Chicago Press; 2008: quotations pp. 117-118, 139, 140, 142, 146.

14. Ray J, Berkwits M, Davidoff F. The fate of manuscripts rejected by a general medical journal. *Am J Med.* 2000;109(2):131-35.

15. Armstrong AW, Idriss SZ, Kimball AB, Bernhard JD. Fate of manuscripts declined by the Journal of the American Academy of Dermatology. *J Am Acad Dermatol.*

2008;58(4):632-35.

16. Gorski D. Does peer review need fixing? *Science-Based Medicine*. August 23, 2010. Available at: http://www.sciencebasedmedicine.org/?p=6523.

17. Weeks G. Facing failure: the use (and abuse) of rejection in political science. *PSOnline*. 2006;39(4):879-82. Available at: http://www.politicalscience.uncc.edu/gbweeks/ Facing%20Failure.pdf.

18. Bedeian AG. Peer review and the social construction of knowledge in the management discipline. *Academy of Management Learning and Education*. 2004;3(2):199-216.

19. Bedeian AG. The manuscript review process: the proper roles of authors, referees, and editors. *Journal of Management Inquiry*. 2003;12:331-38. Available at: http://www. bus.lsu.edu/bedeian/articles/Jmi2589741.pdf.

20. Fairman KA, Motheral BR. Do decision analytic models identify cost-effective treatments? A retrospective look at *Helicobacter pylori* eradication. *J Manag Care Pharm*. 2003;9(5):430-40. Available at: http://www.amcp.org/data/jmcp/Formulary%20 Management-430-440.pdf.

21. Motheral B, Fairman KA. Effect of a three-tier prescription copay on pharmaceutical and other medical utilization. *Med Care*. 2001;39(12):1293-304.

22. Saul S. Doctor accused of leak to drug maker. *New York Times*. January 31, 2008. Available at: http://www.nytimes.com/2008/01/31/business/31censure.html.

23. Boen JR, Zahn DA. *The Human Side of Statistical Consulting*. Belmont, CA: Wadsworth, Inc.;1982: quotation p. 123.

24. Fairman KA, Curtiss FR. What should be done about bias and misconduct in clinical trials? *J Manag Care Pharm*. 2009;15(2):154-60. Available at: http://www.amcp.org/data/ jmcp/154-160.pdf.

25. Fairman KA. Differentiating effective data mining from fishing, trapping, and cruelty to numbers. *J Manag Care Pharm*. 2007;13(6):517-27. Available at: http://www.amcp.org/ data/jmcp/pages%20517-27.pdf.

26. Vickers AJ. Let's dance! The sample size samba. December 16, 2008. Available at: http://www.medscape.com/viewarticle/584026. Vickers acknowledges that the term "sample size samba" was originally coined by trial methodologist Ken Schulz.

27. Rising K, Bacchetti P, Bero L. Reporting bias in drug trials submitted to the Food and Drug Administration: review of publication and presentation. *PLoS Med*. 2008;5(11):1561-70. Available at: http://www.ncbi.nlm.nih.gov/pmc/articles/ PMC2586350/pdf/pmed.0050217.pdf.

CHAPTER 10
Transparency and Clarity: Good Research-Reporting Practices

"Besides it is an error to believe that rigour is the enemy of simplicity. On the contrary ... the rigorous method is at the same time the simpler and the more easily comprehended."—German mathematician David Hilbert[1]

"When you wish to instruct, be brief; that men's minds take in quickly what you say, learn its lesson, and retain it faithfully. Every word that is unnecessary only pours over the side of a brimming mind."—Roman author and politician Marcus Tullius Cicero[2]

"There's nothing to writing. All you do is sit down at a typewriter and open a vein."—American sports columnist Walter Wellesley "Red" Smith[3]

In his delightfully macabre tale, *Lamb to the Slaughter*, master story-teller Roald Dahl writes of fictional protagonist Mary Maloney, who kills her faithless husband by whacking him on the back of the head with a frozen leg of lamb, then cooks up the murder weapon and feeds it to the detectives who come to investigate the crime.[4] In the closing scene of the story, the befuddled policemen, who have spent hours in a fruitless search of the house and surrounding area for the object

---

What You Will Learn in Chapter 10

✓ How using the EQUATOR standards can help you *communicate* with your audience

✓ Why *learning about your target journal* increases the chance that your article will be published and understood by readers

✓ How to *write an accurate title* that will improve your chances of being cited by others

✓ How to use the IMRAD (introduction, methods, results, and discussion) structure to *guide readers through your process of discovery*

✓ How to *enhance your credibility* with those who will read and use your research

used to smash the victim's skull, discuss the case over dinner in Mary's kitchen: "Whoever done it, they're not going to be carrying a thing like that around with them longer than they need," one detective says. "Personally," says another detective, "I think it's right here on the premises." Another agrees. "Probably right under our very noses. What you think, Jack?" Overhearing the men as they talk, "their voices thick and sloppy with meat," Dahl recounts, "Mary Maloney began to giggle."[4]

In its day, *Lamb to the Slaughter* was quite popular. Originally published in 1953, it eventually became a 1958 episode of *The Alfred Hitchcock Hour* and today is available as a YouTube video that has, at this writing, been viewed more than 134,000 times. Perhaps the appeal of the tale lies in Dahl's legendary knack for portraying the flaws inherent in human nature. Improbable as the story is, it nonetheless highlights a characteristic shared by most of us: it is easy to miss information to which we have not explicitly been directed, even if it is "right under our very noses."

As researchers and writers, it is our job to ensure, to the greatest extent possible, that our information users do not miss details that are important to them. For research *results* to be *usable*—a hallmark characteristic of excellence as defined in Chapter 1—*all* aspects of the research project, from the literature review to the methods, findings, and discussion of study limitations and implications, must be completely clear to the target audience.

This chapter reviews research-reporting practices that facilitate that critically important level of clarity. The good news about these practices is that they are not complicated or difficult to understand. Additionally, although many different research-reporting guideline documents exist, all are based on the same basic principles, and all provide similar advice.[5] These documents were originally formulated for written communication. For that reason, I use the term "reader" in this chapter. However, principles of good reporting also apply to other formats, such as poster presentations, scientific conference abstracts, or less formal meetings among colleagues.

Throughout this chapter, I use terms and concepts that were discussed in detail in Chapter 3, such as **internal** and **external validity**, **cross-sectional design**, **observational research**, **confounding**, and **selection bias**. If you are unsure about these terms, please either consult Chapter 3 or review the definitions in the Glossary. This chapter also assumes familiarity with the key concepts described in Chapter 4 on project planning—what is already known about the subject and what the present study is intended to add.

A Note for Information *Users*

If you *use* research information, even if you do not write research reports, an understanding of reporting standards is essential for your work. That is, you should be aware of what to expect from a research report. If a report is substandard, you should view its results skeptically. *Never* trust research findings solely because of the purported expertise or reputation of the investigators. Instead, compare the report with the standards described in this chapter, and make your judgments about its credibility accordingly.

General Principles

Prior to a discussion of specific reporting standards, it is helpful to review key principles of clear communication from researcher to reader.

Consult a reporting guideline. The International Committee of Medical Journal Editors (ICMJE) "Uniform Requirements for Manuscripts Submitted to Biomedical Journals"[6] directs authors to the website of the **E**nhancing the **QUA**lity and **T**ransparency **O**f health **R**esearch (EQUATOR)[7] network for detailed information about effective research reporting—and with good reason. The network, which is "an international initiative that seeks to improve reliability and value of medical research literature by promoting transparent and accurate reporting of research studies," is a *great* source of information about how to write a research report. The EQUATOR website provides links to reporting guidelines for virtually every type of study published in health care today, available in an easily searchable database. Guidelines for common types of health care research are summarized in Table 10A. [8-21]

Facilitate replication. Of all the standards that appear in research-reporting guidelines, the most overarching is that *study methods should be reported with sufficient detail and clarity to enable a knowledgeable reader to replicate the research based solely on the information in the study report.* This is the specific guidance given by the ICMJE for statistical analyses, and it underlies all EQUATOR research-reporting standards.[6,7] Even the United Kingdom's House of Commons has weighed in on this point. In the special report on journal peer review that was discussed in Chapter 9, the House Science and Technology committee described "reproducibility" of research as "the gold standard that all peer reviewers and editors aim for when assessing whether a manuscript has supplied sufficient information to allow others to repeat and build on the experiments."[22] The committee went so far as to recommend that peer reviewers and

Table 10A

Reporting Guidelines for Common Types of Health Care Research

Acronym and Full Name	Authors and Year	Examples of Available Variations
CHERRIES: CHEcklist for **Re**porting **R**esults of **I**nternet **E-S**urveys	Eysenbach (2004)[8]	
CONSORT: CONsolidated **S**tandards **O**f **R**eporting **T**rials	Moher et al. (2010)[9]	RCTs reported in abstracts for scientific meetings and poster sessions; harms in RCTs; noninferiority RCTs; trials for nonpharmacologic interventions and herbals; trials of eHealth interventions
PRISMA: Preferred **R**eporting **I**tems for **S**ystematic Reviews and **M**eta-**A**nalyses	Liberati et al (2009)[10]	MOOSE (**M**eta-analysis **O**f **O**bservational **S**tudies in **E**pidemiology)[11]
SQUIRE: Standards for **QU**ality **I**mprovement **R**eporting **E**xcellence	Davidoff et al. (2009)[12]	
STROBE: STrengthening the **R**eporting of **OB**servational Studies in **E**pidemiology	Vandenbroucke et al. (2007)[13]	ORION (**O**utbreak **R**eports and **I**ntervention studies **O**f **N**osocomial infection);[14] GRIPS (**G**enetic **RI**sk **P**rediction **S**tudies)[15]
TREND: Transparent **R**eporting of **E**valuations with **N**onrandomized **D**esigns	Des Jarlais et al. (2004)[16]	
Cost-effectiveness analyses	Siegel et al. (1996)[17]	
Cost-effectiveness analyses alongside clinical trials	Ramsey et al. (2005)[18]	
Reporting format for economic modeling studies	Nuijten et al. (1998)[19]	
Reporting of comparative effectiveness research using secondary database sources	Berger et al. (2009)[20]	
Reporting considerations for retrospective analyses of claims databases; "checklist" for information users	Motheral et al. (2003)[21]	

Source for references 8-20: EQUATOR network (www.equator-network.org). The list in Table 10A is *not* comprehensive. Readers are strongly encouraged to check the EQUATOR website database for detailed information about their specific study types.

EQUATOR= **E**nhancing the **QUA**lity and **T**ransparency **O**f health **R**esearch; RCT=randomized controlled trial.

editors have "confidential access to relevant data associated with the work" during the peer review process, describing such an arrangement as "essential."[22]

Be specific but not repetitive. In addition to facilitating replication, a good research report presents enough specific information to enable the reader to grasp key concepts quickly without overwhelming the reader with a mind-numbing level of detail. In *The Chicago Guide to Writing about Numbers* and *The Chicago Guide to Writing about Multivariate Analysis*, methodologist Jane Miller describes an excellent approach to achieving this goal—generalization, example, exceptions.[23,24] That is, first describe a *general trend*; then provide a *specific example* that illustrates the trend and has meaning for the reader; then, if there are *exceptions* to the trend, explain what they are.

For example, in writing a literature review, you might say something like the following hypothetical text (including appropriate citations to the source documents, of course): "Numerous studies have found a strong association between a higher level of physical impairment and initial choice of pain medication, with the most physically impaired subjects more likely to receive Drug A than Drug B. For example, in a large-sample (n=35,000) study of patients with at least six visits to one of a nationwide network of chronic pain clinics from 2008-2009, utilization rates among those with the lowest 36-item short-form (SF-36) physical component scores (less than 20, indicating high levels of physical impairment)[25] were 30% for Drug A and 10% for Drug B. However, drug choice is more complex in the presence of comorbidities. In a study of patients diagnosed with both chronic pain and congestive heart failure, utilization rates were 10% and 30% for Drug A and Drug B, respectively."

Use a good reporting example (if necessary). If you are unsure of how to write a clear and effective research article, a learning exercise is helpful. Find a journal that you (or a mentor or colleagues) respect, and read a few articles *about a topic that is unfamiliar to you*. Do not pick a familiar topic, because the point of this exercise is to identify an article that does a good job of explaining unfamiliar material to a reasonably knowledgeable reader. After reading the articles, consider which article most closely meets the following criteria:

1. I can determine to which groups this study does and does not apply. For example, it is clear that this is a study of Medicaid beneficiaries and therefore may not be

applicable to commercially insured enrollees.

2. I can determine whether the study groups adequately represent the intended population (e.g., all Medicaid beneficiaries, all patients taking antidepressant drugs) *or* are a small and/or highly select subgroup of the **sampling frame**. (Note: It does not matter for this purpose whether the groups are representative or nonrepresentative; all that matters is whether the distinction is clear to you from reading the report.)

3. The procedures used in this study are so clearly described that, given access to the study cases (e.g., enrollees, patients, dataset) and necessary resources (e.g., computer programs or programmers; laboratory equipment), I could do this study myself or adequately oversee the work of others doing the study.

4. The findings of this study are so clear to me that I could (a) write a summary that includes specific quantitative findings for the most important study outcomes *and* (b) discuss not only whether the results are *statistically* significant, but also whether the results are *substantively* significant—that is, the report makes the practical meaning of the study results clear.

Once you have identified an article that meets these criteria, use that article as a model when you write your manuscript. Additional helpful sources include EQUATOR "explanation and elaboration" documents, which provide detailed examples of good reporting for each component of a research article,[9,13] and Miller's *Chicago Guide* books, which include helpful examples of "poor," "better," and "best" text.[23,24]

Consider the needs of the unfamiliar reader. As you write, remember that you understand much more about your work than the reader does—especially at the outset of the article, when the reader may know nothing at all about the topic. Ensure that potentially unfamiliar terms are defined as you write about them and that foundational concepts are explained early in the article. For example, beginning the report of a study of the relationship between natural disasters and anxiety treatment rates with a discussion of various anti-anxiety medications would be a poor approach, even if the researcher plans to mention drug treatment options in the results or discussion. A better approach is to begin with a discussion of natural disasters, explaining what was already known about the effects of these disasters on mental health prior to the present study. In *The Craft of Research*, Booth, Colomb, and Williams (2008) issue an important admonition: "Whatever your order [of topics], it must reflect *your readers'* needs, not the order that the material seems to impose on itself (as in an obvious compare-contrast organization), least of all the order in which [the material] occurred to you." (emphasis in original).[26]

Lead the reader step-by-step, in logical fashion. ICMJE standards for manuscripts submitted to biomedical journals suggest that a research report be structured into the following categories, which are familiar to any of us who have read a published research article: Introduction, Methods, Results, and Discussion. The guidelines note that this structure, known in ICMJE as "IMRAD," is "not an arbitrary publication format but rather a direct reflection of the process of scientific discovery."[6] This admonition is helpful, not just because IMRAD is standard but, more importantly, because it reminds us that *a good research article guides its reader through the researcher's learning process.* By the time a reader finishes a research report, he or she should understand, in the following order:

1. Trends that the researcher identified when he or she reviewed previously published work (what was already known about the topic before the project began);
2. Gaps in the knowledge available from previously published work;
3. How the objectives of the present study addressed those knowledge gaps (what the present study adds);
4. Specific methods used in the present study, and how those methods were derived from the literature review (i.e., from an understanding of the methods used in previous research on the topic);
5. Specific findings of the present study, and the implications of those findings for the study objectives, for the topic generally, and for the health care professionals who are the target audience.

Three points about IMRAD are noteworthy. **First**, if you followed the project planning steps described in Chapter 4, you already know the first four items listed above and, if you produced a research proposal, they are written (at least in draft form). **Second**, all these steps should be logically connected in a way that is completely clear to the reader. For example, the report should explain specifically how the implications described in the study report were derived from the study findings. Of course, not every reader will agree with the conclusions that the researcher drew about the study implications— but it should at least be clear to the reader *how* the findings led the researcher to reach those conclusions. **Third,** as described in more detail in Chapter 9, informal and formal peer review obtained throughout the project is of tremendous help in making these points logically clear to readers, because the review process helps to reveal the reader's perspective.

Explain unusual or potentially controversial decisions. Most research projects involve methodological choices, not all of which are straightforward. Sometimes for good reasons, researchers may decide to use a method that differs from those of previous studies. Additionally, as EQUATOR guidelines for randomized trials point out, "it is impossible to predict every possible change in circumstances during the course of a trial."[9] As we saw in Chapter 7, changes to observational analyses of administrative claims databases may be necessary to account for unexpected patterns in the coding of diagnoses and/or procedures in the billing data (e.g., use of a nonspecific code to bill for a newly approved injectable medication because no specific code has been promulgated yet). Thus, researchers may need to change study methods after the *a priori* research plan has been developed and, in some situations, published.

The key to handling these situations is transparency—clear disclosure of any unusual or potentially controversial decisions in the methods section of the article. Additionally, brief explanations of these methodological choices should be provided. This information helps the reader not only to *understand* the study methods but also to *judge* whether they were reasonable.

Understand the target publication. Other than conducting a high-quality research study, the most important step that a researcher can take to maximize his or her chances of publication in the target journal is to *carefully* read *both* the journal's instructions for authors *and* an article on the same or a similar topic that has been published in that journal. Every journal has its own style, both technical and stylistic. For example, some journals present nearly all methodological details in the text; others ask that these details be shown in a table that becomes part of the published research article; and others prefer that they be provided only in appendices that are available to readers online.

The main objective of this exploration is to understand *before* writing your article how your target journal "likes to do things." This step saves both you and the journal staff a great deal of time and effort. A key point in this regard is to pay attention to the journal presentation format *even if* it does not entirely fit with what you were taught in graduate school. For example, most graduate students are taught that when a data distribution is skewed, the median is a more meaningful measure of central tendency than the mean. Although this guidance is absolutely correct, some journals nonetheless require the presentation of multiple measures of central tendency and dispersion, including mean, standard deviation, median, and interquartile range. There is nothing wrong with this requirement, because different measures often provide readers with valuable information. For example, in an analysis of trends in out-of-pocket cost per claim for injectable drugs to treat multiple sclerosis, Kunze et al. (2007) found a large difference between medians ($15 in 2004 and $25 in 2007) and means ($52 in 2004 and $79 in 2007).[27] In fact, in all quarters studied, especially the first quarter of each year, the *mean* value far exceeded the top of the interquartile range (the 75th percentile). These findings provided the important information that mean values were being "driven" by a small proportion of members paying a high share of cost for their medications, particularly early in each calendar year when member contributions to deductibles accrued.

You are, of course, free to disagree with the way that the journal "likes to do things" and to submit a paper that takes a different approach. However, it is important to consider two points in making this decision. **First**, you are likely to have a much easier time explaining your work and convincing editors and peer reviewers of its credibility if you use a format and approach with which they are familiar. **Second**, most journal editors have considerable knowledge of their readers' needs. If a journal editor advises you to present information in a particular way, it is wise to do so—not primarily because it will improve your chances of publication in that journal (although it might), but especially because it will improve your chances of informing the journal's audience. In other words, an understanding of the target journal and its readers helps you fulfill your primary objective in writing the research report—effective communication.

> ### Key Points: Reporting Principles
>
> ❖ Replication—reproducibility is the "gold standard."
> ❖ Specificity—to help the reader understand.
> ❖ Logical progression and explanation.
> ❖ Definitions of terms that may be unfamiliar to the audience.
> ❖ Explanation of unusual decisions.
> ❖ Consideration of the target journal style.

Reporting Guideline Details

In a now very old commercial for a certain brand of spaghetti sauce, family members entered the kitchen expecting to find Mama or Grandma making homemade sauce, only to discover—with considerable dismay—that she was actually pouring the sauce out of a jar. But the "chef" would defend herself, saying that even if her children and grandchildren couldn't see each of their favorite ingredients going into the sauce, they should rest assured: "It's in there."[28]

Although this approach ("it's in there, somewhere") might work well for spaghetti sauce, it is poor practice for research reporting. Readers should not have to spend time searching for essential details, and they certainly should not have to rely on trust that the necessary material is "in there, somewhere." Instead, in a clear study report, information is presented *explicitly* and in a *predictable format and location* that is prescribed by reporting guidelines.

Following is a summary of available standards for each research report component, based primarily on the **CON**solidated **S**tandards **O**f **R**eporting **T**rials (CONSORT), **ST**rengthening the **R**eporting of **OB**servational Studies in **E**pidemiology (STROBE), and related guidelines.[8,9,13,20,21] Because the reporting standards all provide similar guidance, the summary should translate readily into nearly all studies; however, readers are encouraged to consult the guideline specific to their type of research long before writing the study report, preferably in the project-planning stage.[7] Key practices for each report section are summarized in Table 10B and discussed in detail below.

Title: Carefully Worded and Specific

The report title should represent, in a highly abbreviated form, key elements of what the research was about and how it was performed. A title can be "built" in stages by following a few simple instructions. **First**, if the research measured the association between two phenomena or factors, both should be named in the title, typically with the key independent variable named first and the dependent variable named second (e.g., "The Association of Pain Medication Use with Disability").[24] **Second**, if the report studied a specific group, especially if the group is atypical, the title should name the group (e.g., "The Association of Pain Medication Use with Disability in Elderly Low-Income Patients with Osteoarthritis" or "The Association of Pain Medication Use with Disability in Medicaid Enrollees"). **Third**, if the study time period is important to the research topic, it should be named as well (e.g., "The Association of Pain Medication Use

Table 10B
Summary of Research-Reporting Practices

Title: Carefully Worded and Specific
- Identification in article database searches (e.g., PubMed) depends on accurate titles.
- Include the study design, key variables, and study groups.
- Indicate time period if important to topic.
- Indicate novel or especially rigorous statistical methods.
- Never overstate design (e.g., referring to "effect of" in the title of a cross-sectional study report).

Abstract: Specific and Complete
- Many journals have a specific format, typically Background, Objective, Method, Results, and Conclusion.
- To provide sufficient descriptions of methods and findings within word limits, use concise language; consult an experienced abstract writer if necessary.

Introduction: Clearly Based on a Foundation of Previous Work
- Specifically describe previous work to facilitate objectivity and credibility.
- Make gaps in previous work clear so that study objectives make sense to the reader.
- Make clear the present study's causal plausibility.

Methods: Complete and Clear
- Present key elements of study design early in the methods section to facilitate reader understanding.
- Describe study context completely.
- Include specific descriptions of study groups, data sources and quality, and study variables.
- Describe potential sources of bias and methods used to address or adjust for them.
- Describe methods sequentially (in the order in which they were performed).
- Describe statistical methods with sufficient clarity and specificity to enable a knowledgeable reader with access to the data to replicate the results.
- Explain unusual methodological choices.

Results: Practical and Sensible
- Specifically describe sample composition, including *quantitative* effects of each inclusion and exclusion criterion.
- Translate outcomes into practical terms (e.g., number needed to treat).
- If multivariate analysis is used, present both unadjusted (usually bivariate) and adjusted findings.
- Interpret multivariate results considering the substantive (mathematical) meaning of coefficients; consider presenting predicted probabilities or adjusted means.
- Report results of sensitivity analyses, subgroup analyses, and interaction effect analyses, if applicable.
- Consider using "generalization, example, exception" approach when describing results in text.

Discussion: Balance, Caution, and Humility
- Begin by highlighting key results.
- Interpret findings and implications in the context of previous work.
- Interpret nonrandomized designs cautiously, considering alternative explanations for findings and addressing threats to *internal* validity, such as bias and confounding.
- Describe threats to *external* validity.

Ethical Considerations
- Disclose relationships that readers could perceive as influencing the work.
- Explain procedures used to protect patient safety and privacy.

Sources:
Berger et al. Defining, reporting and interpreting nonrandomized studies of treatment effects.[20]
Eysenbach. Improving the quality of web surveys.[8]
Miller. *The Chicago Guide to Writing about Numbers.*[23]
Motheral et al. A checklist for retrospective database studies.[21]
Nuijten et al. Reporting format for economic evaluation.[19]
Moher et al. CONSORT standards.[9]
Vandenbroucke et al. STROBE standards.[13]
CONSORT=**CON**solidated **S**tandards **O**f **R**eporting **T**rials; STROBE=**ST**rengthening the **R**eporting of **OB**servational Studies in **E**pidemiology.

with Disability in Elderly Low-Income Patients with Osteoarthritis After Implementation of Medicare Part D").[24] It is assumed in this example that readers of the target journal understand what Medicare Part D is; if not, the title could be changed to refer to "the Medicare Prescription Drug Benefit."

Fourth, the title should indicate the specific method used,[9,13,24] for example:

- The Effect of a Pain Medication Adherence Program on Disability in Elderly Low-Income Patients with Osteoarthritis: A Randomized Controlled Trial
- Cross-Sectional Analysis of the Association of Pain Medication Use with Disability in Elderly Low-Income Patients with Osteoarthritis
- A Survey of Elderly Low-Income Patients with Osteoarthritis: Opinions about Pain Medication and Disability
- Cohort Analysis of Elderly Low-Income Patients with Osteoarthritis: Change in Disability Associated with Uptake of Prescription Drug Coverage
- Five-Year Budgetary Impact Analysis of Formulary Inclusion of Drug A for Treatment of Chronic Pain

This level of specificity is important not only to indicate the design and sample characteristics to the reader but also to facilitate searches in publication report databases (e.g., PubMed) for your work. If a randomized controlled trial (RCT) is not specifically identified as such in the title, its design may be missed by indexing systems.[9] Thus, a nonspecific or incomplete title may result in the omission of your work from literature reviews conducted by other researchers, especially those who use a "Limits" function within a search algorithm to restrict searches to RCTs. Similarly, an article with a vague title that fails to indicate the specific group in which the research was conducted, such as "Pain Medication Use and Disability," may be missed in a PubMed search conducted using a limit of "Aged: 65+ years."

A final important point about the title is that it should *never* overstate or understate the validity of the design. For example, a study with a cross-sectional design should not be reported with a title that includes the phrases "effect of," "consequence of," or similar language that implies causality, because a cross-sectional association is not sufficient to demonstrate causation.[24] However, if a particularly strong or novel analytic technique was used to investigate an association, the technique should be mentioned in the title (e.g., "The Association of Pain Medication Adherence with Level of Disability in Elderly Patients with Osteoarthritis: Fixed-Effects Analysis").[24]

The key to a good title is to describe in few words what the study *was* and to avoid language that would imply something that it *wasn't*. It may take a few attempts to do this well, and journal peer reviewers and editors often make excellent suggestions in this regard.

Abstract: Specific and Complete

Perhaps more than any other feature of a research article, the abstract should reflect an understanding of readers' needs for *specific* information. In real-world practice, many busy information users will read only the abstract of a research report.[9] Although this reading method is obviously suboptimal, taking it into account in writing the abstract is critical to giving readers an understanding of the internal validity (accuracy of inference) and external validity (applicability) of the work. CONSORT standards provide the guidance that a "journal abstract should contain sufficient information about a trial to serve as an accurate record of its conduct and findings, providing optimal information about the trial within the space constraints and format of a journal."[9] To provide the necessary information despite journal word limits, a good abstract should be specific but concise and tightly written. For example, say "n=90" instead of "Ninety patients were studied" or "Objective: To assess medication adherence …" instead of "We conducted the present study to examine the degree of medication adherence …" (If you have difficulty doing this, consult an experienced abstract writer.)

To encourage informative reporting, most journals require a structured abstract, usually consisting of the categories Background, Objective, Method, Results, and Conclusion. The background is typically a one- or two-sentence summary of what was already known about the subject prior to the present study, and the objective is a single-sentence or single-phrase summary of what the present study was intended to add.

Although brief, abstract descriptions of study methods and findings should be thorough. For example, CONSORT guidelines suggest that the abstract methods section should specify the type of trial design, setting, eligibility criteria for participant inclusion, interventions in each study group, primary outcome, method of randomization, whether participants and/or caregivers were "blinded" to group assignment and, if so, how. The abstract results section should specify, for each study group, the number of participants randomized; the number of participants included in the final analyses; the results for the primary outcome in each study group; the intervention effect size and precision around the estimate; and a description of harms associated with the intervention.

Similarly, the STROBE standards for abstracts say:

> "We advise presenting key results in a numerical form that includes numbers of participants, estimates of associations and appropriate measures of variability and uncertainty (e.g., odds ratios with confidence intervals). We regard it insufficient to state only that an exposure is or is not significantly associated with an outcome."[13]

Although the content of an abstract will vary depending on the type of study, a similar level of specificity should be used regardless of design. For example, the abstract of an observational analysis of a medical claims database will, of course, not indicate a method of randomization; however, it should state clearly the methods for identification and follow-up, including the diagnoses used to select and group subjects for the sample, requirements for continuous health plan enrollment, and the time periods for subject selection and measurement of outcomes. The abstract of a decision analytic model should specify all key input assumptions. This level of specificity enables an abstract reader to assess the strengths and limitations of the work and to apply the results to his or her setting or purpose.

Introduction: Clearly Based on a Foundation of Previous Work

Recall from Chapter 9 the helpful advice of Booth et al. (2008) that a research report is best understood as a conversation with readers. In the conversation, the researcher presents many "claims," that is, assertions of "something that may be true or false and so needs support,"[26] and "reasons," that is, information supporting the claims. "Reasons" are often explanatory sentences. Each "reason," in turn, should be supported by evidence. For example, the following text appeared in the introduction to an article by Delate et al. (2004), which described the results of an RCT of a "dose consolidation program:"*

> "While the concept of dose consolidation is appealing to plan sponsors based
> on the perception that it has a small, negative impact on patients, prescribers,
> and medication access, its cost-effectiveness has not been demonstrated. Only

---

* Dose consolidation programs identify patients receiving multiple tablets or capsules of a medication and attempt to "convert" the regimen to single-pill dosing to simplify the drug regimen and save money.

I peer-reviewed article and I study abstract that evaluated dose consolidation (optimization) programs were identified in a literature search of MEDLINE and HealthStart electronic databases."[29]

This text first made the *claim* that dose consolidation is appealing, then explained the claim (perceived small negative impact). Then the text made a second claim, that dose consolidation has been understudied, and provided evidence to support the claim. After describing the specific programs evaluated in the two previous studies, the text went on:

"While the findings from these studies suggested substantial drug cost savings from a dose consolidation program, these studies had methodological limitations. Both studies utilized nonexperimental study designs that did not account for dose consolidation that would have taken place without the intervention, (e.g., as a result of dose titration). Neither study accounted for administrative costs of the dose consolidation programs that would have offset some of the drug cost savings. Most importantly, neither study took into account that some of the funds for dose consolidation programs are spent to modify medication regimens for which the plan subsequently ceases to have financial liability, either due to member plan disenrollment/coverage termination or drug therapy discontinuation."[29]

This text made the claim that the two previous studies had important limitations, then explained what those were, specifically (evidence supporting the claim). By presenting what was already known about the subject, as well as what was *not* known, the text provided an ideal segue to a study objective.

I selected this example in part because the dose consolidation article was met with opposition by the authors of one of the previous studies, Baldinger and Calabrese (2004), who expressed their concerns in a letter to the editor.[30] Such responses to research publications are not uncommon, although the vast majority of readers' concerns are not expressed in print. The wise researcher understands that *many* readers will ask questions about an article, anticipates those questions, and provides the answers in the article text.[26] Indeed, in responding to the concerns expressed by Baldinger and Calabrese, Delate et al. relied heavily on the content of their original article, using the phrase "as we point out in our report" twice in their brief response.[31] This type of interchange clearly illustrates Booth et al.'s description of a research report as a conversation; in their report, Delate et al. anticipated concerns that might be expressed about their work and incorporated those concerns into the report, facilitating a substantive and informed response when questions arose.

In understanding why the construction of claims based on evidence is essential in research reporting, recognition of two patterns likely to be displayed by readers is foundational. On the one hand, some readers will begin reading an article already disagreeing with its conclusions. In some circumstances, the reader may be disadvantaged by the findings (e.g., the employee of a competing company or an advocate of a particular viewpoint that is refuted by the work). Some readers will even be searching intentionally for a flaw in the study's premise, design, or analysis. Without careful explanations of the rationale for the study's purpose and methods, these readers are unlikely to believe its results. On the other hand, some readers will know little or nothing about the topic. Their greatest need is for education—why the topic is important, what is known about it from previous studies, and how it has been studied in the past. A good research report must speak effectively to *both* of those groups *and*, occasionally, even to a third group consisting of readers who have the unfortunate (and, thankfully, rare) combination of both—strong opinions coupled with little or no knowledge.

The key to effective communication with all these groups is specificity. As Booth et al. observe, "vague claims lead to vague arguments. The more specific your claim, the more it helps you plan your argument and keep your readers on track as they read it."[26] In other words, *specific information* leads the reader through your process of discovery. Note that the text by Delate et al. was effective because it explained the specific limitations of previously published observational research, thereby making it clear why an RCT of dose consolidation was needed—something like groundwork laid for the foundation of a new building.

The best way to lay that groundwork is to use the literature review summary chart and preliminary study plan that were described in Chapter 4. Even if you did not use a literature summary chart in developing your project plan, it is a good idea to read Chapter 4 now, construct a literature summary chart, and base the study introduction on that. Using the summary chart is important for two reasons. **First**, as described in more detail in Chapter 4, it helps you and your readers maintain objectivity. As a sure cure for unsubstantiated opinion—either the researcher's or the reader's—nothing beats an accurate description of the facts about previous work, including an assessment of its limitations, such as weak design or small sample size. **Second**, the literature summary chart facilitates accuracy that, in turn, helps establish your credibility in the minds of knowledgeable readers.

Objectives that reflect gaps in available knowledge. Once the introduction has established what was already known—and what was not yet known—about a topic prior to the research project, stating the objective of the study should be easy. In other words, the introduction has described knowledge gaps, and the objectives of the present study should flow logically from those gaps.[13] Making clear the logical connection between previous work and your work further establishes your credibility.

Establishing this logical connection may also have ethical implications for any research involving human subjects. Specifically, if there is no gap in knowledge, there is no need to conduct the research and therefore no need to expose research subjects to potential harm or inconvenience associated with the study (e.g., adverse effects of experimental surgeries or drugs, answering sensitive or distressing questions on a survey).[9] Referring to the Declaration of Helsinki standards, the explanation of the CONSORT guidelines notes that "some clinical trials have been shown to have been unnecessary because the question they addressed had been or could have been answered by a systematic review of the existing literature." Thus, the guidelines emphasize that "the need for a new trial should be justified in the introduction" to a study report.[9]

Research questions and hypotheses that flow logically from previous work.
In what is typically the last paragraph prior to the methods section, it is important to make clear the specific hypotheses or research questions that guided the study. State hypotheses when the information available prior to the study was sufficient to produce a reasonably informed conjecture about what the study findings would be. State research questions when little or no information was available. For example, in the dose consolidation study report, Delate et al. noted that both of the two previous studies used relatively weak designs. With little information on which to base a hypothesis, Delate et al. described the study objective as exploratory ("to evaluate the effectiveness and financial impact of a drug dose consolidation [optimization] program using letter intervention") and highlighted in the objective the special features of their study design and outcomes:

"The study utilized an experimental study design to examine the (1) 'background rate' of dose consolidation (i.e., the degree to which dose consolidation occurs without intervention); (2) effectiveness of a prescriber, letter-based dose consolidation intervention; (3) effectiveness of supplementing prescriber letters with letters to their patients; and (4) financial impact of the program taking into consideration the program costs."[29]

Plausible causality. In reports of studies that used observational designs, the introduction should make clear the presumed causal mechanism that guided the work. For example, in a claims-based study of outcomes associated with adherence to osteoporosis medications, Halpern et al. (2011) examined rates of fracture, as one might expect.[32] However, Halpern et al. also studied outcomes with a less obvious logical connection to osteoporosis—all-cause medical cost and all-cause hospitalizations. This choice raises a logical question in the mind of the reader: why not limit measurement of the study outcomes to claims with a diagnosis of fracture? Appropriately, Halpern et al. anticipated this question, addressing it effectively in the study introduction with an explanation that included citations to previous research on the clinical consequences of fractures:

"Fractures can result in wide-ranging health care resource utilization and costs beyond the direct costs attributable to acute fracture treatment and follow-up. Osteoporotic fractures may also be associated with depression, functional impairment, cognitive impairment, pain, disability, and decline in lung function. Patients whose fractures are treated in inpatient facilities may require subsequent hospitalization for post-operative complications, such as chest infection, cardiac failure, deep vein thrombosis, or pneumonia."[32]

How best to "make the case" for causal plausibility depends on the study topic. For example, in a study of the association of antidepressant drug choice—initial treatment with first-line versus second-line drugs—with all-cause hospitalizations, the researcher might reasonably establish two plausible causal linkages. First would be the relationship between drug choice and depressive symptoms. This relationship might be established based on previously published RCTs comparing the effects of first- versus second-line antidepressant drug use on Hamilton Rating Scale for Depression (HAM-D) scores.[33] Second would be the relationship between depressive symptoms and all-cause medical utilization. To make this assertion, the researcher might cite previous research regarding the association of depressive symptoms with hospitalizations for causes that might not be diagnosed as depression-related during the hospital stay, such as automobile accidents or unintentional overdose with a nonpsychotropic medication. (And, as discussed in Chapter 6, examining the *actual* diagnoses for which patients were hospitalized is a critically important step in validating causal plausibility in a study of this type.)

Establishing a reasonably plausible causal linkage is important because in health care, and in numerous other fields of study, many factors are statistically associated without being causally related. Thus, for study methods and results to be understandable and credible, plausible causality should be established early in the paper.

Methods: Complete and Clear

Thirty years ago, a small group of biostatisticians in the Harvard School of Public Health (DerSimonian et al., 1982) observed that the descriptions of study methods in research reports of clinical trials appeared to be suboptimal.[34] In what eventually became a seminal project, they set out to quantify the problem by examining the reports of 67 clinical trials in four prominent medical journals—the *British Medical Journal*, the *Journal of the American Medical Association*, *The Lancet*, and the *New England Journal of Medicine* (*NEJM*)—for the degree to which 11 key methodological features were reported accurately and thoroughly. Their findings reflected a shocking lack of critical information in study reports; for example, only 19% indicated the method of randomization, only 37% described the specific eligibility criteria for inclusion in the trial, and only 12% discussed statistical power.

DerSimonian et al. made the importance of their findings clear—and their dismay evident—in their discussion of study results:

> "An author's assurance of random treatment assignment is not convincing unless the method used to generate the random assignment is discussed. ...In scientific usage, 'random' does not mean haphazard. To assure readers that the randomization was done appropriately, the method should be described."

> "If the selection criteria are not clearly stated, a reader is uncertain about who the subjects were and how they were selected. It is difficult to generalize the

findings of such a trial to groups other than the subjects themselves."

"When power is not discussed, the reader has a right to suspect that the study was not large enough to detect important differences. Judging from the frequency with which clinical trials failed to mention power, most investigators seem not to have realized their obligation to report on this item."[34]

Notably, DerSimonian et al. found substantial variation among the journals in the rate of adequate reporting, ranging from a high of 71% in *NEJM* to a low of 46% in the *Lancet*. (Perhaps it is no coincidence that their findings were published in *NEJM*!) DerSimonian et al. concluded, possibly a bit optimistically, that because "editors have the power to control what is published," they "could greatly improve the reporting of clinical trials by providing authors with a list of items that they expect to be strictly reported."[34] This observation gave rise to the CONSORT standards and, ultimately, to the EQUATOR network.[9]

Regardless of study design, the Methods section of a research report should, as stated in the STROBE standards, "describe what was planned and what was done in sufficient detail to allow others to understand the essential aspects of the study, to judge whether the methods were adequate to provide reliable and valid answers, and to assess whether any deviations from the original plan were reasonable."[13] Specific reporting standards for study methods in common health care research applications, which follow from that general guidance, are summarized in Table 10C.

Key elements of study design presented first. STROBE standards recommend providing a summary of the research design early in the methods section "so that readers can understand the basics of the study."[13] The purpose of the overview is to give the reader the "big picture" before delving into details.

Although specific details of the summary description will depend on the design, a few rules of thumb are helpful. For an **observational study**, the overview should specify the basic design and number of groups (e.g., cohort study consisting of two groups); key criteria used to select the study group or groups (e.g., one cohort treated with Drug A and the other treated with Drug B); and the time frame (e.g., during the one-year periods prior to and following Medicare Part D implementation, respectively).[13] An **RCT** summary design statement should specify the type of trial (e.g., parallel group, crossover, pragmatic); the framework (e.g., noninferiority vs. superiority); the unit of randomization

Table 10C
Key Elements of Study Methods to Report for Common Study Types

Reported Element	Administrative Claims Database Analysis	RCT[a]	Decision Analytic Model	Survey
Design summary	• Number of groups • Criteria for group assignment (e.g., Diagnosis X vs. Diagnosis Y or Drug A vs. Drug B) • General description of time frame (e.g., dates of service)	• Type of RCT (e.g., parallel group, pragmatic) • Conceptual framework (e.g., superiority) • Unit of randomization • Allocation ratio	• Model type (e.g., Markov) • Analytic framework (e.g., cost-effectiveness, cost-minimization) • Hypothetical cohort (e.g., patients diagnosed with Disease A) • Time horizon • Perspective • Overview of studies on which the model is based	• Method of administration (e.g., mail, telephone) • Sample design (e.g., probability sample of market research firm list, convenience sample of voters) • General description of survey topics (e.g., opinions about pharmacy benefits)
Context and study groups	• Type of coverage (e.g., commercial, Medicaid) • Restrictions or incentives that affect utilization (e.g., formulary) or reporting (e.g., "carve-outs") • Specific criteria for subject identification, including dates, diagnosis codes and fields (e.g., primary, secondary), and procedure codes • For matched samples, specific procedures for matching; specific details of propensity-score algorithm if applicable • Method of power calculation, if applicable	• Method of recruitment (e.g., physician referral vs. advertisement) • Multiple- versus single-center • Primary, secondary, or tertiary care • Method of randomization • Method of concealing group assignment at randomization • Method of blinding, if applicable • Method of power calculation	• Assumed setting (e.g., MCO, United States) • Specific assumptions about patient groups (e.g., received diagnosis of Disease A and initiated treatment with Drug A or Drug B) • If model is based on one or more previously published studies, key characteristics of those samples	• Location (e.g., physician's office) and/or sampling frame (e.g., likely registered voters) • Type of website if survey was administered by Internet • Qualifications of those who administered survey, if applicable (e.g., nurses made telephone calls to patients) • Method of power calculation, if applicable
Study variables; data sources and quality	• Assessment or indication of data quality or "cleaning" procedures	• For drug study: name, dose, administration method and timing, conditions for dose withholding, and titration regimen	• Table of model inputs, showing specific assumptions, sources for each, and any special calculations or manipulations (e.g., inflated to 2008 dollars using the medical care component of the CPI)	• Use of survey instrument in previous research, if any • Survey instrument development and pretesting processes

Table 10C (continued)
Key Elements of Study Methods to Report for Common Study Types

Reported Element	Administrative Claims Database Analysis	RCT[a]	Decision Analytic Model	Survey
Study variables; data sources and quality (continued)	• For measurement of baseline characteristics and of study outcomes: —Diagnosis codes —Diagnosis fields —Procedure codes —Time periods	• For program intervention: specific intervention type; qualifications of those administering; content of intervention materials, if applicable (e.g., education) • For all: specific description of "usual care," placebo, or active comparator	• Descriptions of ways in which the model differed from the source RCT, if applicable (e.g., RCT duration was 6 months but model time horizon was 20 years) • Descriptions of expert panel composition and use, if applicable • Explanations of reasons for using relatively weak evidence sources (e.g., expert panel), if applicable	• Use of special computerized features (e.g., CATI, automatic randomized ordering of questions or responses) • Copy of survey cover letter and survey instrument included in report or appendix, if feasible
Common sources of bias to be assessed	• Selection bias • Surveillance bias	• None, unless problems occurred in group assignment or concealing group assignment	• Biases in source studies • Application of data from one study population to a different assumed model population	• Nonresponse bias (all surveys) • Nonprobability sample bias (convenience samples) • Computer user bias (Internet surveys)
Statistical methods (all studies)	• Specific description of analytic procedures in sequential order • Specific explanation of all calculations • Specific description of statistical methods used to address problems of bias or confounding (e.g., fixed-effects analysis of observational data, use of two different studies as input data sources in decision analytic model) • Specific methods used to group data and to handle missing values • Specific description of rationale and methods for sensitivity analyses and subgroup analyses • Explanation of which analyses were *a priori* and which were *post hoc*; reasons for performing *post hoc* analyses			

[a] Including pragmatic RCTs; however, these will generally not include some features of a traditional RCT, such as blinding (Chapter 3).

Sources:

Berger et al. Defining, reporting and interpreting nonrandomized studies of treatment effects using secondary data sources.[20]

Eysenbach. Improving the quality of web surveys.[8]

Moher et al. CONSORT standards, explanation and elaboration.[9]

Motheral et al. A checklist for retrospective database studies.[21]

Nuijten et al. Reporting format for economic evaluation.[19]

Vandenbroucke et al. STROBE standards, explanation and elaboration.[13]

CATI=computer-assisted telephone interviewing; CONSORT=**CON**solidated **S**tandards **O**f **R**eporting **T**rials; CPI=consumer price index; MCO=managed care organization; RCT=randomized controlled trial; STROBE=**ST**rengthening the **R**eporting of **OB**servational Studies in **E**pidemiology.

(e.g., whether patients or their physicians were randomized); and the allocation ratio (e.g., 2:1 for a trial in which there was 1 control subject for every 2 subjects assigned to active treatment).[9] **Decision analytic model** summary statements should specify the model type (e.g., Markov, decision tree); the analytic framework (e.g., cost-minimization, cost-effectiveness, budgetary impact); hypothetical subject cohort (e.g., patients diagnosed with type 2 diabetes and treated with either Drug A or Drug B); perspective (e.g., payer, society); and time horizon (e.g., 20 years after treatment initiation, lifetime).[19] The summary of a **survey** should indicate the method of administration (e.g., mail, telephone); key elements of the sample (e.g., probability sample of health plan members identified using eligibility records, convenience sample of visitors to a patient information website); and a general description of the survey topics (e.g., opinions about pharmacy benefits, experience with a recent step-therapy edit).[8]

To enhance the credibility of the work for the reader, the explanation of the study design should reflect an understanding of the principles of internal validity and external validity that were described in Chapter 3. For example, if randomized data on the study topic are already available and the present study is observational, the researcher should explain why this design was chosen. Perhaps previous RCTs of a particular drug excluded a large proportion of potential study subjects prior to randomization, as in the JUPITER (Justification for the Use of Statins in Primary Prevention: an Intervention Trial Evaluating Rosuvastatin) trial. Recall from Chapter 3 that JUPITER investigators excluded 32% of potential subjects for a long list of criteria that included nonadherence and certain common health conditions, such as diabetes and severe arthritis.[35] Although exclusions of this magnitude probably enhance internal validity, they raise concerns about external validity if the patients who will use the drug (rosuvastatin in this example) in clinical practice systematically differ from the RCT subjects. For this reason, the researcher might explain that the observational study was conducted to provide information that is valuable from the perspective of external validity, albeit potentially confounded by selection bias. Similarly, the report of a decision analytic modeling study of Drug A, a new medication to prevent stroke in patients with Diagnosis X, might explain that no data on Drug A's outcomes in routine practice are available, the expected time frame for development of stroke in patients with Diagnosis X is a mean of five years, and health plan decision makers need timely information about the expected clinical and economic effects of Drug A.[19]

Complete description of study context. To understand the applicability of study results for their populations of interest, readers need detailed information about the context in which the research occurred, or was assumed to occur for a decision analytic model. For an observational study, STROBE recommends describing the "setting, locations, and relevant dates, including periods of recruitment, exposure, follow-up, and data collection."[13] Stating specific dates is generally clearer than describing time periods and is recommended by STROBE.[13] For example, it is clearer to say that a cohort was identified from July 2008 through December 2008 and followed from January 2009 through December 2009, than to say that the cohort was identified over a six-month period and followed for the subsequent 12 months.

For analyses of administrative claims databases, several aspects of the setting are especially important. As Motheral et al. (2003) observed in their checklist for retrospective database studies, "any given database represents a particular situation in terms of study population, medical benefits covered, and how services are organized."[21] Thus, details about the type of coverage (e.g., commercial insurance, Medicare, Medicaid) and limitations on coverage (e.g., formulary status of the study drugs, step-therapy protocols, or prior authorization requirements) are important. As we saw in Chapter 7, many factors can affect the degree to which a claims dataset is complete and/or accurate. These include service delivery and coverage arrangements, such as "carve-outs" and financial incentives to code a particular diagnosis; coverage of injectable drugs under either the medical or pharmacy benefit; changes in coding rules for diagnoses and procedures; and data collection methods, such as the use of *superbills*. Although it is unlikely that a researcher can obtain detailed information about all of these factors, he or she should attempt to gather and report as much information as possible. For example, the report might say "During the study period, all study injectable drugs were covered under the pharmacy benefit as nonpreferred with a tier-3 copayment, and J codes for the study drugs were blocked from payment under the medical benefit except for bills submitted by inpatient hospitals." Details of this type reassure the reader that the dataset was reasonably complete and that important coverage rules were taken into account by the researchers.

For RCTs, CONSORT recommends describing the method of recruitment (e.g., physician-referral versus self-referral in response to a television advertisement); whether the trial was conducted in multiple centers versus a single center; and whether the centers provided primary-, secondary-, or tertiary-level care. This information is important because "the environment in which the trial is conducted may differ considerably from the setting in which the trial's results are later used to guide practice and policy,"[9] an issue that arises often in health care research.

For example, in discussing the possible addition of a new diagnosis, "attenuated psychotic symptoms syndrome," to the Diagnostic and Statistical Manual of Mental Disorders, editorialists Cornblatt and Correll (2010) pointed out that the symptomatic standards for the disorder were "generated entirely by specialized research clinics that use highly trained interviewers and raters whose reliability is established and constantly calibrated."[36] They argued that in routine practice, the attempts to diagnose the disorder "by busy clinicians that are not trained in the assessment of attenuated psychotic symptoms" could lead to diagnostic error. This example highlights an important aspect of good research reporting: although a clear explanation of setting is always important, it is especially critical to describe special features of the study context (training and monitoring the symptom raters in this example), so that readers can judge for themselves whether they can adequately replicate and apply the study conditions in their own settings.

Specific definitions of study groups. For all types of research, eligibility criteria for inclusion and exclusion in each study group should be reported specifically.[8,9,13,19] For example, the phrase "patients receiving drug treatment for congestive heart failure" is uninformative. The phrase "patients with at least two medical claims with a primary diagnosis of congestive heart failure (ICD-9-CM code of 428.x) and at least 1 pharmacy claim for an antihypertensive medication (angiotensin-converting enzyme inhibitor, angiotensin-II receptor blocker, beta blocker, digoxin, or a diuretic, identified using Generic Product Identifier [GPI] codes [Medi-Span])" provides the reader with sufficiently specific information. In considering these descriptions, remember that the "gold standard" is reproducibility; readers should be able to replicate your work based on the information that you provide. Thus, if journal space permits, it is extremely helpful to provide specific coding information (the specific GPI codes or code groups in this example), either in the text or in a methodological appendix.

If groups were matched, specific details of the matching process should be provided. These include both the matching variables and any relaxation of matching based on categories (e.g., age in three-year bands: 18 to 21 years, 22 to 24 years, etc.). Additionally, if a propensity-score matching process was used (Chapter 6), all variables entered into the propensity score equation, as well as a summary measure of the score algorithm quality in predicting group assignment (typically a c-statistic), should be described.

For RCT reporting, specification of the method of randomization is critically important, as DerSimonian et al. observed 30 years ago. Elimination of selection bias is considered to be the most important advantage of randomization.[9] Any human intervention in the group assignment process raises the possibility of negating this benefit and biasing study results. For this reason, CONSORT standards indicate that the methods used to ensure "unpredictable [group] allocation sequence and concealment of that sequence until assignment occurs" should be reported in detail.[9] For example, the study report might describe use of a random number generator to assign subjects to groups. Concealment of allocation might be described by specifying the placement of the assignment information in opaque, sealed envelopes, or by describing pre-packaged bottles containing identically appearing active drug and placebo capsules.[9]

Similarly, for decision analytic models that are based on one or more previously published studies, the designs and samples of those studies should be described briefly.[19] Typically, these are RCTs, but sometimes, observational studies of administrative claims data are used. For example, van Staa et al. (2009) modeled the cost-effectiveness of cyclooxygenase-2 (COX-2) inhibitors using data obtained both from RCTs and from the United Kingdom General Practice Research Database and compared the results.[37]

Specific descriptions of data sources, including information about their quality. STROBE standards recommend that study reports should "for each variable of interest, give sources of data and details of methods of assessment (measurement)."[13] Reports of studies that used administrative claims databases should provide an indication of database quality, such as methods used to "clean" the data or the use of the database in previous research.[21] Reports of surveys should provide information about the questionnaire, including whether it has been used and/or tested in previous research and, if not, information about the process used to develop a new questionnaire.[8] For example, the report might describe the use of a focus group or informal discussions to develop an initial list of questions, the pretesting process, and decisions made to modify the survey based on pretest results. Descriptions of computerized surveys (e.g., Internet surveys, computer-assisted telephone interviewing [CATI] surveys) should indicate whether any questions, response choices, or questionnaire sections were randomly ordered to eliminate order effects (Chapter 8).[8] If possible, the survey cover letter or email and the survey instrument should be included as an appendix to the study report.[8] Even if journal space does not permit publication of these materials, they should be provided to reviewers and editors during the peer review process.

Specific descriptions of study variables. STROBE standards recommend that reports "clearly define all outcomes, exposures, predictors, potential confounders, and effect modifiers" and "give diagnostic criteria, if applicable."[13] Specificity is key. For example, in describing an analysis that used diagnoses recorded in a claims database, it is important to indicate the specific diagnosis codes; whether the diagnoses were primary, secondary, or in any position on the claim; and the time period during which diagnoses were measured. For a diagnosis that is sometimes coded incorrectly, such as depression or bipolar disorder (Chapter 7), the rationale for the coding method used in the research should be explained.[21] If space permits, it is extremely helpful to provide text descriptions of each diagnosis code (e.g., tell readers that 296.2x and 296.3x are ICD-9-CM codes for major depressive disorder, single episode and recurrent episode, respectively).

CONSORT guidelines indicate that in a drug intervention study, the information to be reported should include "the drug name, dose, method of administration (such as oral, intravenous), timing and duration of administration, conditions under which interventions are withheld, and titration regimen if applicable."[9] Similarly, the report of a disease management intervention consisting of telephonic education coupled with printed materials might describe the number of scheduled telephone consultations; the qualifications of the professionals performing the consultations (e.g., nurses, pharmacists); the content of the educational materials; and the basis for the education (e.g., treatment guidelines from the American Diabetes Association). For control groups, descriptions of "usual care" should be thorough.[9] Any "stopping rules" that were used in terminating the trial "if an intervention is working particularly well or badly" should be described as well.[9]

In observational studies of medical or pharmacy claims data, it is especially important to make clear the time periods for measurement of the study variables, because these can have an enormous effect on the validity of the work. For example, in examining the association between treatment with Drug A and the occurrence of emergency room (ER) visits, a researcher might explain that both the use of Drug A and the ER utilization were measured during the same one-year time period. This decision should raise questions in the mind of the reader about whether the use of Drug A preceded or followed the ER visits. For this reason, Motheral et al. include the presence or absence of a "clear temporal (sequential) relationship between the exposure and outcome" in their checklist for assessing the quality of database analyses.[21] Additionally, the follow-up time period for measurement of study outcomes should be consistent with the natural history of a disease and its treatment.[21] For example, in measuring the association between adherence with osteoporosis therapies and fracture, Halpern et al. measured only fractures occurring at least six months after initiation of the drug "to provide time for the osteoporosis therapies to achieve their therapeutic effects" as documented in clinical trials.[32] *Regardless of whether the researcher used an optimal or suboptimal method, clear reporting of time periods is essential* **either** *to show the reader that the sequence of events was appropriately considered* **or** *to make clear to the reader the potential flaws in the method used.*

Reports of decision analytic models should include a table of model inputs that presents every assumption (e.g., efficacy rates or probabilities of events for each treatment comparator, costs of specific health care events); the published or unpublished sources for each assumption; and any special calculation methods used, such as inflation of dollars to a common year using a particular component of the consumer price index, method of discounting, or methods of imputing data that were not directly measured or reported in the source publications.[19] If an expert panel was used, the composition of the panel and the method used to obtain the model inputs (e.g., focus group, survey) should be described. Reasons for using an expert panel should be explained as well (e.g., no published information was available) because expert opinion is a weak source of evidence.[19] A good "rule of thumb" for the inputs table is that a knowledgeable reader should be able to calculate "back-of-the-envelope" estimates for the main study findings based on the information provided. Without this ability, the reader is left with the impression that the model is a "black box;" models of this type are often ignored by information users. A good example of an inputs table is available in a report of a decision analytic model by Yuan et al. (2008).[38]

Potential sources of bias and methods used to address them. As discussed in Chapter 3, the primary types of bias in observational health care research are selection bias and, less commonly, surveillance bias. Potential sources of bias should be described specifically. For example, the report of an observational study of a disease management program might cite the Medicare Health Support experiment to indicate the strong likelihood that those who opted into a program may have chosen to do so because they are especially interested in their health and/or likely to engage in healthy behaviors.[39] Then, the report might explain that for this reason, the researchers used a propensity-score matching process, administered a survey assessing health interests and behaviors prior to disease management program entry, or used some other method to control for baseline health and health-related motivation.

Reports of surveys should include an assessment of the likelihood of nonresponse bias, a problem that was discussed in detail in Chapter 8. If Internet survey administration was used, the threat of nonresponse bias is heightened for several reasons: (a) those who use the Internet systematically differ from those who do not;[8,40] (b) Internet users attracted to a particular website may systematically differ from Internet users who didn't visit the website;[8] and (c) noncompletions of Internet surveys are common, making interest in the topic an especially important issue when the opinions of respondents who completed the survey are analyzed.[8]

These factors do not necessarily represent fatal flaws. As the **CHE**cklist for **R**eporting **R**esults of **I**nternet **E**-**S**urveys (CHERRIES) guideline points out, "every biased sample is an unbiased sample of another target population, and it is sometimes just a question of defining for which subset of a population the conclusions drawn are assumed to be valid."[8] However, these potentially biasing factors should be candidly disclosed, and it is especially important to explain procedures used to adjust for them.[8] Companies that specialize in Internet survey administration routinely use numeric weights for this purpose.[40] Common reporting metrics, which ideally should be based on unique user counts (e.g., by measuring unique Internet Protocol [IP] addresses), include (a) the "view rate," the ratio of website visitors to survey page visitors; (b) the "participation rate," the ratio of survey page visitors to those agreeing to survey participation; and (c) the "completion rate," the ratio of those who agree to participate to those who actually complete the survey.[8]

It is readily apparent that a decision analytic model is only as unbiased as its source information—that is, a decision analytic model based on a biased study will produce a biased outcome. However, a more common and complex source of bias arises from the interplay between the design of a decision analytic model and that of the study on which the model is based. Specifically, although the possibility of bias is virtually eliminated by design in an adequately executed RCT,[9] bias in a decision analytic model may occur if the sample or method of one or more of the input studies systematically differed from that of the assumed *hypothetical* model cohort.

For example, the decision tree model by Yuan et al. compared two antiviral medications, entecavir and lamivudine, in the treatment of patients with hepatitis B.[38] In a scenario typical of the sometimes complex world of decision analytic model development, efficacy data for the drugs were based on one trial (Benefits of Entecavir for Hepatitis B Liver Disease [BEHoLD]), but data on long-term disease sequelae were not available in the BEHoLD trial report and had to be derived from a longitudinal observational cohort study of community residents with hepatitis B (Risk Evaluation of Viral Load Elevation and Associated Liver Disease/Cancer-Hepatitis B Virus [REVEAL-HBV]). The problem was that the BEHoLD RCT was based on patients who were seropositive for hepatitis B e antigen (HBeAg), but 85% of the REVEAL-HBV participants were HbeAg-negative. Appropriately, Yuan et al. transparently disclosed the issue in their study abstract and observed that their findings were contingent on the assumption that "liver disease risk levels from the REVEAL-HBV study population (a primarily HBeAg-negative group) adequately represent risk for a treated HBeAg-positive patient group."[38]

The key in all these explanations is not to aim for or portray *perfection* in the study design, which is generally impossible; it is to disclose any factors that could produce *imperfections* and to explain, as transparently as possible, what those might be. An additional purpose of these explanations is to show the reader that the researcher made reasonable efforts to produce valid results given the limitations of the available data.

Sample size. If a power calculation was performed prior to initiating the study (Chapter 4), it should be explained. Report the assumed meaningful effect size or results expected in each study group, the alpha (critical *P* value), and the desired power. It is especially helpful to explain power calculations for small-sample studies because without this information, those that produce nonsignificant results are highly likely to encounter the objection that they were "underpowered." Additionally, explaining power calculations for RCTs and, to a lesser extent, for surveys is important because sample sizes in these studies have potential ethical implications.[9,41] Specifically, an explanation of how the number of study subjects was chosen will facilitate the reader's understanding that the minimum number of cases necessary to meet the study objectives was used in research involving human subjects.

Method and rationale for grouping quantitative variables. Variables measured on a continuous (interval or ratio) scale (e.g., age) may be grouped into categories for several reasons. **First**, although a Pearson correlation shows the strength and direction of a relationship, it does not make the impact of the relationship fully clear to readers. For example, it is much more informative to say "60% of those aged 65 years or older, compared with 30% of those younger than 65 years, had a medication possession ratio (MPR) of at least 80%" than to say "the correlation between age and MPR was 0.43." **Second**, correlation is an inappropriate measure for "U-shaped" or other curvilinear relationships that are common in health care; for example, when the percentages with MPR exceeding 80% are 60%, 30%, and 45% for subjects aged 65 years or older, 45 to 64 years, and 44 years or younger, respectively.

Categorizations should be based on substantive or statistical grounds. For example, for an analysis of the relationship between statin MPR and myocardial infarction (MI), the investigator might examine previous research to see if a cardiovascular study outcome was associated with statin MPR and, if so, what the "cutpoints" were. Additionally, because numerous health care inputs and outcomes change at a threshold age of 65 years, the start of Medicare eligibility for most U.S. residents, nearly all studies of adults will include an age category for 65 years or older. If little or no information is available to base "cutpoints" on substantive grounds, categories might be identified based on common statistical measures, such as quintiles or median and interquartile range.

In making these decisions, the key is to base the decisions on standards that are explained clearly to the reader, with appropriate citations to previously published relevant work. The reader should never be left with a "where did these numbers come from?" feeling.

Statistical methods. Regardless of the study design, the best way to write an effective and clear statistical methods section is to describe the steps in the analysis in the order in which they were performed. Of course, you are writing a summary, not a diary entry; it is not necessary to report every failed programming attempt, for example. However, it is easier for readers to understand and reproduce study procedures—the "gold standard" for the methods section—when steps are presented in sequence.

As discussed in more detail in Chapter 6, statistical methods used to control for bias and confounding, particularly for unmeasured confounders, are often complex. However, even complex methods can be reported clearly using a sequential approach. For example, a study by Bosco et al. (2010), which compared the performance of various statistical adjustment methods in assessing the association between chemotherapy and breast cancer recurrence, included an instrumental variable analysis.[42] In explaining their unusual instrumental variable, Bosco et al. first summarized the variable and rationale for using it, then explained its construction in a step-by-step fashion:

"...we used each patient's surgeon's chronologically preceding patient's receipt of adjuvant chemotherapy ... as the [instrumental variable] ... [because] we did not have information on each patient's medical oncologist (in addition, some patients did not see a medical oncologist). We assigned the [instrumental variable] by stratifying the dataset by surgeon. Within each surgeon, the data were sorted by the patient's date of diagnosis in chronological order. Patients of surgeons who only treated one participant in our dataset were excluded from the [instrumental variable]-like analysis. For surgeons with greater than one patient, the chronologically preceding patient's receipt of chemotherapy was assigned. The chronologically first patient for each surgeon was excluded so that each patient would have an [instrumental variable] defined."[42]

This explanation provided detailed instructions for future researchers who wanted to use a similar technique. Additionally, the explanation made clear the reasons underlying the choice of instrumental variable (i.e., data on treatment choices made by oncologists were unavailable) and the limitations of the analysis (i.e., the variable was based on surgeon and not necessarily on the physician who actually made the choice to prescribe chemotherapy).

Partly because of the related problems of "fishing" and cumulative type I error (Chapter 5), reporting guidelines for RCTs and observational research call for disclosure of the *a priori* analysis plan *and* departures from that plan, including analyses of subgroups and interactions.[9,13,20,21] Specific methods for handling missing data should be described as well.[9,13]

For observational and decision analytic model studies, reporting the methods used in sensitivity analyses is important so that readers can understand "whether or not the main results are consistent with those obtained with alternative analysis strategies or assumptions."[13] For example, an analysis of administrative claims for patients with a primary diagnosis of Disease A might test the effect of basing sample selection on primary, secondary, or tertiary diagnosis.[21] Analyses of this type reassure the reader that results are not dependent on a feature of the study method that could reasonably have been performed in multiple ways and that findings have not been "cherry-picked."

Additionally, recognizing that RCT results may represent only a subgroup of the total patient population using a disease or treatment (e.g., rosuvastatin users in the JUPITER trial), International Society for Pharmaceconomics and Outcomes Research (ISPOR) reporting guidelines for observational studies recommend comparing previously published findings for the RCT subgroup with observational study findings for the same subgroup.[20] For example, a researcher who is performing an observational analysis of all rosuvastatin users might construct a JUPITER-like subgroup by excluding patients with diagnoses of diabetes, certain types of arthritis, or a history of poor compliance with previous medication therapy, then compare JUPITER RCT results with those for the JUPITER-like subgroup in a sensitivity analysis. A finding that the RCT and observational subgroup results are similar would provide assurance about the internal validity of the observational analysis.[20]

Results: Practical and Sensible

Sample composition. Both for RCTs and observational research, among the most important details are the characteristics of those included in the sample and—perhaps even more important—of those excluded. Guidelines suggest reporting the counts of individuals at every study stage from initial identification to final analysis, along with reasons for nonparticipation or dropout. Additionally, both STROBE and CONSORT recommend use of a sample selection flowchart (Figure 10A).[9,13]

This information is essential to help readers understand the degree to which the study sample adequately represented the population in which results may be applied. For example, consider a sampling process that excluded 75% of users of Drug A because they did not have a diagnosis for the U.S. Food and Drug Administration (FDA)-approved indication for Drug A. Although this sampling decision might have been appropriate for internal validity, it raises questions about whether the sample has external validity to represent the users of Drug A.

An additional way to make the sample composition clear is a subject characteristics table; these are recommended in all reporting guidelines and, not surprisingly, included in nearly all published research reports. The subject characteristics table, which is often (although not always) the first table in a research report, should present relevant demographic and clinical characteristics for the sample overall and for each key study group.[9,13] Survey reports should include a characteristics table that compares respondents with nonrespondents. Characteristics should include all factors that might affect the study outcome, including potential confounders. Additionally, in studies in which subjects have been followed for varying lengths of time, the subject characteristics table should include descriptive information on length of follow-up, including mean, median, and interquartile range at a minimum, and perhaps deciles "to show readers the spread of follow-up times," if applicable.[13] A sample characteristics table "shell" (blank table) is in Appendix 10A, Table A.

Figure 10A
Example of a Hypothetical Sample Selection Flowchart

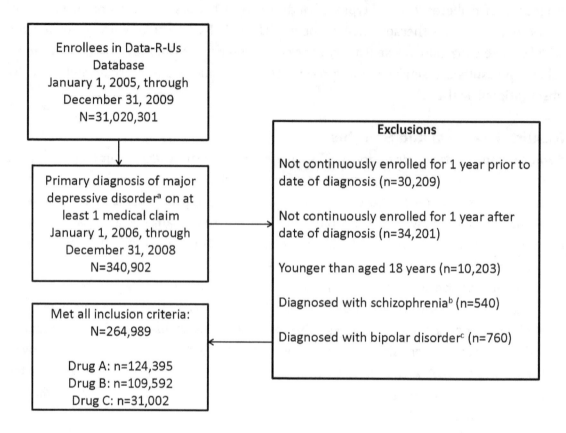

[a] ICD-9-CM codes 296.2x (major depressive disorder, single episode) or 296.3x (major depressive disorder, recurrent episode).

[b] At least 1 medical claim with a primary or secondary diagnosis: ICD-9-CM codes 295.xx (schizophrenic disorders) from January 2006 through December 2008.

[c] At least 1 medical claim with a primary or secondary diagnosis: ICD-9-CM codes 296.0x (bipolar disorder, single manic episode); 296.4x (bipolar disorder, most recent episode manic); 296.5x (bipolar disorder, most recent episode depressed); 296.6x (bipolar disorder, most recent episode mixed); 296.7 (bipolar disorder, most recent episode unspecified); 296.80 (bipolar disorder, unspecified); or 296.89 (bipolar disorder, other) from January 2006 through December 2008.

ICD-9-CM=International Classification of Diseases, Ninth Revision, Clinical Modification.

Outcomes—what your reader "came for." To those who studied advanced statistical methods in graduate school and are aware of their power and effectiveness when used as tools for particular analytic purposes (Chapter 6), it is sometimes surprising to hear that reporting guidelines recommend including a results table of bivariate outcomes in the study report, along with multivariate results if necessary (e.g., because of confounding or for other purposes described in Chapter 6). The data presentation should include counts (e.g., number of patients, number of events), absolute percentages or rates (e.g., number of events per person-year of follow-up), and sometimes a measure of relative risk or hazard (e.g., hazard ratio).[9,13,23,24] Examples of these results tables are easily found in research reports in major medical journals (e.g., *NEJM*). Additionally, table shells for common types of bivariate analyses in observational studies are in Appendix 10A, Tables B and C.

It is extremely helpful for readers, and fortunately common, for results tables to show both primary and secondary outcomes. Reports of secondary outcomes can be used when readers need to make comparisons across studies that used slightly different outcome measures. For example, some studies of statin therapy in primary prevention use all-cause or cardiovascular mortality as the primary outcome measure, whereas others use a combined endpoint of cardiovascular mortality and cardiac events (e.g., nonfatal MI, coronary artery bypass grafting).[43] When one study's primary outcome is another study's secondary outcome, it is relatively easy to make appropriate cross-study comparisons if the authors of both studies have reported all outcomes in results tables.

Reports of decision analytic models should use a similar approach, making it completely clear to the reader how the model "got from" the input values to the final model outputs.[19] For example, consider a study that estimates total medical and drug costs associated with Drug A versus Drug B, assuming that Drug A results in a reduced rate of Surgery X, a negative outcome. The primary results table should show, separately for Drug A and Drug B, estimates of the total counts of people treated, the costs of drug treatment, the counts of those who receive Surgery X, the total costs for Surgery X, and the total net cost taking both drug cost and surgery cost into account. Reporting only final "bottom-line" cost numbers is unacceptable because the reader cannot determine either the estimated effectiveness outcomes or the degree to which the model estimates depend on effectiveness, drug costs, surgery costs, or another model parameter.

Reporting guidelines also recommend that when statistical adjustment methods have been used, both unadjusted and adjusted estimates should be reported to enable readers to "understand the data behind the measures of association" and to "compare unadjusted measures of association with those adjusted for potential confounders and judge by how much, and in what direction, they changed."[13] All statistical estimates should be presented with a measure of precision, most commonly a 95% confidence interval.[9,13,23,24]

Although reporting measures of relative effects, such as odds ratios or hazards ratios, is helpful, sole reliance on these measures is unwise. For example, consider two hypothetical studies of Drug A, one in a primary prevention sample (Study 1), the other in a secondary prevention sample (Study 2). Both studies measured the effect of Drug A on Outcome Q (Table 10D).

Table 10D
Hypothetical Drug Studies: Limitations of Relative Risk Measures

	Study 1 Primary Prevention	Study 2 Secondary Prevention
Baseline risk of Outcome Q	Very low	High
Rate of Outcome Q in patients treated with Drug A	0.25%	5%
Rate of Outcome Q in patients treated with placebo	0.50%	10%
Relative risk reduction with Drug A	50%	50%
NNT	$1 \div (0.0050 - 0.0025) = 400$	$1 \div (0.10 - 0.05) = 20$

NNT=number needed to treat (see Glossary or Chapter 5 for definition).

Clearly, the two studies produced very different outcomes in absolute practical terms despite producing the same result in relative terms. Hence, showing only the relative risk reductions would be extremely misleading. For this reason, guidelines recommend reporting both absolute and relative outcomes.[9,13,23,24]

Text descriptions of multivariate results should be accompanied with a table showing relevant technical details, including coefficients, measures of precision (e.g., confidence intervals around odds ratios), statistical tests, number of cases, and a measure of overall model quality or fit.[24] To describe multivariate results in a way that has practical meaning for readers, first consider the substantive meaning of the coefficients or exponentiated coefficients (Chapter 6). For example, an odds ratio for female, with male as the reference category, should be described as the amount by which the odds are multiplied for females compared with males.

Sometimes, coefficients are less easily interpreted and require a different explanatory approach. For continuous (interval- or ratio-scale) variables, coefficients may be less intuitively meaningful for readers (e.g., the amount of change in Outcome A associated with each one-year increase in age). Additionally, interaction terms should not be interpreted apart from their corresponding main effect terms (i.e., neither the main effect nor the interaction term has a readily interpretable substantive meaning).[24] In these circumstances, predicted values are a great way to make results clear for readers. For any multivariate equation, the predicted outcome for any hypothetical subject with a specific set of characteristics can be calculated. For example, consider this hypothetical linear regression equation to predict MPR:

$$\text{MPR} = \text{Intercept} + (b_1 \times \text{age}) + (b_2 \times \text{female, with male as reference category})$$
$$+ (b_3 \times \text{Drug A, with Drug B as reference category}) + (b_4 \times \text{Drug A} \times \text{female}$$
$$[\text{interaction term}])$$

Assume that the resulting equation is:
$$\text{MPR} = 10.75 + (0.7 \times \text{age}) + (0.2 \times \text{female}) + (2.15 \times \text{Drug A}) + (5.15 \times \text{Drug A} \times \text{female})$$

For a 74-year-old female using Drug A, the predicted MPR is 70.05:
$$\text{MPR} = 10.75 + (0.7 \times 74) + (0.2 \times 1) + (2.15 \times 1) + (5.15 \times 1 \times 1)$$

In contrast, for a 74-year-old female using Drug B, the predicted MPR is 62.75:
$$\text{MPR} = 10.75 + (0.7 \times 74) + (0.2 \times 1) + (2.15 \times 0) + (5.15 \times 0 \times 1)$$

Examples of this type can help make the meaning of coefficients clear for readers. More commonly in the health care literature, the multivariate model can be used to calculate predicted outcomes for a hypothetical group of "average" study subjects. "Estimated marginal means," sometimes called "least-squares means" or "adjusted means" are calculated as the *predicted* (not observed) values for each of the study groups of interest, holding covariates at their mean values.[44] For logistic regressions, the "adjusted predicted probabilities" for study groups can be calculated in a similar manner.[45] Reporting in this way is informative for readers because it presents familiar metrics (means and percentages) while controlling for measured confounders. For example, in the report of a survey study of Medicare beneficiaries, Tseng et al. (2004) calculated the adjusted predicted probabilities of using a variety of strategies to lower drug cost (e.g., stopping a medication, shopping for best price), comparing beneficiaries who had exceeded a "cap" (limit) on their drug benefits with those who had not exceeded the cap, controlling for demographics, health status measures, and the method of survey administration (written vs. telephone).[46]

Figures or tables: which to choose for a journal article? In making an oral presentation (e.g., a poster or speech at a scientific conference), using figures (graphics) rather than tables to convey most quantitative information is obviously essential. But in presenting some study results in an article, researchers may have to choose between figures and tables. Which approach better conveys information to readers? In making this choice, **several factors** may be considered.

First is the *number of data points*. Using a bar graph to present two means on a primary study outcome, one for Group A and the other for Group B, is inefficient; most readers understand means without the visual presentation of the bar size, and the space occupied by the two bars could instead be used in a table to present mean values for multiple primary and secondary outcomes. However, mean values for each year from 1980 through 2009 (30 data points) are best portrayed in a bar graph or line graph so that the reader can easily see trends over time. Similarly, scatterplots of individual subject values and assessments of linear or curvilinear trends are best presented graphically.

A **second** factor to consider is the *nature of the audience*. If your target journal uses graphics only rarely, chances are good that *either* the topics addressed by the journal are best portrayed in tabular format *or* the journal's readers relate better to tabular than graphic presentation. Additionally, it is important to remember that any population of information users will include readers with a variety of learning styles. Visual-spatial learners, who "think in images instead of words," will relate better to graphic than to tabular presentation;[47] thus, it is helpful to include at least one compelling graphic in a study report. **Finally**, a good overall rule of thumb is to consider the main purpose of a graph, as described by Miller: "provide a good general sense of pattern, complementing a prose description by graphically depicting the shape and size of differences between numbers."[23] If the figure does not convey a *pattern*, the data are likely to be more clearly presented in tabular form.

The Chicago Guide to Writing about Numbers includes a helpful list of mistakes commonly made in creating figures. One of these is particularly relevant for health care research—graphs should be presented using zero (0) as the bottom of the Y-axis scale. Using larger minimums (e.g., scale minimum and maximum of 80% and 90%, respectively) makes small differences appear bigger than they are.[23] In fact, statistician Darrell Huff referred to this practice of "truncating" the Y-axis scale as a "gee-whiz" graphing technique in his classic book, *How to Lie with Statistics*.[48] Thus, if a statistical package automatically inserts a nonzero Y-axis minimum, as many packages do, the user should change it. Miller advises that when presenting small differences between large numbers (a common example in health care would be change from an MPR of 0.80 to 0.85), the *change amount* should be shown in the graph and the values stated in the text.[23]

Important details: subgroup analyses, interactions, and sensitivity analyses. Several important findings commonly appear near the end of the results section. In observational analyses and decision analytic models, these generally include sensitivity analyses. Journal space may not permit tabular reporting of all sensitivity analyses; if so, the report should indicate that the results of sensitivity analyses were consistent with the main study findings (if they were) and that detailed information is available from the authors upon request. Analyses of subgroups and interactions should be described as well, again using figures available on request if journal space does not permit detailed reporting.

Describing research findings in the text. Miller's "generalization, example, exceptions" approach is especially helpful in making research findings clear by highlighting both key points and exceptions in the text, while referring readers to tables or figures for most numerical details.[23] For example, in a hypothetical study of medication adherence, one might say something like the following: "In four of five therapy classes studied, MPR declined over time for both intervention and comparison group subjects (Figure 1). For example, during the sixth month after treatment initiation, MPR values in both groups ranged from a low of 60% for antihypertensives to a high of 65% for statins. However, MPRs for antidiabetic drugs were higher for intervention than comparison group subjects throughout the one-year follow-up (e.g., 75% vs. 60%, respectively, at six months and 70% vs. 55%, respectively, at twelve months, both *P* values <0.001)."

Discussion: Balance, Caution, and Humility

Hit the high points—begin with key results. To facilitate understanding of study implications and help readers "assess whether the ... interpretation and implications offered by the authors are supported by the findings,"[13] reporting guidelines recommend opening the discussion section with a *brief* (usually one- to three-sentence) description of *key* study findings.[9,13] The sentence may refer *briefly* to the study method but should focus primarily on results, for example:

> "*We found that patients with moderate kidney disease required lower weekly warfarin doses to maintain therapeutic [international normalized ratio] than matched patients with an [estimated creatinine clearance] greater than 60 [milliliters per minute]. In addition, patients with kidney disease spent significantly less time in therapeutic range. In turn, this decrease in anticoagulation stability resulted in an increase in the clinic management required to maintain therapeutic anticoagulation, as reflected in the proportion of clinic visits with dose manipulations and decreased time between scheduled visits.*"[49]

> "*This large, retrospective, matched comparison cohort study found that patients diagnosed with [hepatitis C virus] infection have [per patient per year] all-cause costs that on average are almost twice as much as those of non-[hepatitis C virus] patients. Furthermore, [per patient per year] costs were higher in patients with [advanced liver disease].*"[50]

The remainder of the discussion section will fall into three main categories: limitations, interpretation, and conclusion. The order of the first two of these categories varies by journal. STROBE guidance cites the order used by the *Annals of Internal Medicine*, which indicates that following "(1) a brief synopsis of key findings," the report should present "(2) consideration of possible mechanisms and explanations; (3) comparison with relevant findings from other published studies; (4) limitations of the study; and (5) a brief section that summarizes the implications of the work for practice and research."[13]

Interpretation of study findings in the context of previous work. Reporting guidelines for study discussion sections sound similar themes regardless of design. STROBE standards call for a "cautious overall interpretation considering objectives, limitations, multiplicity of analyses, results from similar studies, and other relevant evidence."[13] CONSORT guidelines recommend "interpretation consistent with results, balancing benefits and harms, and considering other relevant evidence."[9] Decision analytic model reporting guidelines indicate that study results should be compared with those from other models or expert opinion, "along with the impact of the limitations and level of uncertainty in the modelling study," perhaps concluding with "recommendations to solve any existing uncertainty with regards to the final conclusion."[19] Key points in all these guidelines include *caution*, *balance*, and careful consideration of the results of *previous work*.

With nonrandomized designs, the need for caution in interpretation is amplified because there is *generally*—albeit not always—much more that could "go wrong" in observational than in randomized studies (Chapter 3). Nearly every researcher has been tempted to interpret a cross-sectional association as definitive evidence; it is in this respect that adherence to reporting guidelines can be especially helpful because they prescribe specific steps to help researchers avoid this pitfall.

STROBE standards call for assessment of potential sources of confounding and bias (e.g., selection bias, surveillance bias), including sample attrition and nonparticipation (e.g., survey nonresponse, opting out of a disease management program). For a researcher who has followed reporting guidelines for the methods section, this assessment should be relatively easy to perform. For example, a researcher who has clearly explained in the methods section the use of *primary* diagnosis alone to sample patients with Disease A understands that this method may have resulted in the inadvertent exclusion of patients who had another disorder in addition to Disease A, with Disease A coded as a *secondary* diagnosis. Similarly, a researcher who has carefully delineated the measurement of both exposure and outcome during the same six-month period understands the risk of measuring an outcome that occurred prior to the exposure that "caused" it.

STROBE guidelines emphasize that multivariate analyses do *not* "establish the 'causal part' of an association" because of the possibility of residual confounding or bias; these possibilities should be candidly assessed.[13] Measures of multivariate model quality, such as R-square or c-statistic, are informative in considering these issues.

If differences between the results of the present study and those obtained in previous work have been identified, the discussion section should describe possible reasons for those differences (e.g., different sample characteristics, selection criteria, or follow-up time). If the present study's methodological approach represents a strength compared with previous work, the implications of the change, both for the results of the present study and for future work, should be described.

The interpretation should also consider the external validity of the study results. For a researcher who has followed CONSORT and STROBE guidance to present a sample selection flowchart in the study report, this task is easy because the flowchart clearly shows the quantitative effects of each sample inclusion and exclusion criterion. For example, if 75% of potential study participants were excluded by a sampling rule that was necessary for internal validity, the limitation of the study sample to about 25% of the sampling frame should be candidly acknowledged as a limitation to external validity, using language like the following: "The present study was limited to users of Drug A who were diagnosed with Disease X, Drug A's FDA-approved indication. The study's results may not represent the expected outcomes for patients with Disease Y, who also commonly use Drug A off-label."

Ethical Considerations

ICMJE standards require the disclosure not only of financial conflicts of interest, but also of "any other relationships or activities that readers could perceive to influence, or that give the appearance of potentially influencing, what you wrote in the submitted work."[51] Most journals require that authors advise the editors of these relationships, which are typically summarized in the author information section of the study report. Reports should also explain methods used to protect human subject safety and privacy, including review and approval by an institutional review board, if applicable, and procedures used to obtain subject consent to participate (e.g., in an RCT or survey).[8,9]

Summing Up: What Have We Learned?

In Chapter 1, we noted that *excellence* is not synonymous with *perfection*. The latter is not achievable; the former can be achieved in research with attention—first and foremost—to the needs of the information user. Nowhere is this attention, or lack of it, more evident than in a research report. For this reason, the House of Commons assessment of peer review described scientific reports as "the public face of science; they are the means by which researchers report and explain their findings to the wider world, including other scientists, practitioners, the public, and policy makers."[22]

This observation is the key to understanding the importance of a carefully written, balanced, and appropriately cautious research report. Whether information users find your results useful and credible will depend in large part on what your "public face" says, not only about your specific procedures and findings, but also about *you*—especially your overall attention to detail and willingness to consider alternative interpretations and points of view.[26] Careful attention to good research-reporting practices is the best way to facilitate *both* the reader's understanding of the material that you present *and* his or her trust in you as a source of information.

In the epilogue, our final chapter, we turn to an important question—perhaps *the* question for any researcher who is making the choice between excellence and mediocrity, as described in Chapter 1. Why do methods matter?

Helpful Resources

In addition to the reporting guidelines summarized in Table 10A, the following are helpful sources of information:

- Booth, Colomb, and Williams. *The Practice of Research.* Chapters 7 ("Making Good Arguments: An Overview"), 8 ("Making Claims"), 9 ("Assembling Reasons and Evidence"), 10 ("Acknowledgements and Responses"), 12 ("Planning"), and 13 ("Drafting Your Report").[26]
- Miller. *The Chicago Guide to Writing about Numbers.* Chapters 2 ("Seven Basic Principles"), 4 ("Technical but Important: Five More Basic Principles"), 9 ("Writing about Distributions and Associations"), 10 ("Writing about Data and Methods"), and 11 ("Writing Introductions, Results, and Conclusions").[23]
- The GRACE (**G**ood **R**ese**A**rch for **C**omparative **E**ffectiveness OBSERVED) principles provide a clear and common-sense overview of expectations for comparative effectiveness research; although not a reporting guideline, the GRACE overview may be helpful to those who are preparing results to be used for decision-making purposes.[52]
- The American Association for Public Opinion Research (AAPOR) "Best Practices" guidelines include a helpful list of good reporting practices for surveys in an easy-to-use, bullet-point format.[53]

References

1. Hilbert D. Today in Science History. Available at: http://www.todayinsci.com/H/ Hilbert_David/HilbertDavid-Quotations.htm.

2. Marcus Tullius Cicero. Available at: http://thinkexist.com/quotation/when_you_wish_ to_instruct-be_brief-that_men-s/148606.html.

3. Red Smith quotes. Available at: http://www.goodreads.com/author/quotes/251738. Red_Smith .

4. Dahl R. *The Best of Roald Dahl.* New York, New York: Vintage Books; 1978:108-116.

5. Fairman KA, Curtiss FR. Rethinking the "whodunnit" approach to assessing the quality of healthcare research—a call to focus on the evidence in evidence-based practice." *J Manag Care Pharm.* 2008;14(7):661-74. Available at: http://www.amcp.org/ data/jmcp/661-674_FairmanCurtiss-Final.pdf.

6. International Committee of Medical Journal Editors. Uniform requirements for manuscripts submitted to biomedical journals: writing and editing for biomedical publication. Available at: http://www.icmje.org/urm_full.pdf.

7. EQUATOR network home page. Available at: http://www.equator-network.org/home/.

8. Eysenbach G. Improving the quality of web surveys: the Checklist for Reporting Results of Internet E-Surveys (CHERRIES). *J Med Internet Res.* 2004;6(3):e34.

9. Moher D, Hopewell S, Schulz KF, et al. CONSORT 2010 explanation and elaboration: updated guidelines for reporting parallel group randomized trials. *BMJ.* 2010;340:c869. Available at: http://www.ncbi.nlm.nih.gov/pmc/articles/PMC2844943/?tool=pubmed.

10. Liberati A, Altman DG, Tetzlaff J, et al. The PRISMA statement for reporting systematic reviews and meta-analyses of studies that evaluate health care interventions: explanation and elaboration. *PLoS Med.* 2009;6(7):e1000100.

11. Stroup DF, Berlin JA, Morton SC, et al. Meta-analysis of observational studies in epidemiology: a proposal for reporting. Meta-analysis Of Observational Studies in Epidemiology (MOOSE) group. *JAMA.* 2000;283(15):2008-12.

12. Davidoff F, Batalden P, Stevens D, Ogrinc G, Mooney SE; SQUIRE Development Group. Publication guidelines for quality improvement in health care: evolution of the SQUIRE project. *BMJ.* 2009;338:a3152.

13. Vandenbroucke JP, von Elm E, Altman DG, et al.; STROBE Initiative. Strengthening the Reporting of Observational Studies in Epidemiology (STROBE): explanation and elaboration. *PLoS Med.* 2007;4(10):e297. Available at: http://www.plosmedicine.org/ article/info%3Adoi%2F10.1371%2Fjournal.pmed.0040297.

14. Stone SP, Cooper BS, Kibbler CC, et al. The ORION statement: guidelines for transparent reporting of outbreak reports and intervention studies Of nosocomial infection. *J Antimicrob Chemother.* 2007;59(5):833-40.

15. Janssens AC, Ioannidis JP, van Duijn CM, et al; GRIPS Group. Strengthening the reporting of Genetic RIsk Prediction Studies: the GRIPS statement. *PLoS Med.* 2011;8(3):e1000420.

16. Des Jarlais DC, Lyles C, Crepaz N; TREND Group. Improving the reporting quality of nonrandomized evaluations of behavioral and public health interventions: the TREND statement. *Am J Public Health.* 2004;94(3):361-66.

17. Siegel JE, Weinstein MC, Russell LB, Gold MR. Recommendations for reporting cost-effectiveness analyses. Panel on Cost-Effectiveness in Health and Medicine. *JAMA.* 1996;276(16):1339-41.

18. Ramsey S, Willke R, Briggs A, et al. Good research practices for cost-effectiveness analysis alongside clinical trials: the ISPOR RCT-CEA Task Force report. *Value Health.* 2005;8(5):521-33.

19. Nuijten MJ, Pronk MH, Brorens MJ, et al. Reporting format for economic evaluation. Part II: Focus on modeling studies. *Pharmacoeconomics.* 1998;14(3):259-68.

20. Berger ML, Mamdani M, Atkins D, Johnson ML. Good research practices for comparative effectiveness research: defining, reporting and interpreting nonrandomized studies of treatment effects using secondary data sources: the ISPOR Good Research Practices for Retrospective Database Analysis Task Force Report—Part I. *Value Health.* 2009;12(8):1044-52. Available at: http://www.ispor.org/taskforces/documents/RDPartI.pdf.

21. Motheral B, Brooks J, Clark MA, et al. A checklist for retrospective database studies—report of the ISPOR Task Force on Retrospective Databases. *Value Health.* 2003;6(2):90-97.

22. House of Commons, Science and Technology Committee. Peer review in scientific publications: Eighth report of Session 2010-12. HC856. July 18, 2011. Available at: http://www.publications.parliament.uk/pa/cm201012/cmselect/cmsctech/856/856.pdf.

23. Miller JE. *The Chicago Guide to Writing about Numbers.* Chicago, IL: University of Chicago Press; 2004: quotation p. 129.

24. Miller JE. *The Chicago Guide to Writing about Multivariate Analysis.* Chicago, IL: University of Chicago Press; 2005.

25. Ware JE, Kosinski M. Interpreting SF-36 summary health measures: a response.

Available at: http://www.sf-36.org/news/qolrsupplement.pdf.

26. Booth WC, Colomb G, Williams JM. *The Craft of Research. Third Edition.* Chicago, IL: University of Chicago Press; 2008: quotation p. 122.

27. Kunze AM, Gunderson BW, Gleason PP, Heaton AH, Johnson SV. Utilization, cost trends, and member cost-share for self-injectable multiple sclerosis drugs—pharmacy and medical benefit spending from 2004 through 2007. *J Manag Care Pharm.* 2007;13(9):799-806. Available at: http://www.amcp.org/data/jmcp/JMCPMaga_N-D%2007_799-806.pdf.

28. An agency is like Prego spaghetti sauce. Available at: http://www.margieclayman.com/an-agency-is-like-prego-spaghetti-sauce.

29. Delate T, Fairman KA, Carey SM, Motheral BR. Randomized controlled trial of a dose consolidation program. *J Manag Care Pharm.* 2004;10(5):396-403. Available at: http://www.amcp.org/data/jmcp/Research-396-403.pdf.

30. Baldinger SL, Calabrese D. Dose consolidation can be an effective intervention [letter]. *J Manag Care Pharm.* 2004;10(6):564-65.

31. Delate T, Fairman KA. The authors respond [letter]. *J Manag Care Pharm.* 2004;10(6):565-66.

32. Halpern R, Becker L, Iqbal SU, Kazis LE, Macarios D, Badamgarav E. The association of adherence to osteoporosis therapies with fracture, all-cause medical costs, and all-cause hospitalizations: a retrospective claims analysis of female health plan enrollees with osteoporosis. *J Manag Care Pharm.* 2011;17(1):25-39. Available at: http://www.amcp.org/data/jmcp/25-39.pdf.

33. Hamilton M. A rating scale for depression. *J Neurol Neurosurg Psychiatry.* 1960;23:56-62.

34. DerSimonian R, Charette LJ, McPeek B, Mosteller F. Reporting on methods in clinical trials. *N Engl J Med.* 1982;306(22):1332-37.

35. Ridker PM, Danielson E, Fonseca FAH, et al.; JUPITER Study Group. Rosuvastatin to prevent vascular events in men and women with elevated C-reactive protein. *N Engl J Med.* 2008;359(21):2195-207.

36. Cornblatt BA, Correll CU. A new diagnostic entity in DSM-5? September 3, 2010. Available at: http://www.medscape.com/viewarticle/727682_print. Accessed July 7, 2011.

37. Van Staa TP, Leufkens HG, Zhang B, Smeeth L. A comparison of cost-effectiveness using data from randomized trials or actual clinical practice: selective COX-2

inhibitors as an example. *PLoS Med.* 2009;6(12):e1000194.

38. Yuan Y, Iloeje UH, Hay J, Saab S. Evaluation of the cost-effectiveness of entecavir versus lamivudine in hepatitis BeAg-positive chronic hepatitis B patients. *J Manag Care Pharm.* 2008;14(1):21-33. Available at: http://www.amcp.org/data/jmcp/JMCPMaga_JanFeb%2008_021-033.pdf.

39. Cromwell J, McCall N, Burton J. Evaluation of Medicare Health Support chronic disease pilot program. *Health Care Financ Rev.* 2008;30(1):47-60.

40. Chang L, Krosnick JA. National surveys via RDD telephone interviewing versus the Internet: comparing sample representativeness and response quality. *Public Opin Q.* 2009;73(4):641-78.

41. Babbie E. *The Practice of Social Research. Fourth Edition.* Belmont, CA: Wadsworth Publishing Company; 1986.

42. Bosco JL, Silliman RA, Thwin SS, et al. A most stubborn bias: no adjustment method fully resolves confounding by indication in observational studies. *J Clin Epidemiol.* 2010;63(1):64-74.

43. Curtiss FR, Fairman KA. Tough questions about the value of statin therapy for primary prevention: did JUPITER miss the moon? *J Manag Care Pharm.* 2010;16(6):417-23. Available at: http://www.amcp.org/data/jmcp/417-423.pdf.

44. UCLA Academic Technology Services, Statistical Consulting Group. SPSS Library: MANOVA and GLM. Available at: http://www.ats.ucla.edu/stat/spss/library/sp_glm.htm.

45. UCLA Academic Technology Services, Statistical Consulting Group. SAS FAQ: How can I get 'adjusted' predicted values from a logistic model in SAS? Available at: http://www.ats.ucla.edu/stat/sas/faq/sas_adjust.htm.

46. Tseng CW, Brook RH, Keller E, Steers WN, Mangione CM. Cost-lowering strategies used by Medicare beneficiaries who exceed drug benefit caps and have a gap in drug coverage. *JAMA.* 2004;292(8):952-60. Available at: http://jama.ama-assn.org/content/292/8/952.full.pdf+html.

47. Silverman LK. *Upside-Down Brilliance: The Visual-Spatial Learner.* Denver, CO: DeLeon Publishing; 2002: quotation p. ii.

48. Huff D. *How to Lie with Statistics.* New York: W.W. Norton & Company; 1954: quotation p. 60.

49. Kleinow ME, Garwood CL, Clemente JL, Whittaker P. Effect of chronic kidney disease on warfarin management in a pharmacist-managed anticoagulation clinic. *J*

Manag Care Pharm. 2011;17(7):523-30. Available at: http://www.amcp.org/WorkArea/DownloadAsset.aspx?id=10715.

50. McAdam-Marx C, McGarry LJ, Hane CA, Biskupiak J, Deniz B, Brixner DI. All-cause and incremental per patient per year cost associated with chronic hepatitis C virus and associated liver complications in the United States: a managed care perspective. *J Manag Care Pharm.* 2011;17(7):531-46. Available at: http://www.amcp.org/WorkArea/DownloadAsset.aspx?id=10710.

51. International Committee of Medical Journal Editors. Toward more uniform conflict disclosures: the updated ICMJE conflict of interest reporting form. July 2010. Available at: http://www.icmje.org/updated_coi.pdf.

52. GRACE Initiative. GRACE principles. Good ReseArch for Comparative Effectiveness OBSERVED. April 10, 2010. Available at: https://pharmacoepi.org/resources/GRACE_Principles.pdf.

53. American Association for Public Opinion Research. Best practices. Available at: http://www.aapor.org/Best_Practices1.htm

Appendix 10A
Table A
Study Subject Characteristics: Drug A Versus Drug B[a]

	Drug A	Drug B
Age in years mean [SD]		
	% (n)	% (n)
Age group in years		
18 to 24		
25 to 34		
35 to 44		
45 to 54		
55 to 64		
65 to 74		
75 or older		
Female		
Comorbidity score[b]		
Zero (no comorbidities)		
One		
Two		
Three		
Four or more		
Indications for drug[b,c]		
Diagnosis A		
Diagnosis B		
Diagnosis C		
Other		
Total	100.0% (n)	100.0% (n)
Length of follow-up mean [SD]		
Length of follow-up median (IQR)		

[a] The total number of patients using each drug in this hypothetical analysis is the denominator, using the techniques described for profiling in Chapter 5. Note that often, results are more intuitive and more easily interpretable when the proportion (percentage) value is presented in the table with the n values shown in parentheses; that format is used in all the tables in this appendix.

[b] Comorbidities and indications (diagnoses) in this hypothetical study were measured during the six-month period preceding the start of treatment.

[c] Diagnoses were based on primary or secondary diagnosis, using the codes shown in a hypothetical appendix to this hypothetical table.

IQR=interquartile range; SD=standard deviation.

Appendix 10A
Table B
Association of Cost-Sharing Level with Medication Adherence (MPR)[a]

Cost-Sharing Level Per 30-Day Supply	Total N of Patients	Mean [SD] MPR	Median [IQR] MPR	Adherence % (n)[b]
Generic drugs				
$0-$4.99				
$5-$9.99				
$10-$19.99				
$20 or more				
Brand				
$0-$4.99				
$5-$9.99				
$10-$19.99				
$20-$29.99				
$30-$39.99				
$40-$49.99				
$50 or more				
Patient characteristics				
Age in years				
18 to 24				
25 to 34				
35 to 44				
45 to 54				
55 to 64				
65 to 74				
75 or older				
Sex				
Male				
Female				
Comorbidity score[c]				
Zero (no comorbidities)				
One				
Two				
Three				
Four or more				

[a] This hypothetical bivariate analysis might precede a linear regression of MPR and logistic regression of adherence (binomial) on cost-sharing level and covariates for patient characteristics. For the calculation of the adherence percentage for a given category, the total number of patients in the category is the denominator, using the techniques for assessing predictor or causal relationships as described in Chapter 5. For example, the denominator for the $0-$4.99 category is the number of patients who paid $0-$4.99, the

denominator for the $5-$9.99 category is the number of patients who paid $5-$9.99, and so on.
[b] Adherence in this hypothetical study was defined as MPR of 80% or more.
[c] Comorbidities in this hypothetical study were measured during the six-month period preceding the start of treatment.
IQR=interquartile range; MPR=medication possession ratio; SD=standard deviation.

Appendix 10A
Table C
Drug Utilization and Cost Before and After Policy Change XYZ[a]

	Before Policy Change				After Policy Change			
	Q1 2005	Q2 2005	Q3 2005	Q4 2005	Q1 2006	Q2 2006	Q3 2006	Q4 2006
Company A (Intervention)								
Total number of employees								
Total number of pharmacy claims								
Number of nonpreferred pharmacy claims								
Percent nonpreferred								
Generic drug claims								
Percent generic								
Total pharmacy cost								
Total dispensed days supply								
Pharmacy cost per dispensed day								
Company B (No Intervention)[b]								
Total number of employees								
Total number of pharmacy claims								
Number of nonpreferred pharmacy claims								
Percent nonpreferred								
Generic drug claims								
Percent generic								
Total pharmacy cost								
Total dispensed days supply								
Pharmacy cost per dispensed day								

[a] In this hypothetical study, Policy Change XYZ was implemented to decrease the use of nonpreferred medications, increase the use of generic medications, and lower pharmacy costs. This hypothetical bivariate analysis might precede an interrupted time series analysis using a comparison group.
[b] In this hypothetical study, Company B, the comparison company, was selected to be as similar as possible to Company A on all characteristics except the intervention (e.g., similar industry sector, insurance type, and formulary).

CHAPTER 11
Epilogue: Why Methods Matter

"Never regard study as a duty, but as the enviable opportunity to learn to know the liberating influence of beauty in the realm of the spirit for your own personal joy and to the profit of the community to which your later work belongs."—Physicist Albert Einstein[1]

"The integrity of the peer-review process can only ever be as robust as the integrity of the people involved. ... Ethical and scientific misconduct ... damages peer review and science as a whole."—House of Commons Science and Technology Committee Report on peer review"[2]

"A mistake in the operating room can threaten the life of one patient; a mistake in statistical analysis or interpretation can lead to hundreds of early deaths. So it is perhaps odd that, while we allow a doctor to conduct surgery only after years of training, we give SPSS® (SPSS, Chicago, IL) to almost anyone."—Biostatistician Andrew Vickers[3]

On February 2, 2008, the height of the tourist season in the spectacular Sonoran desert, a 37-year-old Swiss woman arrived in Tucson, Arizona for a vacation—just one of an estimated 30 million visitors to the state each year.[4] The next day, she travelled to Mexico, as many Arizona tourists do, but she became ill there and returned to Tucson on February 9, 2008.[5,6] Three days later, she presented at Tucson's Northwest Hospital emergency room (ER) with breathing difficulties and a fever and was admitted the next day with a diagnosis of "acute viral illness."[5]

Unfortunately, the actual cause of her symptoms was not even suspected by hospital staff until February 15, 2008—she had the measles, against which she had never been immunized. A diagnosis of measles was confirmed on February 20, 2008. Meanwhile, a 50-year-old woman who spent an hour in the ER during the tourist's ER treatment was infected, became ill nine days later, returned to the ER, and was admitted. She, in turn, passed the measles to a 41-year-old health care worker, an 11-month-old boy who was in the same ER for 45 minutes, and two children ages three and five years, who had no contact with her but walked past her hospital room.[5] Events progressed as one might expect, with a sequence of exposures, illnesses, and more exposures; these were detailed in an interesting epidemiological account by Chen et al. in the June 2011 issue of the *Journal of Infectious Diseases*.[5]

By the time that Tucson was "no longer seeing spots," as one news report described it, the damage that had been done in the five months since the tourist's arrival was enormous.[5,6] Arizona Department of Health Services officials had to locate and interview 8,321 potentially exposed people, 6,470 of whom were "exposures to the index case"— including *all* the passengers on the tourist's flight from Mexico to Arizona—at a cost of approximately $400,000 for 13,000 staff hours.[5,6] Two hospitals that treated a total of seven patients with measles spent $799,136 on disease containment, including the cost of furloughing health care workers with unknown vaccination status for a total of 15,120 staff hours.[5] The director of the health department in Pima County, where Tucson is located, later described the episode as "immunization clinics going nonstop, staff needed to maintain the call centers nearly 7 days a week … kind of a nightmare."[6] The humanistic cost was also considerable. Of 14 confirmed cases, six required inpatient care, two in the intensive care unit (ICU), and one of the ICU cases was a two-year-old child hospitalized for six days because of febrile seizures.[5]

The Tucson incident was not isolated. In Minnesota, where there had been zero or one case of measles annually for most of the past ten years, 14 confirmed measles cases were reported in just three months of 2011, one-half of whom were in unvaccinated Somali children who had been exposed to "an unvaccinated Somali infant who returned from a trip to Kenya in February [2011]."[7] Nationwide, 152 cases were diagnosed by June 2011, representing "the biggest outbreak in 15 years," according to the U.S. Centers for Disease Control and Prevention.[8] And the phenomenon is not limited to the United States; case rates are swelling in European countries including France, Belgium, Germany, and Spain.[9]

Measles Resurgence: How Did It Happen?

Public health officials trace the return of what had been a virtually extinct disease to a phenomenon known as "vaccine refusal," a decision made by parents to shun routine immunizations for their children.[8,9] Indeed, all 14 infections in the Tucson outbreak occurred in unvaccinated individuals, and the fourth and fifth transmissions were in two children who were old enough for the measles-mumps-rubella (MMR) vaccine but had not received it "because of parental opposition to vaccination."[5] One of these children, in turn, exposed 130 students to the disease.[5]

In reflecting on the Tucson incident, health officials noted that the area's generally high rate of MMR vaccination coverage overall, estimated at about 91%-96% among Arizona kindergartners, had prevented a more serious outbreak.[5] However, not all regions of the country would fare as well under similar circumstances. Despite high MMR vaccination rates in the United States as a whole, much lower rates are setting the stage for potentially catastrophic levels of disease transmission in small, generally affluent, geographic areas where "like-minded parents" who oppose vaccination "tend to flock together."[8] For example, the rate of vaccine exemption based on "personal belief" is only 2.5% for kindergartners in California overall but more than 6% in wealthier northern coastal counties, such as Marin, Sonoma, and Santa Cruz.[10] On Vashon Island in the Seattle area, the vaccination rate was estimated to be only 85% in one elementary school in 2010—insufficient for "herd immunity" that could protect unvaccinated kids in the event of an outbreak—and the island has three times more children who are not fully vaccinated than does the state overall.[11] In the state of Washington as a whole, the number of counties with more than a 5% rate of vaccine exemption was only "a handful" in 1999 but "more than doubled" by 2004.[12]

Most observers attribute MMR vaccine refusal to concerns about vaccination safety, which, in turn, were the result of an influential study published in the prestigious journal, *The Lancet*, in 1998.[8-11,13] Conducted by then 41-year-old physician Andrew Wakefield and his colleagues, the study was a 12-case series investigation of developmentally disabled children who were referred to a pediatric gastroenterology unit for gastrointestinal disorders (e.g., diarrhea, abdominal pain, and food intolerance). The children "underwent gastroenterological, neurological, and developmental assessment and review of developmental records," as well as a series of invasive and noninvasive tests performed under sedation; these included "ileocolonoscopy and biopsy sampling, magnetic-resonance imaging (MRI), electroencephalography (EEG), and lumbar puncture."[13] Suspicion of a possible association between MMR and "chronic enterocolitis" that "may be related to neuropsychiatric dysfunction" was made by Wakefield et al. based on the reports of eight parents that "the onset of behavioural problems had been linked, either by the parents or by the child's physician," with MMR vaccination and that the "average interval from exposure to first behavioural symptoms was 6.3 days (range 1-14)."[13]

The study would perhaps have gone relatively unnoticed if Wakefield had not taken the unusual and, he now acknowledges, unwise step of holding a press conference in which he raised concerns about the safety of MMR vaccination one day prior to the study's publication.[14,15] As it was, the impact of his allegations was enormous. MMR vaccination rates in the United Kingdom declined precipitously, from 91% in 1997-1998 to 80% in 2003-2004.[16] In the United States, antivaccine sentiment escalated in parent groups, bolstered by the endorsement of a well-known celebrity who has publicly blamed MMR vaccination for her child's autism.[11] In the ensuing years, Wakefield, who now lives in the United States, has developed a vocal and loyal cadre of followers, mostly parents of autistic children, one of whom described him in an April 2011 *New York Times* interview as "Nelson Mandela and Jesus Christ rolled up into one ... a symbol of how all of us feel."[14]

Poor-Quality Evidence of the "Risks" of MMR Vaccination

Such adulation, certainly unusual for the field of medical research, appears especially inappropriate in light of the results of a seven-year investigation by British journalist Brian Deer, which revealed a number of unsavory details about Wakefield's work. Deer reported that eight months *prior to* Wakefield's public expression of concern about the safety of the MMR, he had filed a patent on his "safer" measles vaccine.[17] The *Lancet* study children were *not* consecutively referred to the pediatric service as stated in the article, but were instead "pre-selected through MMR campaign groups," and "most" were clients of a lawyer who was in the process of assembling a class-action lawsuit against vaccine manufacturers.[17,18] Although the study hospital was located in London, none of the children lived there, and one had been flown in for the consultation from California.[17,18] Information provided to Deer by the study parents refuted information presented in the report by Wakefield et al., particularly with respect to one element critical to study validity, the timing of vaccine exposure relative to behavioral symptom onset.[19] Worst of all, although Wakefield et al. reported in *The Lancet* that their project—which involved *five days* of testing—had been approved by the hospital's ethics review board, the board actually was not provided with full information about the project and did not approve of its protocol.[16,18]

After a 197-day professional standards trial, the Fitness to Practise Panel of the United Kingdom's General Medical Council ruled in January 2010 that "Wakefield had acted unethically and had shown 'callous disregard' for the children in his study."[16,18,20] Wakefield lost his right to practice medicine in the United Kingdom, and *The Lancet* retracted the study in February 2010, 12 years after its publication.[20]

Although it is clear that important details about the study were not reported to

The Lancet during the peer review process, it is instructive to step back from Deer's investigation and look at the study methods *as originally reported.* The sample n was 12, of whom only eight were even reported to have a link between MMR and behavioral problems. The purported link was based solely on the retrospective recall of parents. No verification of the parental reports was made. There was no autism-free control group, as in the classic and powerful case-control design. And, perhaps most important, the findings of Wakefield et al. were inconsistent with years of vaccine safety experience. A commentary by Chen and DeStefano, published simultaneously with the Wakefield et al. report, noted that "hundreds of millions of people worldwide ... have received measles-containing vaccine without developing either chronic bowel or behavioural problems since the mid-1960s."[21] Yet, the commentary also said that "it is important ... to examine" the report, "critically and with an open mind."[21]

One might reasonably wonder why it was appropriate to give it any credence at all. As we saw in Chapter 9, peer review has sometimes been criticized for stifling innovation, but perhaps a bit more stifling would have been appropriate in this instance. Just weeks following the study's publication—about a decade before emergence of information about the ethical problems with the research—knowledgeable observers expressed concern about its poor-quality methodology and likely negative impact on public health in letters to the editor of *The Lancet.*[22] In 2010, one pediatrician and clinical professor of medical genetics observed in an interview with the *Canadian Medical Association Journal:* "Why *The Lancet* published it is completely beyond me."[20]

Methodological Quality and Public Health

In health care and in other fields, many professionals view study methods as esoteric detail. Methods must be reported, perhaps as bothersome afterthought, but they are far less interesting and important than the interpretation and promulgation of findings by the experts who conduct and report research.

Nothing could be further from the truth—or more dangerous to patients. The events that followed the publication of the study by Wakefield et al. demonstrate with troubling clarity that study methods, which lie at the heart of the internal and external validity of research, have the power to affect the lives and well-being of the patients and families whom the health care system serves. High-quality methods produce accurate findings and sometimes important, maybe even lifesaving, scientific developments. Suboptimal methods usually lead to erroneous results and may result in decades of harm. The commentary by

Chen and DeStefano, described in one letter to the editor as "perhaps the only saving grade [sic]"[23] in *The Lancet*'s publication of the study by Wakefield et al., noted that without *high-quality* epidemiological research, "vaccine-safety concerns such as that reported by Wakefield and colleagues may snowball into societal tragedies when the media and the public **confuse association with causality** and shun immunization." (emphasis added)[21]

Thus, although the study by Wakefield et al. reflects an extreme instance of what one journal editor described as a "deeply shocking" breach of public trust,[24] it also makes what is perhaps an even more important point far more clearly than any textbook description of methodological principles ever could. Methods matter.

Choosing Excellence: What Makes It Happen?

In this book, I tried to provide tips and techniques to make it easier for researchers to pursue excellence. I tried to show that a researcher does *not* have to choose between excellence and efficiency, and that many resources—not just this book, but others cited in its chapters—are available to help in that endeavor. In the end, though, the choice to pursue excellence is left to the researcher alone. And, as helpful as these resources are, that choice takes more than techniques, tips, or tools. It takes *love*.

It may seem strange to talk about love in a methods textbook, but the idea did not originate with me. The "father of quality assurance" in health care, the late Avedis Donabedian, had this to say about how to improve the health care system in a speech that he gave in 1986:

> "Systems awareness and systems design are important for health professionals, but are not enough. They are enabling mechanisms only. It is the ethical dimension of individuals that is essential to a system's success. Ultimately, the secret of quality is love. You have to love your patient, you have to love your profession, you have to love your God. If you have love, you can then work backward to monitor and improve the system."[25]

Donabedian, who grew up as a refugee in Palestine after his parents fled the Armenian holocaust that had killed his sisters, perhaps understood from his own life experiences—better than many of us with easier personal circumstances—both the difficulty and the value of making tough choices. He understood that excellence is a *decision* that is made when we are willing to put aside personal, political, or economic agendas and pursue accuracy in our work. All of us fail, to some extent, in this pursuit. All of us must try to succeed.

Most authors place a dedication in their book's foreword or acknowledgements page. I am putting mine here. To those who wish to pursue excellence, who are willing to invest the extra time and effort that accuracy may require, who want to place the needs of information users at the center of every decision made throughout the course of every research project—I hope that this book is helpful. It is dedicated to you.

References

1. Albert Einstein. *Famous Quotations Network.* Available at: http://www.famous-quotations.com/asp/acquotes.asp?author=Albert+Einstein+%281879%2D1955%29&category=Science+%2F+Research.

2. House of Commons, Science and Technology Committee. Peer review in scientific publications: Eighth report of Session 2010-12. HC856. July 18, 2011. Available at: http://www.publications.parliament.uk/pa/cm201012/cmselect/cmsctech/856/856.pdf.

3. Vickers A. Interpreting data from randomized trials: the Scandanavian Prostatectomy Study illustrates two common errors. *Nat Clin Pract Urol.* 2005;2(9):404-05.

4. Greater Phoenix Convention & Visitors Bureau. Fun facts.

5. Chen SY, Anderson S, Kutty PK, et al. Health care-associated measles outbreak in the United States after an importation: challenges and economic impact. *J Infect Dis.* 2011;203(11):1517-25.

6. Media accounts of this incident include the following:
    - No authors listed. Hospitals more prepared for measles outbreak. May 16, 2011. The Main Stream. Available at: www.kvoa.com/news/hospitals-more-prepared-for-measles-outbreak/.
    - McKenna M. What vaccine refusal really costs: measles in Arizona. Superbug. April 29, 2011. Available at: http://www.wired.com/wiredscience/2011/04/cost-vaccine-refusal/.
    - Gargulinski R. County measles outbreak ends after 13 cases. Tucson Citizen Morgue (1992-2009). July 22, 2008. Available at: http://tucsoncitizen.com/morgue/2008/07/22/91569-county-measles-outbreak-ends-after-13-cases/.

7. Karnowski S. Autism fears, measles spike among Minn. Somalis. MPR News. April 2, 2011. Available at: http://minnesota.publicradio.org/display/web/2011/04/02/somali-autism-vaccines/.

8. Szabo L. Childhood diseases return as parents refuse vaccines. *USA Today.* July 15, 2011. Available at: http://yourlife.usatoday.com/health/medical/story/2011/06/Childhood-diseases-return-as-parents-refuse-vaccines/48414234/1.

9. Ropeik D. Public health: Not vaccinated? Not acceptable. *Los Angeles Times.* July 18, 2011. Available at: http://articles.latimes.com/2011/jul/18/opinion/la-oe-ropeik-vaccines-20110718.

10. No authors listed. Thousands in California started school without vaccines. USAtoday.com. September 26, 2011. Available at: http://yourlife.usatoday.com/health/healthcare/story/2011-09-26/Thousands-in-Calif-started-school-without-

vaccines/50553202/1.

11. Riemer S. One woman's campaign: confronting Vashon's low vaccination rates. *Vashon-Maury Island Beachcomber.* April 29, 2010. Available at: http://www.pnwlocalnews.com/vashon/vib/news/92239334.html.

12. Ostrom CM. More parents resisting vaccines for kids. *Seattle Times.* July 16, 2006. Available at: http://seattletimes.nwsource.com/html/health/2003130272_resisters16m.html.

13. Wakefield A, Murch SH, Anthony A, et al. Ileal-lymphoid-nodular hyperplasia, non-specific colitis, and pervasive developmental disorder in children. *Lancet.* 1998;351(9103):637-41.

14. Dominus S. The crash and burn of an autism guru. *New York Times.* April 20, 2011. Available at: http://www.nytimes.com/2011/04/24/magazine/mag-24Autism-t.html?pagewanted=all.

15. Press release from the Royal Free Hospital School of Medicine. New research links autism and bowel disease. 26 February 1998: embargoed until 0001 27 February 1998. Available at: http://briandeer.com/mmr/royal-free-press-1998.pdf.

16. Leask J, Booy R, McIntyre PB. MMR, Wakefield, and *The Lancet:* what can we learn? *Med J Aust.* 2010;193(1):5-7.

17. Deer B. Secrets of the MMR scare. How the vaccine crisis was meant to make money. *BMJ.* 2011;342:c5258.

18. Exposed: Andrew Wakefield and the MMR-autism fraud. Brian Deer's award-winning investigation. Available at: http://briandeer.com/mmr/lancet-summary.htm.

19. Deer B. How the case against the MMR vaccine was fixed. *BMJ.* 2011;342:c5347.

20. Eggertson L. Lancet retracts 12-year-old article linking autism to MMR vaccines. *CMAJ.* 2010;182(4):E199-200.

21. Chen RT, DeStefano F. Vaccine adverse events: causal or coincidental? *Lancet.* 1998;351(9103):611-12.

22. Autism, inflammatory bowel disease, and MMR vaccine [multiple letters]. *Lancet.* 1998;351:905-08.

23. Lindley KJ, Milla PJ. Autism, inflammatory bowel disease, and MMR vaccine. *Lancet.* 1998;351(9106):907.

24. Godlee F. The fraud behind the MMR scare. *BMJ.* 2011;342:d22. Available at: http://www.bmj.com/content/342/bmj.d22.full.

25. Best M, Neuhauser D. Avedis Donabedian: father of quality assurance and poet. *Qual Saf Health Care.* 2004;13(6):472-73.

Glossary

All-cause—Refers to use of health care services for any diagnosis or condition, rather than for the specific disease or condition of interest (e.g., a hospitalization for cancer in a study of patients with diabetes).

Allocation concealment—Hiding information about group assignment from investigators and their assistants to eliminate human intervention in the group assignment process in a *randomized controlled trial*. For example, allocation might be concealed by placing group assignment information in opaque, sealed envelopes so that those who are processing subjects for study entry cannot see or act upon the allocation.

Alpha—See "*P* value, critical."

A priori—Refers to decision rules and analysis plans established at the start of a research project, prior to beginning the study.

Binomial—A variable with only two possible values, e.g., yes versus no, or Candidate A versus Candidate B in a two-person election.

Bivariate—Refers to a two-variable analysis, such as a crosstabulation of disease incidence by age or a comparison of mean health care costs by sex.

Blinding—The practice of concealing group assignment from study subjects, investigators, and/or those who assess subject outcomes, typically in the context of a randomized controlled trial. For example, study subjects may receive capsules with identical appearance and taste; however, the treatment group receives active drug, whereas the control group receives placebo.

Budgetary impact analysis—A type of decision analytic model that estimates the impact of a change in treatment or policy on overall expenditures.

Case-control study—A study in which "cases" are selected based on having a particular outcome (e.g., a diagnosis of lung cancer) and their potential risk factors are compared with those of "controls" (e.g., those who do not have a diagnosis of lung cancer).

CATI (computer-assisted telephone interviewing)—pronounced "catty"—(1) A computerized system for survey administration that permits extremely complex skip and contingency patterns, such as tailoring the response choices for an item based on the response to a question asked several minutes previously; (2) Behavior of some 13-year-old girls at junior high social events.

Censoring—The situation in which a study outcome of interest occurs after the end of observation. For example, in a three-year study of mortality following Surgery A, subjects who die less than three years after Surgery A are *uncensored* (i.e., their outcome was observed), and subjects who live longer than three years after Surgery A are *censored* (i.e., the study ended before the outcome was known).

Cluster sampling—The selection of study subjects in "clusters" (groups), for example, selecting a probability sample of physicians, then selecting for study all or a sample of patients treated by each sampled physician.

Cohort study—A study in which one or more study groups (cohorts) are selected and their outcomes analyzed throughout a follow-up period. Cohort studies can be performed prospectively (e.g., the Framingham Heart Study) or retrospectively (e.g., an analysis of administrative claims data performed in 2011 in which the researchers select patients who had a new diagnosis or new drug start [index event] during 2009 and follow them for 12 months post-index to measure health care events, such as emergency room visits, hospitalizations, and health care costs).

Comparison group—A group to which results for an intervention group will be compared. *JMCP* uses this term, rather than "control group," for *observational* designs.

Competence to answer—The ability of a respondent to provide the requested information; in health care surveys, competence to answer should be considered in light of the roles played by consumers in the medical care system.

Comprehensiveness (in sampling)—The degree to which a sampling process yields a sample that adequately represents the target population.

Confounding—The process by which the relationship between two variables is influenced by one or more additional variables, sometimes creating statistical associations that can be misleading rather than causal. For example, the number of fire trucks at a fire is highly associated with the amount of damage, but trucks do not cause fire damage; the size of the fire is the confounding factor that causes both the number of fire trucks and the amount of damage.

Confounding by indication—The situation in which health status factors affect both the selection of the treatment and the patient's outcome. The factors might or might not be measurable; for example, a physician may select a surgical treatment for a patient based on the patient's comorbidities (measurable) or on the physician's perceptions of the patient's social supports for the surgical recovery period (usually not measurable).

Contingency question—A survey question that is asked of only a subgroup of respondents, not all respondents, and therefore requires a *skip pattern*.

Control group—(1) In a *randomized controlled trial*, the group that was not assigned to receive the intervention of interest. In a drug study, the control group may receive either placebo or an alternative drug; in a programmatic study (e.g., of a disease management program), the control group typically receives "usual care." (2) In a *case-control* study, the group that does *not* have the disease or condition of interest.

Convenience sample—A sample for which the probability of selection is unknown because the sampling process was based at least partially on the convenience of study subjects or investigators.

Critical *P* value—See "*P* value, critical."

Cross-sectional association—A relationship between two factors, measured at a brief or single point in time (e.g., gray hair is associated with mortality, the number of fire trucks at a fire is associated with the amount of fire damage); does *not* indicate a causal relationship but may lead to hypotheses that can be tested using more rigorous methods.

Cross-sectional design—A simple comparison of one group versus other(s) over a brief or single point in time.

Decision analytic modeling—The calculation of expected outcomes of an intervention or treatment based on a set of input assumptions, usually performed using specialized software and techniques, such as Markov chain modeling or decision tree analysis.

Dependent variable—The outcome that a study is designed to predict or explain.

Detection bias—Sometimes called "*surveillance bias*;" a situation in which the *reporting* of an outcome (but not the outcome itself) is influenced by one or more factors thought to influence the outcome; for example, one might find an association between diabetes and glaucoma partly because patients with diabetes are more likely to have regular eye examinations.

Difference-in-difference—The measurement of change in an outcome from before versus after an intervention/treatment, followed by a comparison of the change amount for a group exposed to the intervention/treatment versus an unexposed group.

Disease-specific—Refers to use of health care services for only the specific disease or condition of interest; opposite of *all-cause* analysis.

Distribution—Refers to the way in which observations are arrayed when plotted in two-dimensional space, for example, a bell-shaped curve (normal distribution) versus a skewed curve. Distributions are important because they help to determine the statistical technique necessary to analyze the data appropriately.

Double-barreled items—Survey questions that address more than one topic in the same question, thereby confusing and/or annoying respondents.

Effect size—A mathematical measure of the degree to which the independent variable affects or is associated with the dependent variable; Cohen's d, the mean difference divided by the standard deviation, is a commonly used measure.

Efficiency (in sampling)—The degree to which a sampling process identifies a sample with the least possible amount of effort on the part of study subjects and investigators.

Exclusion criteria—The specific requirements for exclusion from a research sample; these should be established in as much detail as possible in an *a priori* analysis plan.

Exposure—The treatment or intervention of interest in a study; for example, in a randomized study of an "opt-in" disease management program, the exposure might be a letter of invitation to participate in the program.

External validity—See "validity, external."

Hypothesis—A statement, established by investigators prior to beginning a research study, about what the investigators expect to find; should be based on information obtained from a review of previous work.

Inclusion criteria—The specific requirements for inclusion in a research sample; these should be established in as much detail as possible in an *a priori* analysis plan.

Independent variable—A variable that is hypothesized to predict or explain the dependent variable.

Instrumental variable analysis—A multivariate technique that uses an "instrument" (a covariate) intended to control for the effects of unmeasured confounding factors. The "instrument" should meet the following criteria: (1) no systematic relationship with either *measured or unmeasured* confounders; (2) a strong systematic association with the treatment or independent variable of interest (exposure); and (3) no direct effect on the outcome (i.e., no association with the outcome except through the exposure).

Intention-to-treat analysis—An analytic approach in which the outcomes for *all* those who are assigned to the treatment or intervention of interest are included in the analysis, in contrast with a *per protocol* approach, in which only those who successfully complete the treatment are analyzed.

Interaction—A statistical relationship in which the effect of one independent (predictor) variable on a dependent variable depends on another independent variable; for example, in the New Hampshire Medicaid study described in Chapter 4, the association between the cap and nursing home admission depended on the degree of chronic disease as measured by medication use.

Internal validity—See "validity, internal."

Interrupted time series—See "time series."

Intervention group—The group that receives the treatment or policy change of interest in a research study.

Interviewer effect—A suboptimal situation in which the behavior or appearance of an interviewer affects survey responses, either by attracting particular demographic groups or by encouraging particular answers to survey questions.

Loss to follow-up—Termination of measurement for a study subject prior to the end of the planned data collection time frame; examples include subjects in a drug trial who stop treatment because of adverse drug effects and patients in an analysis of administrative claims data who leave the study health plan prior to the study end date.

Marginal effect—In a multivariate model, the effect of an independent variable on the dependent variable, controlling for (holding constant) the effects of other independent variables included in the model.

Misclassification of exposure—A problem in measurement that occurs when a subject who has not been exposed to an independent variable (e.g., intervention, treatment, risk factor) is erroneously classified as exposed, or vice versa. For example, a study of the effects of aspirin use in cardiovascular disease that examines only pharmacy claims data would incorrectly classify users of over-the-counter aspirin as unexposed to aspirin, when in reality their aspirin use was unobserved.

Mixed mode—Term used to describe a survey process in which potential respondents who fail to complete a survey using one mode (e.g., mail) are invited to complete the survey using a different mode (e.g., telephone).

Multicollinearity—A situation in which two or more independent variables in a multivariate model are so highly correlated (i.e., share so much variance) that it is impossible to determine their individual marginal effects, resulting in unstable or unreliable regression coefficients.

Multistage sampling—The selection of study subjects using a process of selecting multiple clusters and/or sampling within clusters, for example, selecting a sample of health plans, then selecting a sample of primary care providers within each health plan, then selecting a sample of patients for each primary care provider.

Multivariate—Refers to a type of statistical analysis in which the effects of multiple variables are assessed simultaneously, such as an analysis of health care cost controlling for age, sex, comorbidities, and inclusion in the intervention versus comparison group of a study.

Nonparametric test—A statistical test that does not assume that the population has a specific distribution, especially the normal distribution. Common examples include the Mann-Whitney U test, a nonparametric alternative to the Student's t test for independent samples, and the Wilcoxon signed-rank test, a nonparametric alternative to the t test for related samples.

Nonresponse bias—A situation in which those with particular points of view are more likely to respond to a survey, thereby providing misleading information about the opinions of the population as a whole.

Null hypothesis—The hypothesis that the relationship between or among the study variables is *not* as hypothesized by the investigators; tests of statistical significance assess the probability that the observed results would have been obtained if the null hypothesis were true.

Number needed to treat (NNT)—Used in assessing the practical interpretation of the differences between two or more groups; calculated as the mathematical reciprocal of the estimated benefit of the treatment. For example, if the treatment reduces an outcome by two percentage points, the NNT is $1 \div 0.02 = 50$.

Observational research—General term encompassing numerous study designs and data sources, referring to research in which the investigator performs no interventions but instead observes events, either prospectively or retrospectively.

Observational study groups—Study groups that were not randomly assigned by the investigator but were observed by the investigator; for example, customers who chose to use Pharmacy A versus Pharmacy B, patients who met clinical criteria for a disease management program versus those who did not, or patients who were adherent to medication versus those who were not. Subject to *confounding* and *selection bias*.

Odds—The ratio of the probability of an event occurring to the probability of the event not occurring, that is $p \div (1-p)$, where p=probability.

Odds ratio—The amount by which the odds are multiplied for one group relative to another. For example, if the odds ratio for males compared with females is 3.0, then the odds for males are three times those for females.

Operationalize—Translate from a concept to one or more specific decision rules—for example, if the concept is "new user of Drug A," the specific decision rules might be: (1) filled at least one prescription for Drug A during 2010, (2) continuously eligible for health care benefits for the 12 months prior to the first prescription for Drug A (baseline period), and (3) no claims in Drug A's therapy class during the baseline period.

Order effect—A situation in which a respondent's answers to a question are affected, at least in part, by the question's placement in the survey or by the order of response choices (e.g., Excellent, Good, Fair, Poor **vs.** Poor, Fair, Good, Excellent).

Oversampling—(1) A situation in which one subgroup of a population has a higher probability of selection than another subgroup, for example, sampling 200 patients with multiple sclerosis and 200 patients without multiple sclerosis (when, of course, the proportion of people with multiple sclerosis in the general population is far less than 50%); oversampling is appropriate for many purposes but requires the use of **weighting** in analysis. (2) Eating too many cookies at the office holiday party; this situation requires **unweighting**.

P value, critical—The *P* value threshold, established *a priori* by the researcher, below which a result will be deemed statistically significant, usually 0.05 or 0.01. Also called the *alpha*.

P value, observed—The probability that the observed result for a sample would have been obtained if the *null hypothesis* were true.

Panel—In Internet surveys, a group of people who agree to respond to a certain number of surveys over a certain period of time on an ongoing basis, sometimes in exchange for the use of computer equipment necessary for survey completion.

Per protocol analysis—An analytic approach in which only those who successfully complete the treatment or intervention of interest are studied, in contrast with an *intention-to-treat* approach, in which the outcomes for *all* those who are assigned to the treatment are studied.

Perspective—The viewpoint from which a decision analytic model is conducted. For example, a model to assess a health plan's costs for treating Disease X is from the "payer perspective," whereas a model to assess not only treatment costs but also caregiver time, burden on family members, and lost work time is from the "societal perspective."

Post hoc— Refers to decision rules or changes in analysis plans made after the start of a research project.

Power—See "statistical power."

Pragmatic randomized trial—A study that combines the key design feature of a randomized trial (randomization to eliminate threats to internal validity, such as selection bias and confounding by indication) with design features intended to enhance external validity (e.g., minimizing the number of sample exclusion criteria, imposing no limits on treatment decisions made after randomization).

Pretest—A test in which a survey is given to a small sample of potential respondents to identify and correct problems (e.g., questions that are confusing or offensive) prior to full-scale survey administration.

Probability of selection—For any given potential member of a sample, refers to the likelihood of being selected for that sample. For example, if I in 2,000 health plan members without multiple sclerosis and 250 of 500 with multiple sclerosis are selected, the probability of selection is 0.05% for members without multiple sclerosis and 50% for members with multiple sclerosis.

Probability sampling—A sampling method in which each study subject has a known probability of selection. See "random sampling."

Propensity score—A mathematical algorithm that is derived from logistic regression analysis and commonly used in observational research to adjust for selection bias; the propensity score represents a calculated score in a logistic regression analysis predicting membership in a particular group, such as a group of patients who receive a treatment versus those who do not. Scores are commonly entered into multivariate analyses as covariates or used for matching.

Quasi-experimental—Generally refers to an observational design with methodological features intended to approximate an experiment as closely as possible; more specifically, often refers to a pre-post with comparison group or time series with comparison group design (e.g., calculate pre-to-post change amounts or trends for a group that was subject to the intervention versus a group that was not subject to the intervention).

Randomized controlled trial—A test of an intervention or treatment that is performed using randomized, rather than human-selected (e.g., physician-assigned or self-selected) groups; compares one or more treatment or intervention groups (e.g., Drug A, Drug B, disease management program) with one or more control groups (e.g., placebo, Drug C, "usual care").

Randomized design—A study design in which subjects are assigned to groups using mathematical methods that assure a known probability of selection (e.g., using a random number generator to assign 70% of potential study subjects to an intervention and 30% to a control group that does not receive the intervention). Relies upon the absence of human involvement in the group allocation process. If properly implemented, this design virtually eliminates the possibility of *confounding* or *selection bias*.

Random sampling—A process in which mathematical methods (e.g., use of a random-number generator) or other procedures (e.g., selecting every Nth case in a list that has been sorted using a random number generator) have been used to give each member of a group a known probability of selection for a study. Different groups within a sample (e.g., males vs. females, people with versus without a certain medical condition) can be given different probabilities in a random sampling process (e.g., select 10% of males and 20% of females), as long as all of the cases *within* each group have an equal probability of selection.

Regression to the mean—A mathematical phenomenon in which high values tend to decline over time and low values tend to increase over time; one of the main reasons why simple pre-post study designs without an adequate comparison or control group often produce erroneous findings.

Reliability—(1) The ability of an instrument or measure to produce consistently the same answer under the same circumstances (e.g., of 100 respondents with the same opinion, 95 would give the same answer on the survey). (2) Highly desirable quality in a babysitter.

Reliability, internal—The degree to which a group of items on a survey that are intended to measure a similar concept actually yield similar results; typically assessed using Cronbach's alpha.

Reliability, inter-rater—The degree to which different individuals, using the same instrument and metric, will reach the same conclusion or result; commonly assessed using kappa or weighted kappa statistics.

Reliability, interviewer—The degree to which different interviewers achieve the same results (e.g., response rates, specific responses) using the same survey instrument in the same pool of respondents.

Reliability, test-retest—The degree to which repeated measures of the same metric on the same subject yield the same result.

Residual confounding—Confounding that continues to affect the results of an analysis even after statistical adjustment, often because of unmeasured confounding factors that affect the study outcomes, such as social support or motivation.

Response rate—The proportion of those asked to complete a survey who actually do so. The numerator in the calculation is the number of completed surveys. The denominator is the total count of potential respondents for whom contact was attempted *minus* the count of potential respondents who are determined to be ineligible for the study (e.g., no longer eligible for the health plan conducting the survey).

Sample screening—The process of asking questions (usually in a survey) to determine if a potential respondent is or is not a member of the sampling frame.

Sample size—The number of cases included in a sample.

Sampling frame—The intended target population, which should then become the group from which the sample is derived.

Selection bias—A type of confounding in which factors that are systematically related to choice of group membership are also systematically related to the study outcome. For example, those with healthy lifestyles may be more likely to "opt into" a health-improvement program, and healthy lifestyles may also produce better health outcomes.

Sensitivity—The percentage of cases with a diagnosis or condition who are correctly identified by a test (e.g., laboratory test, screening mammogram, pap smear).

Skip pattern—(1) A technique in which survey respondents to whom a question does not apply are "skipped" around the question using a simple instruction. (2) Small boy's response when asked to travel directly from home to the school bus stop.

Slow start—(1) A survey scheduling process in which few interviews are done initially, often used to monitor respondent reactions to a survey because of a controversial or difficult-to-understand topic. (2) Reaction of a teenager who has just been asked to get up at 6AM on a school day.

Social desirability—The tendency of survey respondents, especially in telephone or face-to-face surveys, to give the answer that the respondent believes the interviewer wants to hear.

Specification error—The situation in which an assumed multivariate model structure and/or assumptions are inconsistent with the data. Common types of specification error in health care research include (a) misspecification of the form of the relationship (e.g., assuming linearity when the relationship between the independent and dependent variable is actually curvilinear); (b) misspecification of direction of causation (e.g., assuming that A causes B when B causes A); (c) omission of one or more relevant independent variables from the model, often because they are not measurable; and (d) misspecification of the distribution of the independent and/or dependent variables (e.g., assuming a normal distribution for ordinal data or for count data that have a Poisson distribution).

Specificity—The percentage of cases without a diagnosis or condition who are correctly identified by a test (e.g., laboratory test, screening mammogram, pap smear).

Staggered or phased implementation—A process of implementing an intervention to one or more subgroups initially, then to other subgroup(s) at a later time (e.g., six months after initial implementation), often used when randomization of all study subjects at the start of the intervention is impossible for practical or business reasons.

Statistical power—The probability of detecting a statistically significant relationship when a true relationship exists; the probability of rejecting the null hypothesis when it is false.

Stratified sampling—See "oversampling."

Superbills—(1) Preprinted billing forms used by physician offices; important in health care research because they can influence the diagnoses for which physicians bill, which in turn become the diagnoses reported on administrative health care claims data. (2) What parents of college students receive in the mail when the tuition is due.

Surveillance bias—See "detection bias."

Survey instrument (sometimes called survey tool)—Questionnaire; refers to surveys administered by any method (e.g., mail, telephone, Internet).

Target population—The intended group; for example, in a survey intended to predict the outcome of an election, the target population is voters.

Time-dependent or time-varying independent variables—Predictor or explanatory variables for which the value may change over time; for example, adherence to bisphosphonate therapy for osteoporosis prevention in a study with an outcome of fracture.

Time horizon—The period of time during which outcomes are predicted by a decision analytic model. For example, a model that assesses a hypothetical cohort of patients for 20 years after initiation of treatment with Drug A has a 20-year time horizon.

Time series analysis—Analysis of trends in an outcome that is measured in a regular series over a period of time (e.g., monthly). Subtypes include **interrupted time series**, a design that compares trends before versus after an event or policy change, and **time series with comparison group**, a design that compares the trends in one group versus other(s), such as a group that is subject to an intervention versus a group that is not.

Total survey design—A general approach to survey research that emphasizes the quality of the project overall, incorporating the reliability and validity of questions, the pretesting process, the professionalism of materials and personnel presented to potential respondents, and the accuracy of data collection methods.

Type 1 error—Rejecting the null hypothesis when the null hypothesis is actually true; also known as "false positive." For any single statistical test, the probability of type 1 error equals the critical P value (*alpha*).

Type 2 error—Failing to reject the null hypothesis when the null hypothesis is actually false; also known as "false negative." The probability of type 2 error equals 100% minus the statistical power (e.g., if the power of a test is 85%, the probability of type 2 error is 15%).

Underpowered—(1) Term used to describe a study that has an insufficient sample size to produce a significant result, even if the null hypothesis is false. (2) Term used to describe a child who didn't eat enough breakfast before going to school.

Validity, construct—Accurate measurement of the intended concept. For example, in a study of major depressive disorder, the use of antidepressant drug claims to indicate the presence of major depression has very limited construct validity because antidepressant drugs are commonly used for other conditions (e.g., anxiety, obsessive compulsive disorder).

Validity, content—Measurement of all important dimensions of a concept; for example, a survey intended to assess mathematics skills should not be limited to addition but should also include subtraction, multiplication, and division.

Validity, criterion—The degree to which a measure is consistent with an external criterion or benchmark. For example, patient-reported health status might be compared with subsequent morbidity and mortality.

Validity, external—Applicability of research results to the group(s), purpose(s), and/or circumstance(s) in which they will be applied.

Validity, internal—Accuracy of inference about the causality of relationships between or among study variables.

Validity, predictive— See "validity, criterion."

Weighting—(1) The calculation and application of numbers in a statistical calculation for a stratified, multistage, or cluster sample to produce a result mathematically equivalent to that which would have been obtained from a simple random sample of the population. Simple weights are based on mathematically inverting the probability of selection. More complex weights account for unequal probability of selection as well as homogeneity within clusters (e.g., similar treatment of patients by the same physician). (2) What Vladimir and Estragon did for Godot.

What is already known and **what the present study is intended to add**—Two important concepts in research design that reflect the need for every research study to build upon the foundation of previously published work. Before beginning a research project, the investigator should be aware of the methods, findings, and limitations of previous studies, especially work that is considered important and/or frequently cited.

Sources:

- Babbie E. *The Practice of Social Research. Fourth Edition.* Belmont, CA: Wadsworth Publishing Company; 1986.

- Ballinger GA. Using generalized estimating equations for longitudinal data analysis. *Organizational Research Methods.* 2004;7(2):127-50. Available at: http://orm.sagepub.com/content/7/2/127.full.pdf+html.

- Cook TD, Campbell DT. *Quasi-Experimentation: Design & Analysis Issues for Field Settings.* Boston, MA: Houghton Mifflin Company; 1979.

- Greenland S. An introduction to instrumental variables for epidemiologists. *Int J Epidemiol.* 2000;29(4):722-29.

- Kalton G. *Introduction to Survey Sampling.* Newbury Park, CA: Sage Publications; 1983.

- Mann CJ. Observational research methods. Research design II: cohort, cross sectional, and case-control studies. *Emerg Med J.* 2003;20(1):54-60.

- Motheral BR, Fairman KA. The use of claims databases for outcomes research: rationale, challenges, and strategies. *Clin Ther.* 1997;19(2):346-66.

- Norušis M. *SPSS Advanced Statistics 6.1.* Chicago, IL: SPSS Inc.; 1994.

- Ostrom CW. *Time Series Analysis: Regression Techniques. Second Edition.* Newbury Park, CA: Sage Publications; 1990.

- Pedhazur EJ. *Multiple Regression in Behavioral Research: Explanation and Prediction. Second Edition.* New York: CBS College Publishing; 1982.

- Vandenbroucke JP, von Elm E, Altman DG, et al. Strengthening the Reporting of Observational Studies in Epidemiology (STROBE): explanation and elaboration. *PLoS Med.* 2007;4(10):e297. Available at: http://www.ncbi.nlm.nih.gov/pmc/articles/PMC2020496/?tool=pubmed.

Index of Tables, Figures, and Appendices

Index of Tables, Figures, and Appendices (*continued*)

Index of Topics

Index of Topics *(continued)*

Index of Topics *(continued)*

Index of Topics (continued)

About the Author

Kathleen Fairman, who has been Associate Editor and Senior Methodology Reviewer for the *Journal of Managed Care Pharmacy* (*JMCP*) since 2006, is an experienced principal investigator who has authored or coauthored numerous peer-reviewed articles, including more than 50 Medline-indexed publications. Fairman has developed and taught seminars on a wide variety of subjects, including appropriate use of administrative data for research purposes, opinion surveys on complex medical and clinical issues, and systems of documentation to facilitate accurate work. Fairman is especially experienced at using medical claims data and in 2005 designed an automated system that uses procedure and revenue codes recorded in medical bills to categorize raw claims data for thousands of medical services into meaningful service groupings for research analysis. Prior to her tenure at *JMCP*, she was a research consultant for Express Scripts, Inc., a large pharmacy benefits management company, and in that capacity developed "crash course" classes to bridge the gap between the formal training provided in graduate school curricula and the practical skills needed to conduct and publish research projects in "real-life" practice.

Fairman also served AHCCCS, Arizona's Medicaid Agency, for eight years. During that time, she oversaw the design and implementation of a new statewide hospital reimbursement system, was the lead negotiator in reimbursement rate discussions with nursing home representatives worth $0.5 billion annually, supervised calculations of the rates paid to the state's contracted providers, managed the calculation and monitoring of the agency's then $1.2 billion budget, testified in rate-setting cases in civil court, and provided analytic support for negotiations with top federal officials.

Fairman was a co-recipient of the Academy of Managed Care Pharmacy's "Award for Excellence" for the best article published in *JMCP* in both 2003 and 2004 and received an honorable mention in the same competition in 2009. A *Phi Beta Kappa* graduate of Wellesley College, she earned both Sociology Departmental Honors and Durant Scholar (magna cum laude) status while employed more than half-time in local hospitals to work her way through college. She earned a Master's Degree in Sociology with *Phi Kappa Phi* distinction from Arizona State University, concentrating in multivariate statistics.

Fairman spends part of each month working as a music minister with bed-bound and terminally ill nursing home patients. She and her husband, Michael, have been married for more than 20 years and have three active boys and two even more active dogs, including an eccentric, large-eared terrier named "Yoda." Their home is almost always joyful, rarely completely clean, and never quiet.

CPSIA information can be obtained
at www.ICGtesting.com
Printed in the USA
BVHW07s2221030918
526283BV00004B/34/P